Functional Cerebral SPECT and PET Imaging

Third Edition

Functional Cerebral SPECT and PET Imaging

Third Edition

Editors

Ronald L. Van Heertum, M.D.
Professor of Clinical Radiology and Vice Chairman
Department of Radiology
Columbia University College of Physicians and Surgeons
New York, New York

Ronald S. Tikofsky, Ph.D.
Associate Professor of Clinical Radiology
Department of Radiology
Columbia University College of Physicians and Surgeons
Harlem Hospital Center
New York, New York

LIPPINCOTT WILLIAMS & WILKINS
A **Wolters Kluwer** Company
Philadelphia · Baltimore · New York · London
Buenos Aires · Hong Kong · Sydney · Tokyo

Acquisitions Editor: Joyce-Rachel John
Developmental Editor: Sara Lauber
Production Editor: Janice G. Stangel
Manufacturing Manager: Tim Reynolds
Cover Designer: David Levy
Compositor: Maryland Composition

Printed and bound in China

Library of Congress Cataloging-in-Publication Data

Functional cerebral SPECT and PET imaging / editors, Ronald L. Van Heertum, Ronald S. Tikofsky.—3rd ed.
     p. ; cm.
   Rev. ed. of: Cerebral SPECT imaging. 2nd ed. New York: Raven Press, c1995.
   Includes bibliography references and index.
   ISBN 0-7817-1870-8 (alk. paper)
    1. Brain—Tomography. 2. Tomography, Emission. I. Van Heertum, Ronald L. II. Tikofsky, Ronald S.
   [DNLM: 1. Brain Diseases—diagnosis—Atlases. 2. Tomography, Emission-Computed—methods—Atlases. WL 17 F979 2000]
   RC386.6.T65 C47 2000
   616.8'047575—dc21
                           99-057557

10   9   8   7   6   5   4   3   2   1

To Rita Tikofsky and our children,
Andrew, Richard, Beth, Jonathan, and Kristin.
To the memory of Melissa Jo Tikofsky.
To a special friend.

Contents

Contributing Authors

Ariela Berman   *Medical Student, New York Medical College, Valhalla, New York 10595*

H. Branch Coslett, M.D.   *Professor, Department of Neurology, Temple University School of Medicine, 3401 North Broad Street, Philadelphia, Pennsylvania 19140*

David L. Daniels, M.D.   *Professor, Department of Radiology, Medical College of Wisconsin, 8700 West Wisconsin Avenue, Milwaukee, Wisconsin 53226*

Michael D. Devous, Sr., Ph.D.   *Professor, Department of Radiology, Associate Director, Nuclear Medicine Center, The University of Texas Southwestern Medical Center, 5323 Harry Hines Boulevard., Dallas, Texas 75235-9061*

Peter D. Esser, Ph.D.   *Professor of Clinical Radiology, Department of Radiology (Physics), Columbia University; and Chief Physicist of Nuclear Medicine and PET, Columbia Presbyterian Medical Center, New York Presbyterian Hospital, 177 Fort Washington Avenue, New York, New York 10032*

Robert S. Hellman, M.D.   *Associate Professor, Department of Radiology, Medical College of Wisconsin; Staff Physician, Division of Nuclear Medicine, Froedtert Memorial Lutheran Hospital, 9200 West Wisconsin Avenue, Milwaukee, Wisconsin 53226*

Dolores Malaspina, M.D.   *Associate Professor of Clinical Psychiatry, Columbia University; Associate Attending Physician, Department of Psychiatry, The Presbyterian Hospital; and Research Psychiatrist, New York State Psychiatric Institute, 1051 Riverside Drive, New York, New York 10032*

Leighton P. Mark, M.D.   *Professor of Radiology, Department of Diagnostic Radiology, Medical College of Wisconsin; and Neuroradiologist, Department of Radiology, Froedtert Memorial Lutheran Hospital, 9200 W. Wisconsin Avenue, Milwaukee, Wisconsin 53226*

Charles R. Noback, Ph.D.   *Professor Emeritus, Department of Anatomy and Cell Biology, Columbia University College of Physicians and Surgeons, 630 W. 168th Street, New York, New York 10032*

Alan B. Rubens, M.D.   *Professor, Department of Neurology, University of Arizona College of Medicine, 1501 North Campbell, Tucson, Arizona 85724*

Ronald S. Tikofsky, Ph.D.   *Associate Professor of Clinical Radiology, Department of Radiology, Columbia University College of Physicians and Surgeons, Harlem Hospital Center, 506 Lenox Avenue, New York, New York 10037*

Ronald L. Van Heertum, M.D.   *Professor of Clinical Radiology, Vice-Chairman, Department of Radiology, Columbia University College of Physicians and Surgeons, 177 Fort Washington Avenue, New York, New York 10032*

Preface to the Second Edition

Significant advances in functional brain imaging using single photon emission tomography (SPECT) have taken place since the original publication of *Advances in Cerebral SPECT Imaging: An Atlas and Guideline for Practitioners* in 1989. These advances include the introduction of new radiopharmaceuticals and instruments for performing SPECT brain imaging studies. As a result of these developments, members of the nuclear medicine community are increasingly being called upon to perform rCBF/SPECT studies.

In addition, there has been an explosion of papers focusing on the clinical applications of rCBF/SPECT. It is now nearly impossible to provide readers with a complete and comprehensive compilation of references pertaining to rCBF/SPECT brain imaging. Findings pertinent to the clinical application of rCBF/SPECT brain imaging are being published in an increasingly diverse range of scientific journals. This has led to greater awareness of the role of rCBF/SPECT brain imaging as a viable tool for the evaluation of patients with a wide range of neurologic and psychiatric disease states.

This new edition, while containing many of the original cases, has been greatly expanded. We have increased the number of cases to enable the imaging physician to see the variety of patterns that can occur within a given disease state. There is also a wide representation of imaging instruments and laboratories included in the text. Both color and black and white images are presented. Wherever possible, data pertinent to the method of image acquisition and processing is included with the case studies. Images obtained with single-head, multi-detector, and dedicated imaging systems are presented. Studies using IMP, HMPAO, and ECD (not yet FDA approved) are included. Interpretation of the studies are drawn from the reports provided by the contributing laboratories.

In addition to the greatly increased number of case studies included in Chapters 5–10, the text has also been expanded. A chapter on instrumentation, radiopharmaceuticals, and processing has been included. The chapters introducing the illustrations of the disease states have also been expanded. These emendations to the original text should provide those new to functional brain imaging, and the more experienced imaging clinician, with a broad-based foundation from which to approach the interpretation of rCBF/SPECT studies. This revised text should also provide nonimaging referring clinicians (neurologists, psychiatrists, neurosurgeons, physiatrists, and psychologists) with a better understanding of how they might better utilize this nuclear medicine procedure in their practice.

rCBF/SPECT brain imaging is a dynamic component of nuclear medicine practice and research. It is anticipated that developments in the area of receptor imaging, activation, and assessment of various forms of treatment will require future revisions of the present text. The authors hope that the present revision will serve to further enhance the practice and development of rCBF/SPECT brain imaging.

Ronald L. Van Heertum
Ronald S. Tikofsky

Preface

In the few short years since the publication of the second edition of *Cerebral SPECT Imaging,* significant progress has occurred in the field of functional brain imaging. Most significant is the increased utilization of positron emission tomography (PET) in the clinical setting. There have also been significant advances in the areas of radiopharmaceutical development and instrumentation. In response to the rapid changes in brain imaging, we decided to change the scope (and, hence the title) of the book.

Cerebral SPECT and PET Imaging now has a new chapter pertaining to PET physics, instrumentation, and the basics of radiopharmaceuticals. The chapter on single photon emission tomography (SPECT) instrumentation, radiopharmaceuticals, and technical factors has been significantly revised. This chapter summarizes the current state of the field of clinical cerebral SPECT imaging. The entire book has been thoroughly revised and all of the clinical chapters have undergone critical review to reflect an appropriate balance between SPECT and PET applications. We have also expanded the presentation of clinical indications and case materials in all areas.

Many of the developments that were anticipated at the writing of the second edition of this atlas have now entered routine clinical practice. We look forward with great optimism to continued advances in the field of functional nuclear brain imaging particularly in the areas of receptor imaging, activation, and functional image analysis.

Ronald L. Van Heertum, M.D.
Ronald S. Tikofsky, Ph.D.

Acknowledgments

We would like to express our sincere appreciation and thanks to our colleagues, residents, fellows, and technical staff who over the years have submitted case studies, offered suggestions, comments, and critically reviewed various portions of this book. This book would never have come to fruition without these contributions.

We would also like to express special thanks to Joyce-Rachel John, Sara Lauber, and Janice Stangel of Lippincott Williams & Wilkins. Their prodding and continuous support made it possible to publish this work in a timely fashion.

Functional Cerebral SPECT and PET Imaging

Third Edition

SECTION I

General Aspects of SPECT/PET Imaging

Functional Cerebral SPECT and PET Imaging, Third Edition, edited by R.L.Van Heertum and R.S. Tikofsky, Lippincott Williams & Wilkins, Philadelphia © 2000.

CHAPTER 1

SPECT Instrumentation, Radiopharmaceuticals, and Technical Factors

Michael D. Devous, Sr.

Functional brain imaging refers to that set of techniques used to derive images reflecting biochemical, physiologic, or electrical properties of the central nervous system (CNS). The most developed of these techniques are single-photon-emission computed tomography (SPECT), positron-emission tomography (PET), and topographic electroencephalography (TEEG). Of these, SPECT may offer the most widely available *and* widely applicable measure of neuronal behavior. Some recent reviews may be of interest to the reader (1–9). Though PET still provides the highest-resolution tomographic images of brain function, modern SPECT images have similar resolution, making any differences relatively inconsequential in clinical application. Also, while the breadth of radiopharmaceuticals available for brain SPECT is not as great as that for PET, the variety SPECT tracers is expanding rapidly. SPECT perfusion tracers are Food and Drug Administration (FDA)-approved and available for wide distribution, while FDA approval for nationally distributable PET tracers for brain function remains elusive. The lack of a direct SPECT measure of metabolism remains a limitation. Since cerebral perfusion and metabolism are tightly coupled under most normal and pathologic circumstances, this difference may also be of no great clinical relevance.

This chapter provides an overview of the technical aspects of SPECT functional brain imaging, referring primarily to the most common SPECT brain function measure, regional cerebral blood flow (rCBF). SPECT images of rCBF are influenced by a number of factors separate from pathology, including (a) the quality of the tomographic device; (b) the radiopharmaceutical employed; (c) environmental conditions at the time of radiotracer administration; (d) characteristics of the subject (e.g., age, gender, handedness, etc.); (e) the

format used for image presentation; and (f) image processing techniques. All but the last aspect are reviewed in this chapter. Image processing per se is not covered, since the considerable variety in the details of various methods (e.g., filter choices, methods of reconstruction, attenuation and scatter correction schemes, etc.) is beyond the scope of this chapter. The reader is referred to available reviews (4,10–14). However, a brief overview of the essential components of image processing necessary to the achievement of high-quality SPECT brain images has been added. In addition, two new sections have been provided: an intercomparison of available techniques for the quantitative measurement of rCBF and a brief description of relevant radiation safety issues.

INSTRUMENTATION

Tremendous growth in instrumentation over the last two decades has resulted in commercially available, very high quality tomographs for SPECT brain imaging and very sophisticated image-processing hardware and software. SPECT instruments developed by university-based research paved the way for current devices, but industry has led the computational hardware-development process. SPECT brain imaging is now a mature clinical entity, with ongoing commercial tomograph development as well as cooperative ventures between academic centers and industry. SPECT instruments fall into two categories: non-camera-based and camera-based systems, although the latter dominate both academic and commercial development.

Non-Camera-Based Systems

Non-camera-based systems include rotating detector arrays, multidetector scanners, and fixed rings. Rotating detector array devices include the Tomomatic two-, three-, and five-slice machines (Medimatic, Inc) and the Hitachi four-head

---

M. D. Devous, Sr.: Nuclear Medicine Center and Department of Radiology, The University of Texas Southwestern Medical Center, Dallas, Texas 75235-9061.

system. The Tomomatic's most characteristic attribute is the capacity for xenon 133 (^{133}Xe) SPECT imaging, which requires very high sensitivity and rapid dynamic sampling (i.e., complete tomographic studies every 10 seconds) (11, 15). Figure 1.1 shows a typical ^{133}Xe SPECT study from this device for a normal volunteer, with low flow in the cool end of the color scale increasing to high flow in the warm end. The advantage of ^{133}Xe SPECT is that it yields absolute quantitation of rCBF in ml/min/100 g tissue without arterial blood sampling. The Tomomatic, by changing collimators, can also produce moderate resolution (9–10 mm) rCBF images using iodine 123 (^{123}I) or Tecnetium 99m (^{99m}Tc)-labeled radio tracers. The Hitachi rotating detector array system is also capable of both ^{133}Xe and high-resolution (8–10 mm, Fig. 1.2) static imaging (16).

The original fixed-detector research systems were the SPRINT (17), the HEADTOME (18), and the MUMPI (19). They were designed with fixed detectors or a circular annulus of sodium iodide with an internally rotating collimator. The Shimadzu (HEADTOME) system, available only in Japan, is capable of high-sensitivity ^{133}Xe studies and moderate-resolution (10–12 mm) imaging using ^{123}I or [99m]Tc. The most widely available fixed-ring system is the CERASPECT (20), first of the fixed sodium-iodide annulus/rotating collimator machines to come to commercial production. It yields high resolution images (8–10 mm) and is the only fixed-ring system still commercially available in the United States.

The original multidetector scanner was developed by Stoddart et al. (21). It was later known as the Harvard multidetector scanner (22) and was commercially available from Strichman, Inc. This is a slice-based tomograph—as are the Hitachi, Shimadzu, and Tomomatic—but it is built with very thick crystals that operate much like pinhole cameras as they traverse through space to obtain tomographic data. Hill et al. (23) have demonstrated that this device can image [18]fluorodeoxyglucose ([18]FDG) in a single-photon (not PET) mode as well as ^{99m}Tc and [123]I. It cannot perform ^{133}Xe SPECT.

Gamma-Camera-Based Systems

Both single- and multihead gamma camera–based systems are vastly more prevalent than dedicated tomographs, primarily because they can do both head and body SPECT. Modern single-head tomographs have overcome many of the limitations of the original systems, such as poor head alignment, magnetic field aberrations, and inadequate uniformity and linearity for tomography. A few systems have also been designed to circumvent shoulders, so that minimal radius scanning is possible. Most of these systems provide high-resolution images with static tracers (7–10 mm). Unfortunately, single-head systems suffer from poor sensitivity and prolonged imaging times.

A collaborative team from the University of Texas Southwestern Medical Center at Dallas and the nuclear engineering division of Technicare developed the first three-head gamma camera–based SPECT system to address the limited sensitivity of single-head systems (24). This collaboration yielded a system capable of both head and body SPECT at high resolution with static tracers and with adequate sensitivity and rotation speed for dynamic tomography with [133]Xe. The first three-head system (PRISM) was installed in Dallas in late 1987 under the sponsorship of Ohio Imaging, now a division of Picker. Additional three-head SPECT instruments have been produced by Trionix (also as a by-product of the collaboration mentioned above), Toshiba, General Electric, and Siemens. Three-head SPECT systems currently are the most sophisticated instruments for brain SPECT.

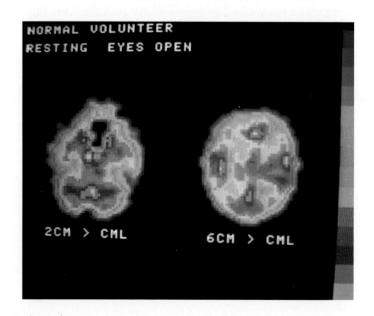

FIG. 1.1. Transverse regional cerebral blood flow (rCBF) images obtained by ^{133}Xe single-photon-emission computed tomography (SPECT) and the Tomomatic 64 (Medimatic A/S, Copenhagen). Images are obtained 2 and 6 cm above and parallel to the canthomeatal line. The 16-shade color scale displays rCBF in ml/min100 g. Images are displayed with subject's left on viewer's left, while images from all other scanners used in this chapter are in the more conventional left-on-right format.

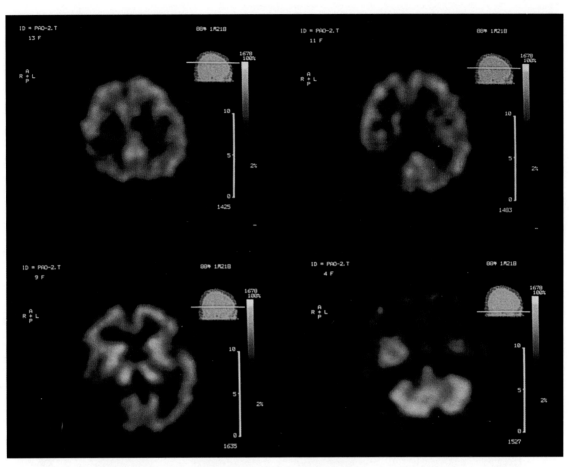

FIG. 1.2. High-resolution rCBF images obtained in a stroke patient with the Hitachi four-head dedicated SPECT unit using ^{99m}Tc HMPAO. (Images provided courtesy of Hitachi.)

There are more than 1,000 such units installed, indicating wide acceptance of this technology. The first ^{133}Xe SPECT images in humans from a three-head system (PRISM) were produced in late 1992 by the Dallas group (Fig. 1.3) and have also been produced by Toshiba.

Image-Processing Essentials

State-of-the-art SPECT systems can be expected to provide high-resolution imaging of statically distributed brain radiopharmaceuticals with patient imaging times of 10–20 min (Fig. 1.4). All of the currently available three-head systems offer excellent spatial resolution: 6-mm resolution in the cortex and about 7 mm at the center of the brain, with appropriate collimators and ^{99m}Tc hexamethylpropyleneamine-oxime (HMPAO) (exametazime or Ceretec, Amersham International) or ethyl cysteinate dimer (^{99m}Tc ECD) (bicisate or Neurolite, DuPont).

To achieve such resolution, a few simple principles should be followed. First, it is necessary to reconstruct nearly motion-free data. A key instrumentation feature to facilitate collection of motion-free data is the capability of sequential image acquisitions. That is, it should be possible to acquire multiple short studies back to back and subsequently discard segments degraded by patient motion (e.g., collecting five 4-min studies to achieve a 20-min total acquisition time). While a 20-min acquisition on a three-head system provides completely adequate data density, studies with less acquisition time may be acceptable for some clinical purposes, as illustrated in Fig. 1.5.

Next, data must be filtered in three dimensions simultaneously. This can be accomplished by either filtering projection data prior to transverse reconstruction (which is automatically 3D), or by filtering reconstructed data if the manufacturer offers true 3D postfiltering. The postreconstruction filtering option has the advantage of being able to view the effects of filter choices on final images and is therefore generally preferred. It is also important to use spatially invariant filters, such as Butterworth, exponential, or similar lowpass filters, thus optimizing cutoff frequency and order (slope) to maximize resolution while minimizing noise (graininess). Spatially varying filters (e.g., Metz or Weiner) can be used only if they are carefully calibrated for brain, which is seldom done. Without such calibration, they can artificially enhance the already substantial contrast present in SPECT brain images [such as that found between gray and white matter or between either of these and cerebrospinal fluid (CSF)] and lead to incorrectly reconstructed rCBF distributions (Fig. 1.6) and even to creation of "false" lesions.

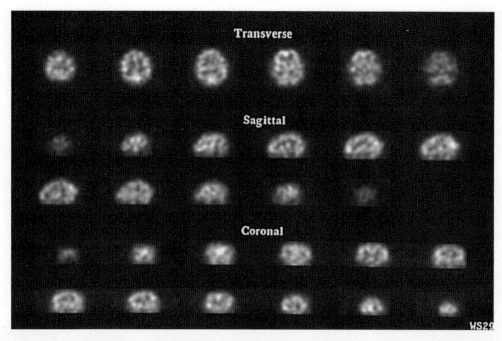

FIG. 1.3. Quantitative (ml/min/100 g) dynamic rCBF images obtained using Xenon 133 (^{133}Xe) and the PRISM 3000S. Images were obtained in 4 min, including 1 min of washin and 3 min of washout of the inert gas tracer.

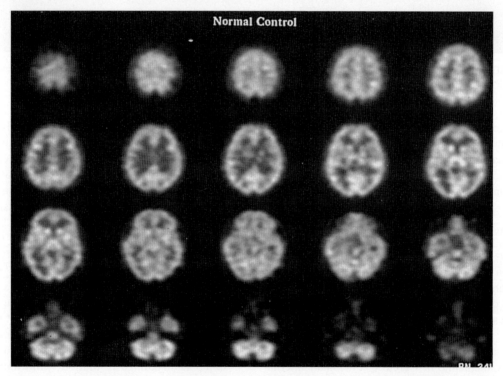

FIG. 1.4. Typical high-resolution rCBF SPECT images obtained using ^{99m}Tc HMPAO and the PRISM 3000S tomograph in a normal volunteer.

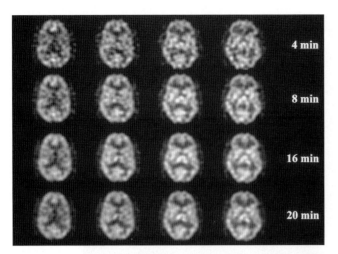

FIG. 1.5. Effect of acquisition time on image quality. Subject was imaged for 20 min in five 4-min sequential blocks using a three-headed gamma camera (Picker 3000S). Either a single projection set was used ($t = 4$ min), or several sets were summed. (Time on the right side of each row indicates total summed acquisition time for that image set). Each row was reconstructed and filtered in exactly the same manner. Note that ideal image quality is obtained at 20 min, but acceptable quality is obtained at 16 min; for rough clinical assessments (such as the presence of a severe acute stroke), even a 4-min acquisition may be adequate.

Transverse reconstruction should be done at single-pixel thickness, so that later processing of oblique angle views (sagittal and coronal) will be unhindered by limited sampling errors. Further, no filtering should be conducted during reconstruction, as this is by definition a 2D (within-slice) filtering process. ("No filtering" is often referred to as a "ramp reconstruction".) After reconstruction and filtering, the next step should be attenuation correction. Here several basic principles need to be applied. First, use an attenuation-correction coefficient that has been calibrated for your system. This can be done by simply imaging a phantom that is an unstructured uniform container of ^{99m}Tc and adjusting the attenuation-correction coefficient until it leads to a flat profile through a cross section of the phantom. Second, be sure that the brain is aligned, so that its long axis (anterior to posterior) is parallel to the long axis of the correction ellipse. Third, it is important to apply an ellipse shape that conforms to the changing shape of the skull (assuming that you use an approximation for attenuation correction, such as the Chang method, instead of a direct measurement). Thus, each transverse slice requires unique ellipse. This process is now automated on most systems through the use of threshold-based edge-detection techniques and takes only a few seconds.

Following reconstruction, filtering, and attenuation correction, the next step is to create oblique multiple-angle views. The brain has a complex and convoluted anatomy, and it is not possible to fully evaluate all components from a single (classically transverse) view. At a minimum, transverse, coronal, and sagittal images should be created. Most modern software will allow you to dynamically alter all three angles, correcting for tilt and yaw as well as choosing the transverse angle of interest. For example, you can orient brain to the canthomeatal line or to some angle relative to it such as might be used for computed tomography (CT) or magnetic resonance imaging (MRI), without prepositioning your patient to a specific anatomic orientation (see discus-

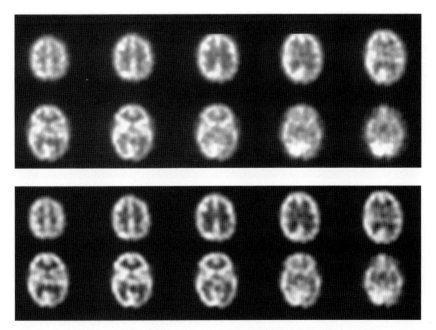

FIG. 1.6. Effect of spatially varying filters on image contrast. Upper images, while appearing to have better definition, have had midfrequency data boosted and high-frequency data removed using a Wiener filter. Lower images have had high-frequency noise removed using a lowpass filter (Butterworth), but the midfrequency data have not been altered. Wiener filtering produced a gray/white ratio of 3.7, while lowpass filtering produced a gray/white ratio of 2.3. The true gray/white ratio of HMPAO (used here) is approximately 2.8, suggesting that the Weiner filter produced a 32% false contrast enhancement.

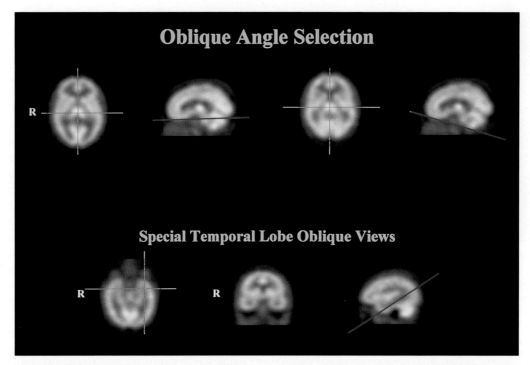

FIG. 1.7. Modern SPECT image-processing software can reformat images at any angle. Top left quadrant shows a sagittal section for reference with an angle selected that is approximately that of the AC–PC line (red) and the resulting transverse image at the level of the marker in the sagittal image. Right upper quadrant shows an angle approximating the canthomeatal line (red) and the associated transverse slice. Bottom row indicates a cross section obtained parallel to the long axis of the temporal lobe (red), providing, in transverse views, a complete image of the mesial temporal wall, including hippocampus and amygdala. These latter images are particularly useful for the evaluation of temporal lobe epilepsy and memory disorder patients.

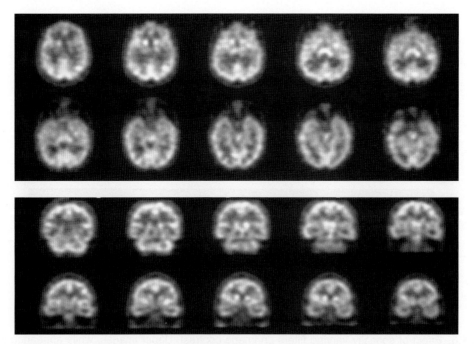

FIG. 1.8. Images derived from orienting along the long axis of the temporal lobe in order to more clearly assess mesial temporal (hippocampus and amygdala) pathology. Top two rows are normal "transverse" sections cut parallel to the long axis of the temporal lobe; bottom two rows are "coronal" sections cut perpendicular to this same axis. See further explanation in Fig. 1.7.

sion below). In fact, oblique reformatting is now so fast that you can make various sets of images for the same patient to facilitate interpretation relative to several axes if you wish (Fig. 1.7). Last, some special orientations can be of interest. One particular view, cut parallel to the long axis of the temporal lobe, is especially useful for evaluating medial temporal lobe structures such as the hippocampus, often the site of abnormalities in epilepsy and memory disorders (Figs. 1.7 and 1.8).

In summary, image-processing software should support dynamic filtering, surface-variable attenuation correction, multiple-angle (oblique) reconstructions, and 3D as well as conventional cross-sectional displays (Fig. 1.9). While numerous permutations of reconstruction algorithms, filter choices, and attenuation methods can be pursued, the general guidelines offered above should result in optimal image generation for your system.

Dual-Isotope Imaging

Dual-isotope imaging permits simultaneous imaging of ^{99m}Tc- and ^{123}I- (or Thallium 201 (^{201}T1) labeled brain radiopharmaceuticals administered to a single subject. Modern SPECT systems should have adequate energy resolution (≤9%) and multiple-energy-window capability in order to separate ^{99m}Tc and ^{123}I radiotracers in the same patient. We

examined the effect of dual-isotope imaging on isotope discrimination as a function of window width and position and on quantitative count recovery (25). Simultaneous dual-isotope imaging of phantoms separated isotope distributions for 10% asymmetric and for 15 or 10% centered ^{99m}Tc windows when combined with a 10% asymmetric ^{123}I window. Isotope concentrations were recovered as accurately from asymmetric dual-isotope windows as from conventional or asymmetric single-isotope windows.

We applied this technique to the simultaneous measurement of resting rCBF and changes induced by vasodilation (1 g acetazolamide) in 10 subjects with cerebrovascular disease (26). Resting and vasodilated ^{133}Xe SPECT images were compared to resting (^{99m}Tc HMPAO) and postacetazolamide (^{123}I IMP or HIPDM) dual-isotope images (Fig. 1.10). There was a linear relationship between ^{133}Xe SPECT and dual-isotope SPECT measurements of lesion/cerebellum ratios in baseline, vasodilated data, and rest–minus vasodilated data. A further advantage of the dual-isotope technique is that ^{99m}Tc and ^{123}I images obtained through dual-isotope imaging are by definition in perfect anatomic registration. Unfortunately, rCBF tracers labeled with ^{123}I are not currently commercially available. Additional applications for dual-isotope rCBF imaging included ictal/interictal seizure imaging, monitoring of acute therapeutic interventions, and single-session evaluations of cognitive or pharmaceutical

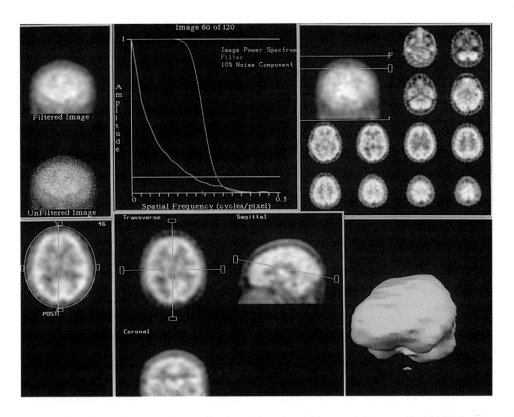

FIG. 1.9. Typical image-processing applications that should be available on all SPECT instruments. **Upper row, Left:** Fourier-space filtering, **Center:** patient-specific filter design. **Right:** backprojection reconstruction. **Lower row. Left:** Adjustable attenuation correction. **Center:** Oblique angle reconstruction. **Right:** 3D display.

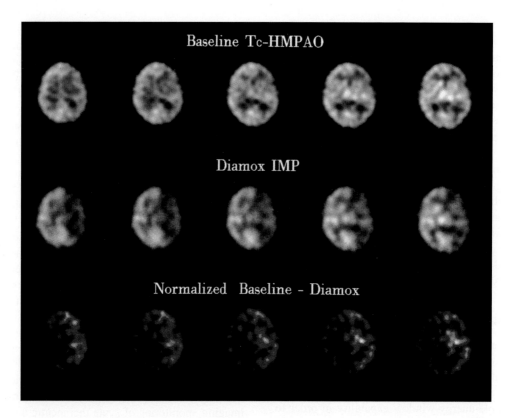

FIG. 1.10. Dual-isotope rCBF images in a patient with transient ischemic attacks demonstrating failed vasodilator reserve. Baseline study (^{99m}Tc HMPAO, *top row*) shows only mild left frontal hypoperfusion, while extensive reserve failure ^{123}I IMP, *middle row*) is seen after vasodilation with acetazolamide (Diamox). The distribution of failed reserve is seen in the subtraction images (*bottom row*), which are easily obtained since the dual-isotope technique produces image sets that are in perfect anatomic registration.

challenge tests. Similarly, it would be possible to use this technique in receptor modeling studies by directly measuring rCBF (normally deduced by assumption) with a ^{99m}Tc-labeled flow tracer, while simultaneously using an ^{123}I-labeled receptor ligand. Several receptor imaging ligands labeled with ^{123}I are in clinical trial.

RADIOPHARMACEUTICALS

Several ^{99m}Tc-labeled and ^{123}I-labeled radiopharmaceuticals for the SPECT measurement of rCBF have been developed. It is also possible to measure regional cerebral blood volume (rCBV) using SPECT techniques. Receptor imaging with SPECT is still primarily a research tool, although at least one agent for D2 receptor studies is commercially available in Europe (^{123}I IBZM). SPECT agents for dopaminergic, serotonergic, noradrenergic, cholinergic, and GABAergic receptor systems are in various stages of clinical trial or preclinical testing. At this moment, there is no tracer for the measurement of cerebral metabolism by SPECT. However, two metabolism-related SPECT measurements can be made. The rCBF/rCBV ratio can be measured directly and is related to regional oxygen extraction. Also, several groups have tested a class of [99m]Tc- and ^{123}I-labeled agents that permit detection of hypoxic cerebral tissues.

Diffusible Tracers

A diffusible tracer is one that passes through the circulation without engaging in metabolism or catabolism. Its concentration in tissue (brain) is therefore dependent only on the concentration gradient between arterial supply and tissue and on the rate of delivery (perfusion). By measuring (directly or indirectly) the arterial concentration, usually known as the input function, and by imaging the rate of brain uptake and clearance, reasonably standard models of diffusible tracer clearance can be used to provide a quantitative measure of rCBF (11). Xenon 133 is the original noninvasive brain blood-flow marker (27–29). It has been in clinical use for several decades and still has significant value (4, 11). The cerebral transit of ^{133}Xe is very rapid, requiring complete tomographic scans every 10 sec to obtain accurate reconstructions (15). It undergoes no chemical interaction in the brain because it is an inert gas. Therefore, its kinetics provide very high fidelity to true rCBF across a broad range of perfusion values and consequently yields superb lesion contrast. The input function can easily be measured by placing a scintillation probe over the lungs. SPECT studies of the transit of ^{133}Xe, when combined with a measure of the input function, can be fit to a mathematical model yielding quantitative estimates of brain blood flow (11, 30–32). Unfortunately, the high sensitivity required for dynamic scanning is usually obtained by sacrificing spatial resolution. Since ^{133}Xe has a short *biological* half-life, you can repeat examinations about every 15 min. For example, in Fig. 1.11 are shown ^{133}Xe rCBF scans in resting and post-Diamox (acetazolamide) states from an elderly woman with transient ischemic attacks (TIAs). Images are relatively normal at baseline, but the scan obtained 15 min later, after vasodilation with Diamox, identifies an extensive area of failed vasodilatory reserve. Short imaging times and rapid isotope clearance greatly facilitate rest and stress brain imaging. In addition, the entire SPECT acquisition process is accomplished in 4 min—an important feature for difficult, uncooperative patients.

Xenon 127 is not currently commercially available in the United States; therefore, it has not enjoyed the extensive use as an rCBF tracer that has occurred for ^{133}Xe. However, it has several potential advantages (see later), including more optimal photon energy (204 keV vs. 81 keV for ^{133}Xe) and reduced radiation dose, since its decay does not include the emission of a soft beta, in contrast to ^{133}Xe. These factors should combine to provide improved spatial resolution, likely exceeding that available for the static tracers at a reduced radiation burden. Kromium 81m (^{81m}Kr) has also been proposed as an rCBF tracer, though its extremely short half-life (13 sec) would require the use of a steady state model rather than the clearance models used for the Xe tracers for quantitation. It has been successfully used for measurements of cardiac blood flow.

Static Tracers

All SPECT rCBF agents other than ^{133}Xe or ^{127}Xe (e.g., IMP, HIPDM, HMPAO, and ECD) were designed for use

with rotating gamma cameras, which have low sensitivity. Consequently, rCBF tracers for use with such systems must be relatively stable *in vivo* (at least 60 min). Unlike the diffusible tracers, these radiopharmaceuticals are extracted by the brain on first arterial pass after intravenous injection and are then retained for several hours. Brain retention (or at least hindered diffusion from brain) is due to some trapping mechanism, such as metabolic degradation or conformational alteration. Agents such as IMP, HIPDM, HMPAO, and ECD are commonly referred to as *chemical microspheres*. Their stable distribution permits prolonged imaging times (as long as the patient does not move), so that specialized collimators can be used to produce high-resolution images. While count ratios among brain regions correctly represent relative rCBF, most retention mechanisms do not lend themselves to simple mathematical models to provide absolute quantitation.

The original tracer microsphere model works reasonably well for IMP and HIPDM but not for ECD or HMPAO. More sophisticated models have been proposed. Unfortunately, these models depend on knowing the input function, which requires arterial blood sampling (not a routine practice in most nuclear medicine laboratories). If a simple method of measuring the input function is devised, then the microsphere-like compounds can be used to measure absolute rCBF as quantitatively as any other noninvasive modality, including PET (see additional comments under "Quantification," below).

^{123}I rCBF Tracers

The first rCBF agent for use on rotating gamma cameras was ^{123}I IMP, followed almost immediately by ^{123}I HIPDM. IMP

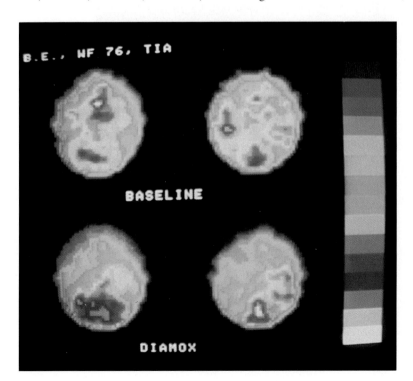

FIG. 1.11. Failed vasodilator reserve illustrated using ^{133}Xe SPECT and the Tomomatic 64 scanner in a 76-year-old woman suffering from transient ischemic attacks (TIAs). Upper images (2 and 6 cm above the CML) obtained in the resting state are nearly normal, while the lower images, obtained after vasodilation with acetazolamide, show middle and anterior cerebral artery reserve failure. Postacetazolamide were obtained 30 min after the resting study.

(Spectamine) was developed by Winchell et al. (33) at MediPhysics and HIPDM was developed by Kung et al. (34) at the State University of New York. Both are iodinated amines with fairly rapid brain uptake and good extraction. HIPDM has a 6-h brain retention half-life. IMP has a much shorter brain retention half-life (on the order of 60–90 min). Both IMP (35–38) and HIPDM (39) follow higher cerebral blood-flow levels more accurately than either HMPAO or ECD. Unfortunately, neither agent is commercially available in the United States, though IMP remains the most widely used rCBF tracer in Japan.

Some investigators have compared initial (early) to delayed IMP images (usually a 4-hr delay) to determine if changes in distribution over time relate to tissue status (3,6,7,40). This procedure is commonly referred to as *redistribution imaging*. Some reports suggest that filling in (redistribution) of lesions seen in early images is indicative of salvageable tissue. Current literature is contradictory, neither clearly supporting nor refuting the value of redistribution imaging with IMP.

⁹⁹ᵐTc rCBF Tracers

Investigators at Amersham (39,41) and Volkert et al. (42) at the University of Missouri developed the first of the technetium agents approved by the FDA for use in humans, ⁹⁹ᵐTc HMPAO (Ceretec). ⁹⁹ᵐTc-ECD (Neurolite) is of a class suggested by Kung et al. (43) and was developed and commercialized by DuPont (44,45). Both agents have good brain uptake. The extraction of ECD is slightly lower, but the contrast (the ratio of gray to white matter) is higher than for HMPAO. Both tracers image defects similarly, although there are suggestions that, during luxury perfusion following stroke, HMPAO will follow perfusion, while ECD will continue to show a defect at the site of injury. There is also a growing body of literature (mostly from Japan) that HMPAO and IMP mark somewhat different territories of damage in cerebrovascular disease. (HMPAO underestimates IMP lesion size.) There are few data directly comparing ECD and IMP.

ECD initially proved easier to use because HMPAO was unstable *in vitro* and required freshly eluted ⁹⁹ᵐTcO₄⁻. However, Amersham refined a stabilized version of HMPAO (Fig. 1.12) that subsequently achieved FDA approval. ECD may be used for up to 6 hr after reconstitution, and HMPAO may be used for up to 4 hr. ECD clears from the blood and the body faster, consequently producing less radiation exposure per millicurie administered than HMPAO. In general, image contrast with ECD is superior to that with HMPAO, but recent studies with HMPAO obtained 90 min after injection demonstrate the potential for equivalent contrast (Fig. 1.4).

In separate studies in human subjects, we compared "derived" rCBF for either ⁹⁹ᵐTc-ECD (46) or ⁹⁹ᵐTc HMPAO (47) to absolute rCBF. "Derived" rCBF refers to whole-brain-normalized ROI data converted to absolute rCBF values by equating ECD or HMPAO whole-brain counts to whole brain rCBF (¹³³Xe) for each subject. On the left of Fig. 1.13 is a regression analysis of "derived" ECD rCBF vs. true rCBF indicating a strong linear relationship and demonstrating that ECD follows rCBF up to at least 80 ml/min/100 g. On the right side of Fig. 1.13 are the data comparing ⁹⁹ᵐTc

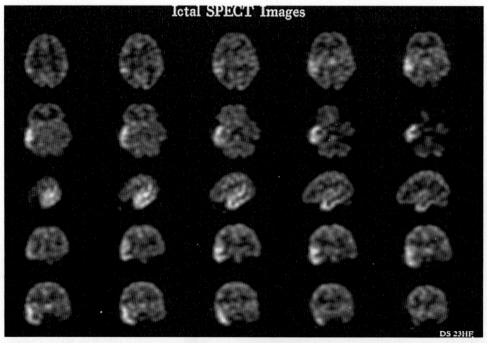

FIG. 1.12. Ictal rCBF SPECT images obtained in a epilepsy patient with complex partial seizures of temporal lobe origin using the stabilized form of ⁹⁹ᵐTc HMPAO.

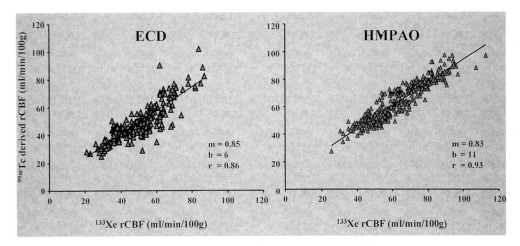

FIG. 1.13. Comparison of the "derived" rCBF for ^{99m}Tc ECD *(left)* or ^{99m}Tc HMPAO *(right)* relative to rCBF determined by quantitative ^{133}Xe SPECT. "Derived" rCBF refers to whole-brain-normalized ROI data converted to absolute rCBF by equating ECD or HMPAO whole brain counts to whole brain rCBF (^{133}Xe) for each subject. Regression analysis *(right)* of "derived" ECD rCBF vs. true rCBF. There is a strong linear relationship and ECD follows rCBF up to at least 80 ml/min/100 g. Data comparing ^{99m}Tc HMPAO to ^{133}Xe SPECT *(right)* show similar results. ECD and HMPAO mildly underestimated high rCBF and mildly overestimated low rCBF.

HMPAO to ^{133}Xe SPECT, illustrating similar results. Both ECD and HMPAO mildly underestimated high rCBF and mildly overestimated low rCBF.

Regional Cerebral Blood Volume

Under most circumstances, rCBF is tightly coupled to tissue metabolism. However, rCBF is not the only hemodynamic parameter that affects tissue metabolism. Regional cerebral blood volume (rCBV) and the extraction of oxygen can be important determinants of nutrient availability. Although direct measures of oxygen metabolism or extraction are not available by SPECT, the ratio of rCBF to rCBV is related to the regional oxygen extraction ratio (rOER). Thus, an estimate of the rOER can be obtained from the rCBF/rCBV ratio (48). rCBV imaging is conducted in a manner analogous to that of cardiac blood pool imaging: Red cells are labeled with ^{99m}Tc, followed by static SPECT of the head.

Quantitative values are obtained by SPECT imaging of a reference blood sample drawn from the subject at the time of rCBV imaging (49–51). The dual-isotope technique can be used to image rCBF and rCBV simultaneously (Fig. 1.14).

Receptor Imaging

Although neuroreceptor imaging currently has no proven clinical role, early clinical trials and extensive PET experience suggest that SPECT imaging using specific receptor binding agents may soon find major clinical application. Radioligands are currently under study in human trials for quantitating adrenergic, dopaminergic (transporter, D1 and D2) (52), serotonergic (transporter, 5-HT$_2$ and 5-HT$_{1A}$), benzodiazepine and GABA (53), muscarinic cholinergic (54,55), and opioid systems. Neurotransmitter values obtained include distribution volume, receptor density, receptor or transporter occupancy, and binding constants. Most

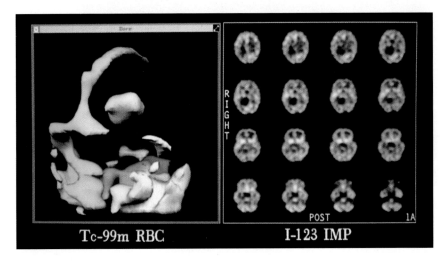

FIG. 1.14. Dual-isotope images of regional cerebral blood volume (rCBV) obtained with ^{99m}Tc-labeled red blood cells (*left image*: 3D right posterior oblique view) and rCBF obtained using ^{123}I IMP (*right image*: transverse cross sections) in a patient with an arteriovenous malformation (AVM). The AVM appears as a large mass just anterior to the descending sagittal sinus in the regional cerebral blood volume (rCBV image), while it appears as a defect in the rCBF images, since it does not retain the perfusion tracer.

such agents rely on ^{123}I as the radiolabel, although a few ^{99m}Tc labeled ligands are under investigation. While these compounds differ structurally from their native analogs, their affinity for the specific receptor site often exceeds that of the native compound. In addition to their high affinity for the receptor site, many of these agents also have high total brain uptake (on the order of 10%). Such uptake is comparable to that seen with blood-flow agents.

Potential clinical applications for receptor imaging would include the diagnosis of specific neurodegenerative diseases, quantitative assessment of therapeutic interventions designed to alter receptor function, assessment of toxic effects of substances of abuse, and evaluation of interventions capable of producing prophylaxis. Such applications, in combination with or separate from perfusion imaging, may be particularly of interest in the study of psychiatric disorders, which are so commonly responsive to neurotransmitter-active pharmaceuticals. Areas for further investigation necessary to make receptor imaging a practical clinical tool include the establishment of correlations between the binding-site concentration and the disease process as well as the development of more accurate methods for absolute quantitation of the distribution of brain radioactivity. Combined use of receptor, perfusion, and structural imaging in a coregistration paradigm may also greatly enhance quantitation. Fortunately, Innis et al. have demonstrated that at least receptor affinity can be determined from data reflecting only relative count density (56). Initially, advances in receptor imaging were hampered by the fact that many neurotransmitters bind to a family of receptors; recently, more specific ligands have been developed.

Metabolism

Metabolic aspects of neuronal function cannot be directly imaged with SPECT. We do not have, even on the horizon, an oxygen analog. Glucose metabolism has been monitored with great success by PET with [18F] fluorodeoxyglucose (FDG), it has been suggested that it might be possible to iodinate glucose analogs for SPECT that would behave like [18]FDG. While there have been two promising preliminary reports, neither has come to fruition at this time.

In summary, SPECT measures of rCBF are well developed, perhaps even better than those for PET. Both dynamic and static techniques are effective. SPECT can also be used to image rCBV, though clinical application of this technique has been minimal. There is great potential for receptor imaging, which has now moved out of the basic science laboratory and into clinical research. Interest in ^{201}Tl as a SPECT brain agent has also developed because it has been shown to be useful in distinguishing recurrent brain tumor from radiation necrosis after radiation therapy (57–59) and in staging brain tumors (60–62). Last, progress is being made with glucose metabolic imaging at the animal level.

FACTORS THAT AFFECT IMAGE APPEARANCE

Environmental Conditions

These include conditions experienced by subjects during radiotracer administration that play a significant role in determining the observed rCBF distribution. The coupling of rCBF to regional metabolism has frequently been demonstrated not only under resting conditions but also during cognitive or motoric activation (63–69). Thus, visual, auditory and somatosensory stimuli can all be expected to affect the regional level of neuronal activity and thus rCBF (Fig. 1.15). Unfortunately, there are no clearly established standards describing the ideal conditions for any of these environmental parameters. Most investigators use an "eyes and ears open" imaging environment in which subjects are seated during radiotracer injection. Supportive of this choice are data from our group and others indicating that quantitative flow or metabolism values are less variable under such conditions

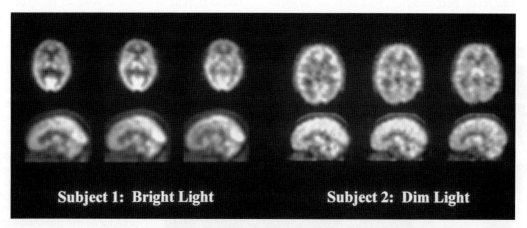

FIG. 1.15. The effect of visual stimulation on rCBF in a normal volunteer. Left images were obtained from subject during stimulation with bright white light. Right images were obtained in a subject with eyes and ears open sitting in a dimly lit room. Note that perfusion decreases in the "dim light" condition relative to the "bright light" condition not only in primary visual cortex but also in associative cortices.

than in the "eyes and ears closed" setting (11,70). Room lights are often dimmed to provide a minimum and relatively standard visual stimulus. The degree to which surrounding personnel provide both auditory and visual stimuli should be (though seldom is) carefully controlled.

The duration of steady-state conditions necessary to ensure minimal variability induced by environmental conditions is also not well established. To some degree, this is a radiotracer-dependent issue. For example, ^{99m}Tc HMPAO has very rapid first-pass extraction, while a component of ^{123}I IMP is retained by lung and likely affects brain tracer distribution for 5–10 min after injection. Xenon 133 is a dynamic tracer that must be imaged during administration. In each case, the requirements vary for how long environmental conditions must be constant both before and after tracer administration. As a general rule, we require steady-state environmental conditions for 10 min prior to and after tracer administration for injectables. No requirement after administration is needed for ^{133}Xe.

Subject Characteristics

Age, gender, handedness, anxiety, time of day (diurnal variations), blood pressure, arterial carbon dioxide levels, cognitive involvement (attention), and other factors are subject-specific determinants of rCBF. While it is clear that there are both age (65,71–76) and gender (71,77–80) effects on whole-brain blood flow, regional effects are somewhat less well characterized (71,73,74,77,78,80). Further, recent studies suggest that these two factors affect rCBF in complex ways. For example, the decline in rCBF seen with age is not as marked in active elderly individuals as it is in age-matched inactive subjects (76). Also, gender effects seem dependent even on gender dominance within a particular gender (e.g., males with more feminine characteristics have higher flow than males with more masculine characteristics) (78).

Challenge Studies

Pharmacologic challenges induce alterations in rCBF, which can provide both useful tools for the discrimination of disease and conundrums for image interpretation. For example, acetazolamide is a cerebral vasodilator commonly used in the determination of vasodilatory reserve (Figs. 1.10 and 1.11) (81–84). However, the consistency with which it alters or preserves regional patterns from a "resting" state is not well known. Caffeine, which may be present in subjects in various quantities, can lead to reductions in both global and rCBF (85). The impact of other pharmacologic factors (e.g., antidepressants, antiepileptics, etc.) is only now being elucidated. It is advisable to eliminate all such complicating factors for as long as possible preceding a study. For caffeine, 24 hr may be effective. For antidepressants, drug clearance may not be complete for up to 14 days (86).

Cognitive challenges are also sources of valuable discrimination and unwanted variability. For example, mild visual stimulation (dimly lit room) seems to minimize variability among normals relative to deprivation of visual stimuli (11,70). Auditory stimuli must similarly be carefully controlled and evaluated (66,87). However, specific sensory stimuli can induce asymmetry (Fig. 1.16) and lead to activation not only of primary and associative sensory cortices but even of remote cortical and subcortical sites (67,88). In general, consistency is the greatest asset. That is, study all subjects under as identical a set of conditions as possible.

Image Presentation

Recent advances in image processing instrumentation and SPECT have afforded the opportunity to present image data in a wide variety of formats. The degree to which conventional transverse cross-sectional images provide adequate information for image interpretation is being appropriately challenged. Sagittal, coronal, and other oblique-angle reconstructions are readily produced by most computer systems. Experienced observers recognize that certain brain structures are more readily appreciated in nonconventional display orientations. For example, evaluation of the medial aspect of the orbital frontal cortex is more readily performed from sagittal cross sections than from transverse. Evaluation of mesial temporal lobe hypoperfusion in epilepsy is easiest in special oblique views designed to highlight the mesial tem-

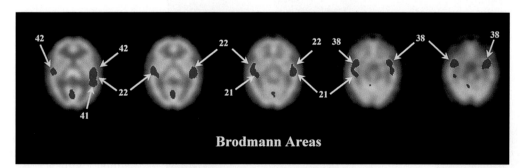

FIG. 1.16. Cognitive activation from speech perception results in (contralateral) rCBF asymmetry. Parametric images representing areas of significant change (red) in 13 normal controls overlaid on a SPECT Talairach atlas-based registration model (gray scale) and labeled according to the responding Brodmann areas. Images are arranged in order to correspond *(from left to right)* to Talairach levels of 12, 4, −1, −8, and −16 mm above/below the AC-PC line.

poral wall (Fig. 1.8) than in classic coronal, sagittal, or transverse views. It is wise to review studies in at least three orthogonal orientations.

Similarly, the modality employed for image review has significant impact on interpretation. Conventional film-and-lightbox formats require the reviewer to consider all image data over a similar contrast range and often with a fixed degree of background subtraction. In contrast, direct viewing from a video display affords the opportunity for gray-scale manipulation and dynamic background subtraction. Choosing between gray-scale image displays and color-image displays presents the viewer with yet another poorly defined dilemma. In general, most reviewers of high-resolution images prefer gray scales. The human visual system is better suited to gray-scale discrimination across structural boundaries than it is to the same discrimination using a color-based scheme. However, with poorer resolution systems or foreshortened image data sets (minimum pixel density), color scales can provide enhanced interpretation of abnormalities. Similarly, parametric displays in which color can be used to portray functional information may provide enhanced opportunities for lesion detection (Fig. 1.16).

Recently, 3D surface-rendered displays have become commonplace (Fig. 1.17), while more sophisticated 3D displays of "see-through" or "smoked-glass" images are not as available (Fig. 1.18). The "dial-a-lesion" format of most surface-rendered images currently limits their routine applicability. Established standards for count-density threshold settings have not been published. Cinematographic displays of projection data also provide a certain 3D quality. Their primary use is in monitoring patient motion as a source of image degradation.

Six conclusions can be drawn regarding image presentation. (a) SPECT rCBF studies should be presented in at least

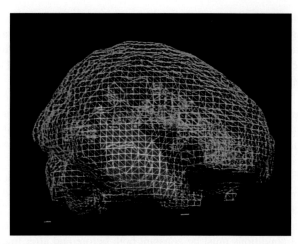

FIG. 1.18. Some "see-through" 3D rCBF SPECT images combine multiple surfaces. In this case, a "wire-cage" surface is used to outline the brain, while a solid body is used to define the location of an area of high flow in an ictal study of rCBF in a seizure patient (same patient as shown in Fig. 1.11).

transverse, coronal, and sagittal cross sections. (b) The conditions under which subjects are studied should be established as a laboratory standard and maintained for all clinical and research studies. The most common standard is eyes and ears open in a dimly lit environment with minimal auditory "white noise." (c) The normal distribution of rCBF in such a setting shows symmetric flow distribution between homologous regions. (d) Both age and gender effects can be noted. They are only well characterized for whole-brain blood flow, which is not readily measured by conventional SPECT techniques. (e) Among brain stress tests that could be employed to enhance discrimination of disease, the only well-estab-

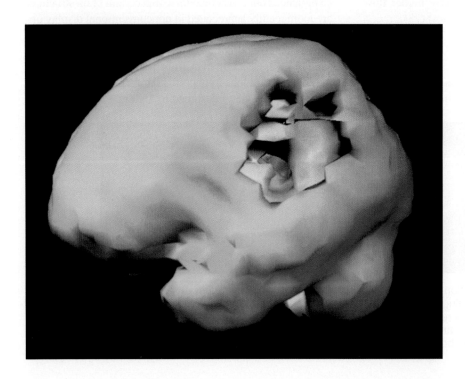

FIG. 1.17. 3D surface-rendered rCBF SPECT image in a patient with a left parietal stroke. Surface-rendered images are useful to assess the distribution (vascular territory) of cortical defects but do not allow visualization of either defect magnitude (count density) or of subcortical abnormalities.

TABLE 1.1. *Brain SPECT—imaging principles*

1. Patient preparation
   a. Quiet reproducible environment
      eyes/ears open; dimly lit room
   b. Intravenous line placed approximately 10 min before injection
      quiet approximately 10 min after injection
2. Radiopharmaceuticals
   a. rCBF tracers
      ^{99m}Tc HMPAO   Ceretec (Amersham)
      ^{99m}Tc ECD   Neurolite (DuPont)
   b. Delay imaging for best results
      90 min for Ceretec
      45 min for Neurolite
3. Imaging Systems
   a. High-resolution collimators
      UHR and fan beam when possible
   b. Minimum radius (heads in close)
   c. "Motion-free" positioning
      patient comfort first
      multiple sequential acquisitions
   d. Single pixel reconstruction
      no filtering during reconstruction
   e. 3D lowpass filtering
   f. Attenuation correction
      shape-conforming ellipse
   g. Oblique reformatting
      transverse, sagittal, coronal, special views

SPECT, single-photon-emission tomography; rCBF, regional cerebral blood flow; ^{99m}Tc, Technetium 99; HMPAO, hexamethylpropyleneamine-oxine; ECD, ethylcysteinate dimer.

lished technique is the acetazolamide vasodilator test. Under most circumstances, it reveals striking asymmetries in disease states of vascular origin. Its regional effects independent of global flow changes have not yet been established in normal controls. (f) Future research should focus on the establishment of normative databases and the effect of environmental variations on regional cerebral blood flow.

In summary, factors reviewed above that significantly influence the final quality of your SPECT brain images fall broadly into three categories: patient preparation, radiopharmaceuticals, and imaging systems. These key factors are summarized in Table 1.1.

INTERCOMPARISON OF NEUROIMAGING TECHNIQUES FOR THE QUANTIFICATION OF rCBF

The two most commonly reported imaging procedures for measuring rCBF are SPECT and PET. In addition, functional measures that are related to rCBF (though indirectly) can be obtained with either functional MRI (fMRI) using the blood oxygenation level determination (BOLD) technique or by obtaining a signal that is heavily dependent on water diffusion characteristics (diffusion-weighted MRI). The latter two techniques are still under development, while SPECT and PET are well established for both research and clinical applications.

The current literature suggests that both global and focal effects on neuronal metabolism and CBF are observed in a variety of neurologic and psychiatric disorders; it may therefore be important to use imaging procedures that can quantify both global and regional CBF. This is possible with both SPECT and PET but is not currently possible with either fMRI or diffusion-weighted MRI. Key characteristics of the most commonly used functional brain imaging procedures are outlined in Table 1.2. Many aspects of SPECT and PET techniques are similar, but important differences should be carefully considered when choosing the appropriate imaging tool for a particular investigation. For this discussion, we restrict ourselves to a description of those characteristics of interest to the measurement of rCBF.

PET rCBF Imaging

Advantages

A principal advantage of PET for rCBF measurement lies in the tracer H_2O^{15}, which functions as a diffusible tracer. Because O^{15} has a short (2-min) physical half-life, the tracer is rapidly removed from the subject by decay and so an additional advantage is that repeat imaging can be performed as quickly as 10 min after the initial scan. Also, the rapid image-acquisition process permits detection of rather transient phenomena (rCBF changes as brief as 30 sec in duration can be detected, though 2 min is more typical.) This is in contrast to regional cerebral glucose metabolism (rCGM) PET imaging, for which tracer uptake occurs over about 30 min and the resulting image represents the integral of brain activity over that time period (Table 1.2). Radiation dose is quite low, and many scans can safely be conducted in one session (see "Issues of Radiation Risk," below).

Disadvantages

Unfortunately, the 2-min half-life of O^{15} requires that one use an on-site cyclotron to produce the tracer and perform rapid chemical procedures to make the chemical entity of interest (in

TABLE 1.2. *Key parameters of the most common functional brain imaging procedures*

Imaging procedure	Parameter measured	Spatial resolution	Temporal resolution	Test environment
PET (^{18}FDG)	rCGM	4 mm	30 min	Scan room
PET (H_2O^{15})	rCBF	10 mm	2 min	Scanner
SPECT (^{99m}Tc)	rCBF	7 mm	20 sec	Anywhere
SPECT (^{133}Xe)	rCBF	12 mm	2 min	Scanner
fMRI	$\propto$ rCBF and rCBV	3–8 mm	100 msec	Loud scanner

PET, positron-emission tomography; ^{18}FDG, ^{18}fluorodeoxyglucose; rCGM, regional cerebral glucose metabolism; rCBF, regional cerebral blood flow; SPECT, single-photon-emission tomography; ^{133}Xe, Xenon 133; fMRI, diffusion-weighted magnetic resonance imaging; rCBV, regional cerebral blood volume.

this case water). Further, the subject to be imaged must be fully prepared and in the scanner when the tracer is compounded for use. Therefore, imaging results can be confounded by cognitive effects of anxiety in the scanner or by visual or auditory stimuli present therein. Also, as a consequence of the short half-life of O^{15} and the rapid transit of H_2O^{15}, the PET scanner must be operated in a data-acquisition mode that maximizes sensitivity to emitted radiation and minimizes the duration of the image acquisition. So while the spatial resolution of PET scanners can be as good as 4 mm when long imaging times can be used (such as in imaging rCGM), when PET scanners are used for rCBF imaging, this resolution is typically degraded to about 10 mm (Table 1.2). Next, while ^{15}O offers minimal radiation exposure per dose to the subject being imaged, its short half-life requires the cyclotron production of substantial quantities, so that enough is left after radioactive decay to provide a reasonable dose to the subject. This means that radiation safety for PET technologists, chemists, and physicists can be challenging. Last, PET tomographs and cyclotrons are expensive, and this technique requires a considerable capital investment. Though this is a complex process, these details are well developed, and PET rCBF imaging can readily be performed in properly equipped facilities with experienced personnel.

PET Quantitation

PET rCBF imaging with H_2O^{15} can be fully quantified using a mathematical model that relies principally on the diffusible tracer technique. It is worth noting that water is not completely freely diffusible across the blood-brain barrier; therefore, H_2O^{15} is not a perfect rCBF tracer, yielding values that somewhat underestimate true rCBF, especially at higher perfusion rates. Full quantitation requires arterial catheterization and blood sampling during the scan, subsequent counting of the acquired samples, and cross-calibration of the scanner and counting equipment. This process, once established in a laboratory, is straightforward though time-consuming and permits precise intercomparison of global CBF values within subjects across conditions and between subjects. The value of absolute rCBF determination varies with the desired study. In most of the reported literature, the substantial intersubject variance in *normal* absolute global CBF has served primarily as a confound; therefore, it is removed by calculating relative rCBF values either through normalization to global CBF or rCBF in a reference brain region such as cerebellum or occipital lobe or by use of analysis of variance or a related statistical procedure. However, in the circumstance where a task, pharmacologic challenge, disease process, or treatment is expected to affect absolute CBF values, full quantitation may be important for within-subject across-condition assessments.

SPECT rCBF Imaging

As described above, SPECT rCBF imaging can be accomplished with either of two classes of radiopharmaceuticals: the diffusible tracers ^{133}Xe or ^{127}Xe, or the static tracers ^{99m}Tc HMPAO or ^{99m}Tc ECD. General characteristics common to both classes and specific characteristics unique to each are outlined below.

General Advantages

SPECT is widely available (approximately 2,500 installed systems in the United States compared to about 50 for PET), and the tracers used are FDA-approved. (No PET tracer for the imaging of neuronal function has received FDA approval for national distribution.) SPECT is the only functional brain-imaging technique in common clinical use. SPECT is generally considered to be less complicated than PET, often only because less rigorous approaches to its use are employed. The radiopharmaceuticals are commercially available and relatively inexpensive (though there is a substantial difference between the classes, ^{133}Xe being about one-fourth the cost of the ^{99m}Tc-labeled tracers). As also previously described, the instrumentation has matured, so that distinctions between SPECT and PET spatial resolution are not substantial (Table 1.1).

Advantages of ^{133}Xe and ^{127}Xe

As described above, Xe SPECT tracers are freely diffusible tracers and are in a sense the SPECT equivalent of ^{15}O for PET. Both ^{133}Xe and ^{127}Xe have short biological half-lives because they are inert gases and are exhaled from the body within a few minutes of the completion of their administration. Therefore, as with ^{15}O, repeat imaging can be performed as quickly as 15 min after the initial scan. The inert gas chemical form makes these the purest of the diffusible tracers yielding the best fidelity to true rCBF; it also permits administration either by inhalation or intravenous injection of dissolved gas, which can be helpful with patients for whom intravenous placement is challenging. Also, the rapid image-acquisition process (about 4 min compared to about 2 min for H_2O^{15}) also permits detection of transient phenomena (Table 1.1). Radiation dose is also low (the dose of ^{127}Xe is similar to that of ^{15}O, but ^{133}Xe requires a higher dose per scan due to the emission of a low-energy β particle) and several scans can safely be conducted in one session (see "Issues of Radiation Risk," below). Only ^{133}Xe is commercially available in the United States at this time and can be obtained in bulk for frequent use. (One vial will last about a week, since ^{133}Xe has a 5.3-day half-life.) A commercial system for the distribution and recycling of ^{127}Xe (which has a 36.4-day half-life) has been proposed but is not yet in production. This would be an important development, as ^{127}Xe affords much higher spatial resolution than ^{133}Xe (approximately 6 mm compared to 12 mm).

Advantages of ^{99m}Tc Static Tracer

^{99m}Tc HMPAO and ^{99m}Tc ECD function as "static" rCBF tracers, or chemical microspheres. The fact that they are retained in brain for several hours provides the unique opportunity to inject subjects away from the scanner and obtain a "snapshot" of rCBF at the time of injection in an environment completely under investigator control; imaging can then occur up to 6 hr later.

Because the tracer distribution is stable *in vivo* for such a long time, advanced high-resolution scanning techniques can be used to acquire data. Thus, these tracers yield rCBF images with better spatial resolution than those of any technique.

General Disadvantages

It is generally agreed that the spatial resolution for SPECT scanners is inferior to that of PET scanners for comparable tracers. For example, for diffusible tracers, the resolution of ^{133}Xe is a little worse than for H_2O^{15}, and the same would be true for a comparison with ^{99m}Tc tracers if there were a "chemical microsphere" PET radiopharmaceutical. (The closest comparator for this purpose would be ^{18}FDG.) This difference is typically only a few millimeters, and differences may be nonexistent for specific instrument comparisons. If ^{127}Xe becomes available, it would have the best resolution of the diffusible rCBF tracers for either SPECT or PET and would be comparable to or slightly better than that for the ^{99m}Tc agents. In addition to inferior resolution, SPECT is generally regarded as having poorer quantitative properties. For example, attenuation correction is usually accounted for by direct measurement with PET and only by mathematical approximation for SPECT. This is of importance only for static tracers, since the models for quantifying diffusible tracers with SPECT do not rely on attenuation correction. (This is not the case for the bolus H_2O^{15} PET method.)

Disadvantages of ^{133}Xe and ^{127}Xe

As with H_2O^{15}, the subject to be imaged with the Xe tracers must be in the scanner when the tracer is administered. Again, imaging results can be confounded by cognitive effects of anxiety when the patient is in the scanner or by visual or auditory stimuli present therein. Further, as a consequence of the short biological half-life of the Xe tracers, as with the short physical half-life of O^{15}, the SPECT scanner must be operated in a data-acquisition mode that maximizes sensitivity to emitted radiation and minimizes the duration of the image acquisition, leading to significant reductions in spatial resolution. Xenon 133 has a relatively low gamma-ray energy (80 keV), making it difficult to obtain good count statistics and further degrading image resolution. While the 5.3-day half-life is useful for "off the shelf" use, it does present a radiation safety complication for both storage and disposal. Even though ^{127}Xe would have many advantages over ^{133}Xe—including superior spatial resolution, minimal attenuation artifact, and reduced radiation dose to the subject—its longer half-life further complicates the storage and disposal issues, and these are not yet thoroughly solved.

Disadvantages of ^{99m}Tc Static Tracer

The principal disadvantage of the static tracers is a consequence of one of the advantages—long *in vivo* residence time. In addition to the multihour biochemical half-life, the 6 h physical half-life of ^{99m}Tc means that one must wait four to six half-lives before the radioactive background of an initial scan is below detectable limits. While this feature affords superb control over the imaging environment, it also means that one must wait at least a day, and preferably 2 days, before repeating the imaging sequence. Several means to address this problem have been explored, including split-dose techniques and dual-isotope imaging, but in most settings simply waiting for the decay of the first injection is the preferred solution. Additionally, neither ^{99m}Tc HMPAO nor ^{99m}Tc ECD are perfect chemical microspheres; consequently, they underestimate rCBF values above about 60 ml/min/100 g, with the error increasing in proportion to rCBF (Fig. 1.13).

SPECT Quantitation

As with H_2O^{15}, SPECT rCBF imaging with the Xe tracers can be fully quantified using a mathematical model that relies principally on the diffusible tracer technique. Fortunately, full quantitation does not requires arterial catheterization but only measurement of the Xe concentration curve over time in the lungs (i.e., the input function), which can be accomplished with a simple radiation detector placed above the chest. This process is also straightforward and can readily be performed in most nuclear medicine departments. Full quantification of ^{133}Xe rCBF actually preceded that by PET, since this procedure was developed for 2D nonimaging measurement techniques as early as the 1950s.

Models used to quantitate rCBF for static tracers differ from those for diffusible tracers and are not as well developed. In fact, earlier studies using these tools to examine rCBF used only the semiquantitative relative measures mentioned above. While this method provides a useful index of regional rCBF relationships, it cannot be used to measure absolute change in CBF. Several fully quantitative approaches have been explored, including complete modeling with arterial sampling. These approaches are effective but have not been popular, since they remove from SPECT its advantage of relative simplicity. It is also possible to measure a quantity known as the brain perfusion index (BPI) that is closely related to global CBF (89,90). This process is not substantially more complicated than that required for Xe tracer rCBF modeling but does require that the subject be physically in the scanner at the time of tracer administration. Thus, both classes of SPECT rCBF tracers can be used either for relative or absolute rCBF measurement with differing degrees of complexity and accuracy, neither of which exceeds those required for PET modeling with H_2O^{15}.

ISSUES OF RADIATION RISK

There is a general view that radiation is harmful at any level and that, consequently, medical imaging procedures that involve exposure to any radiation whatsoever are associated with some level of risk (91,92). Great efforts (and costs) are extended to minimize radiation exposure for patients, research volunteers, and workers. With the advent of functional measures based on MRI imaging sequences, it is sometimes suggested that these techniques should be used in favor of PET or SPECT imaging whenever possible to avoid the perceived radiation risk of the radioactive tracer techniques. Much of this impression has been fostered by the widespread regulatory use of the "linear no-threshold theory" regarding the assessment of radiation risk (93–95). The purpose of this section is to briefly describe the data regarding low-level radiation and risk and to clarify that, in fact, SPECT and PET procedures pose no more risk than MRI-based procedures.

The linear no-threshold theory assumes that measures of mortality, disease induction, or tissue injury caused by very high levels of radiation exposure either in nuclear accidents, atomic bomb exposures, or via intentional radiation therapy treatments can be extrapolated over many orders of magnitude to the much lower levels of radiation exposure incurred in diagnostic imaging procedures by a simple linear interpolation. That is, the injury caused by high-level radiation is lowered in linear proportion based on the assumption that the only "zero risk" state is in fact zero exposure. A single gamma ray stopping in the human body would therefore be associated with at least some risk. However, most data indicates that this is not the case, but actually that risk asymptotes to zero at radiation exposure levels well above those incurred in diagnostic procedures for both adults and children (96–98).

In 1996, the Health Physics Society (99) issued a policy statement indicating that while there is substantial and convincing scientific evidence for health risk at high dose "health risks are either too small to be observed or are nonexistent" for exposures below 10 rem. The whole-body dose of a typical SPECT brain-imaging procedure is about 0.1 rem. In its assessment of risk to children for diagnostic imaging procedures used in clinical and research investigations, the Office of the Clinical Director of the National Institutes of Health stated:

> The risk of increased rates of cancer after low-level radiation exposure is not supported by population studies of health hazards from exposure to background radiation, radon in homes, radiation in the workplace or radiotherapy. Compared to the frequency of daily spontaneous genetic mutations, the biologic effect of low-level radiation at the cellular level seems extremely low. Furthermore, the potentiation of cellular repair mechanisms by low-level radiation may result in protective effect from subsequent high-level radiation. (100)

They concluded their risk review by saying: "Health risks from low-level radiation could not be detected above the "noise" of adverse events of everyday life. In addition, no data were found that demonstrated higher risks with younger age at low-level radiation exposure."

Indeed, there are no data that have ever demonstrated any harm to humans by radiation exposure at diagnostic imaging levels. In fact, current data support the presence of radiation hormesis: that low levels of radiation exposure induce beneficial effects of cellular repair and immune system enhancement (101–103). This certainly makes sense, since we evolved as a race in a background radiation environment

many times higher than is currently present. Further, current background radiation levels vary by an order of magnitude across geographic regions without any indication that those living in lower-background regions have less cancer prevalence than those in higher-background areas. Data from studies in the United States, China, India, Austria, and the United Kingdom show that populations in higher-background areas have *increased* longevity and *decreased* cancer death rates (98,101). Therefore, it should be concluded that neither PET nor SPECT brain imaging procedures are associated with any particular risk over activities of daily living and certainly should not be considered to be any more "risky" than MRI or any of its associated functional imaging derivatives.

CONCLUSIONS

SPECT functional brain imaging is a powerful clinical and research tool. Several clinical applications are now documented, a substantial number are under active investigation, and an even larger number are yet to be studied. Instrumentation continues to improve, although current SPECT tomographs yield excellent image quality. There is a rapidly expanding armamentarium of radiopharmaceuticals. Challenge tests, well-developed only in cerebrovascular disease (the acetazolamide test for vasodilatory reserve), offer great promise in elucidating the extent and nature of disease as well as predicting therapeutic responses. Some standards regarding the imaging environment and image presentation are emerging. However, much is yet to be learned about the ideal circumstances for the performance and evaluation of SPECT functional brain imaging. Finally, we must keep in mind that SPECT will achieve its full potential as a clinical tool for the management of patients with cerebral pathology only through close cooperation between the nuclear medicine community and our colleagues in neurology, psychiatry, or neurosurgery.

ACKNOWLEDGMENTS

Many individuals have made important contributions to this chapter through their collaborative efforts. However, one stands out above the others for his patience and long-standing, unswerving support: Frederick J. Bonte, M.D. I would also like to acknowledge three extremely talented members of my staff: J. Kelly Payne, M.S.; James L. Lowe, M.S.; and Thomas S. Harris, M.S.

REFERENCES

1. Alavi A, Hirsch LJ. Studies of central nervous system disorders with single-photon emission computed tomography and positron emission tomography: evolution over the past 2 decades. *Semin Nucl Med* 1991;21:58–81.
2. Bonte FJ, Hom J, Tintner R, Weiner MF. Single-photon tomography in Alzheimer's disease and the dementias. *Sem Nucl Med* 1990;20:342–352.
3. Brass LM, Rattner Z. Single photon emission computed tomography in cerebral vascular disease. In Weber DA, Devous MD, Tikofsky RS, eds. *Workshop on brain SPECT perfusion imaging: optimizing imaging acquisition and processing.* DOE CONF-9110368, 1992;77–88.

4. Devous MD Sr. Imaging brain function by single-photon emission computed tomography. In: Andreasen N, ed. *Brain imaging: applications in psychiatry,* Washington, DC: American Psychiatric Press, 1988;147–234.

5. Devous MD Sr, Leroy RF, Homan RW. Single photon emission computed tomography in epilepsy. In: LM Freeman, MD Blaufox, eds. *Sem Nucl Med.* 1990;325–341.

6. Hellman RS, Tikofsky RS. An overview of the contributions of regional cerebral blood flow studies in cerebrovascular disease: is there a role for single photon emission computed tomography? *Sem Nucl Med* 1990;20:303–324.

7. Holman BL, Devous MD Sr. Functional brain SPECT: the emergence of a powerful clinical method. *J Nucl Med* 1992;33:1888–1904.

8. Tikofsky RS, Hellman RS. Brain single photon emission computed tomography: New activation and intervention studies. *Sem Nucl Med* 1991;21:40–57.

9. VanHeertum RL, O'Connell RA. Functional brain imaging in the evaluation of psychiatric illness. *Sem Nucl Med* 1991;21:24–39.

10. Devous MD Sr. Image presentation and normal SPECT rCBF. In Weber DA, Devous MD, Tikofsky RS, eds. *Workshop on brain SPECT perfusion imaging: optimizing image acquisition, processing, display and interpretation.* DOE CONF-9110368, 1992:56–62.

11. Devous MD Sr, Stokely EM, Bonte FJ. Quantitative imaging of regional cerebral blood flow in man by dynamic single-photon tomography. In: BL Holman, ed. *Radionuclide imaging of the brain.* New York: Churchill Livingstone, 1985;135–162.

12. Hoffer PB, Zubal G. A guide to SPECT equipment for brain imaging. In: Weber DA, Devous MD, Tikofsky RS, et al., eds. *Workshop on brain SPECT perfusion imaging: image acquisition, processing, display and interpretation.* DOE CONF-9110368, 1992:21–27.

13. Links JM. Optimization of acquisition parameters for brain SPECT. In: Weber DA, Devous MD, Tikofsky RS, et al., eds. *Workshop on brain SPECT perfusion imaging: image acquisition, processing, display, and interpretation.* DOE CONF-9110368, 1992:28–32.

14. Todd-Pokropek A. Image reconstruction in tomography: Basics. In: Weber DA, Devous MD, Tikofsky RS, et al., eds. *Workshop on brain SPECT perfusion imaging: image acquisition, processing, display, and interpretation.* DOE CONF-9110368, 1992:33–41.

15. Stokely EM, Sveinsdottir E, Lassen NA, Rommer P. A single photon dynamic computer assisted tomograph (DCAT) for imaging brain function in multiple cross-sections. *J Comput Assist Tomogr* 1980;4:230–240.

16. Kimura K, Hashikawa K, Etani H, et al. A new apparatus for brain imaging: four-head rotating gamma camera single-photon emission computed tomograph. *J Nucl Med* 1990;31:603–609.

17. Rogers WL, Clinthorne NH, Stamos J, et al. Performance evaluation of SPRINT, a single-photon ring tomograph for brain imaging. *J Nucl Med* 1984;25:1013–1018.

18. Kanno I, Uemura K, Miyura S, Miyura Y. HEADTOME: A hybrid emission tomograph for single-photon and positron emission imaging of the brain. *J Comput Assist Tomogr* 1981;5:216–226.

19. Logan KW, Holmes RA. Missouri University Multiplane Imager (MUMPI): a high-sensitivity rapid dynamic ECT brain imager. *J Nucl Med* 1984;25:PI05.

20. Smith AP, Genna S. Imaging characteristics of ASPECT, a single-crystal ring camera for dedicated brain SPECT. *J Nucl Med* 1989;30:796.

21. Stoddart HF, Stoddart HA. A new development in single-gamma transaxial tomography. Union Carbide focused collimator scanner. *IEEE Trans Nucl Sci* 1979;26:2710–2712.

22. Kirsch C-M, Moore SC, Zimmerman RE, et al. Characteristics of a scanning, multidetector, single-photon ECT body imager. *J Nucl Med* 1981;22:726–731.

23. Hill TC, Stoddart HF, Doherty MD, et al. Simultaneous SPECT acquisition of CBF and metabolism. *J Nucl Med* 1988;29:876.

24. Devous MD Sr, Bonte FJ. Initial evaluation of cerebral blood flow imaging with a high-resolution, high-sensitivity three-headed SPECT system (PRISM). *J Nucl Med* 1988;29:912.

25. Devous MD Sr, Lowe JL, Payne JK. Dual-isotope brain SPECT imaging with ^{99m}Tc and ^{123}I: validation by phantom studies. *J Nucl Med* 1992;33:2030–2035.

26. Devous MD Sr, Payne JK, Lowe JL. Dual-isotope brain SPECT imaging with ^{99m}Tc and ^{123}I: clinical validation using ^{133}Xe SPECT. *J Nucl Med* 1992;33:1919–1924.

27. Glass HI, Harper AM. Measurement of regional blood flow in cerebral cortex of man through intact skull. *Br Med J* 1963;2:1611.

28. Mallett BL, Veall N. The measurement of regional cerebral clearance rate in man using Xe^{133} inhalation and extracranial recording. *Clin Sci* 1965;29:179–191.

29. Obrist WD, Thompson HK, King CH, Wang HS. Determination of regional cerebral blood flow by inhalation of xenon-133. *Circ Res* 1967;20:124–135.

30. Kanno I, Lassen NA. Two methods for calculating regional cerebral blood flow from emission computed tomography of inert gas concentrations. *J Comput Assist Tomogr* 1979;3:71–76.

31. Celsis P, Goldman T, Henriksen L, Lassen NA. A method for calculating regional cerebral blood flow from emission computerized tomography of inert gas concentrations. *J Comput Assist Tomogr* 1981;5:641–645.

32. Smith GT, Stokely EM, Lewis MH, et al. An error analysis of the double-integral method for calculating brain blood perfusion from inert gas clearance data. *J Cereb Blood Flow Metab* 1984;4:61–67.

33. Winchell HS, Baldwin RM, Lin TH. Development of ^{123}I-labeled amines for brain studies: localization of ^{123}I iodophenylalkylamines in rat brain. *J Nucl Med* 1980;21:940–202.

34. Kung HF, Tramposh K, Blau M. A new brain imaging agent: (I^{123}) HIPDM: N,N,N′-trimethyl-N′-(2-hydroxy-3-methyl-5-iodobenzyl)-1,3-propanediamin e. *J Nucl Med* 1983;24:66–72.

35. Lassen NA, Henriksen L, Holm S, et al. Cerebral blood-flow tomography: xenon-133 compared with isopropyl-amphetamine-Iodine-123: concise communication. *J Nucl Med* 1983;24:17–21.

36. Kuhl DE, Barrio JR, Huang SC, et al. Quantifying local cerebral blood flow by N-isopropyl-p-[^{123}I] iodoamphetamine (IMP) tomography. *J Nucl Med* 1982;23:196–203.

37. Nishizawa S, Tanada S, Yonekura Y, et al. Regional dynamics of N-isopropyl-(^{123}I)p iodo-amphetamine in human brain. *J Nucl Med* 1989;30:150–156.

38. Nakano S, Kinoshita K, Jinnouchi S, et al. Comparative study of regional cerebral blood flow images by SPECT using xenon-133, iodine-123 IMP, and technetium-99m HMPAO. *J Nucl Med* 1989;30:157–164.

39. Leonard J-P, Nowotnik DP, Neirinckx RD. Technetium-99m-d,1-HM-PAO: a new radiopharmaceutical for imaging regional brain perfusion using SPECT—a comparison with iodine-123 HIPDM. *J Nucl Med* 1986;27:1819–1823.

40. Defer G, Moretti JL, Cesaro P, et al. Early and delayed SPECT using N-isoprophyl p-iodoamphetamine iodine 123 in cerebral ischemia: a prognostic index for clinical recovery. *Arch Neurol* 1987;44:715–718.

41. Neirinckx RD, Canning LR, Piper IM, et al. Technetium-99m d,1-HM-PAO: a new radiopharmaceutical for SPECT imaging of regional cerebral blood perfusion. *J Nucl Med* 1987;28:191–202.

42. Volkert WA, Hoffman TJ, Seger RM, et al. Tc^{99m}-propylene amine oxime (Tc^{99m}-PnAO); a potential brain radiopharmaceutical. *Eur J Nucl Med* 1984;9:511–516.

43. Kung HF, Guo YH, Yu C-C, Billings J, et al. New brain perfusion imaging agents based on ^{99m}Tc-bis(aminoethanethiol) complexes: stereoisomers and biodistribution. *J Med Chem* 1989;32:437–444.

44. Walovitch RC, Hill TC, Garrity ST, et al. Characterization of technetium-99m-1,1-ECD for brain perfusion imaging: Part 1. Pharmacology of technetium-99m ECD in nonhuman primates. *J Nucl Med* 1989;30:1892–1901.

45. Leveille J, Demonceáu G, De Roo M, et al. Characterization of technetium-99m-1,1-ECD for brain perfusion imaging: Part 2. Biodistribution and brain imaging in humans. *J Nucl Med* 1989;30:1902–1910.

46. Devous MD Sr, Payne JK, Lowe JL. Comparison of ^{99m}Tc-ECD to ^{133}Xe SPECT in normal controls and in patients with mild to moderate rCBF abnormalities. *J Nucl Med* 1993;34:754–761.

47. Payne JK, Trivedi MH, Devous MD Sr. Comparison of 99mTc HM-PAO to 133Xe for the measurement of regional cerebral blood flow by SPECT. *J Nucl Med* 1996;37:1735–1740.

48. Gibbs JM, Wise RJS, Leendersbs KL, et al. Cerebral hemodynamics in occlusive carotid artery disease. *Lancet* 1985;1:933–934.

49. Buell U, Stirner H, Ferbert F. Cerebral blood flow-to-volume imaging by SPECT. *J Nucl Med* 1986;27:1938–1939.

50. Knapp WH, Kummer RV, Kubler W. Imaging of cerebral blood flow-to-volume distribution using SPECT. *J Nucl Med* 1986;27:465–470.

51. Toyama H, Takeshita G, Takeuchi A, et al. Cerebral hemodynamics in patients with chronic obstructive carotid disease by rCBF, rCBV, and rCBV/rCBF ratio using SPECT. *J Nucl Med* 1990;31:55–60.

52. Kung HF, Alavi A, Chang W, et al. In vivo SPECT imaging of CNS D-2 dopamine receptors: initial studies with iodine-123-IBZM in humans. *J Nucl Med* 1990;31:573–579.

53. Schubiger PA, Hasler PH, Beer-Wohlfahrt H, et al. Evaluation of multi-centre study with iomazenil: a benzodiazepine receptor ligand. *Nucl Med Commun* 1991;12:569–582.

54. Holman BL, Gibson RE, Hill TC, et al. Muscarinic acetylcholine receptors in Alzheimer's disease: in vivo imaging with iodine-123-labeled 3-quinuclidinyl-4-iodobenzilate and emission tomography. *JAMA* 1985;254:3063.

55. Weinberger DR, Gibson R, Coppola R, et al. The distribution of cerebral muscarinic acetylcholine receptors in vivo in patients with dementia: a controlled study with [123]IQNB and single photon emission computed tomography. *Arch Neurol* 1991;48(2):169–176.

56. Innis RB, Al-Tikriti MS, Zoghbi SS, et al. SPECT imaging of the benzodiazepine receptor, feasibility of in vivo potency measurements from stepwise displacement curves. *J Nucl Med* 1991;32:1754–1761.

57. Kim KT, Black KL, Marciano D, et al. Thallium SPECT imaging of brain tumors: methods and results. *J Nucl Med* 1990;31:965–969.

58. Mountz JM, Stafford-Schuck K, McKeever PE. Thallium-201 tumor/cardiac ratio estimation of residual astrocytoma. *J Neurosurg* 1988;68:705–709.

59. Schwartz RB, Carvalho PA, Alexander III E, et al. Radiation necrosis vs high-grade recurrent glioma: differentiation by using dual-isotope SPECT with ^{201}Tl and [99m]TC-HMPAO. *AJNR* 1991;12:1187–1192.

60. Kaplan WD, Takvorian T, Morris JH, et al. HL. Thallium-201 brain tumor imaging: a comparative study with pathological correlation. *J Nucl Med* 1987;28:47–52.

61. Brismar T, Collins VP, Kesselberg M. Thallium-201 uptake relates to membrane potential and potassium permeability in human glioma cells. *Brain Res* 1989;500:30–36.

62. Black KL, Hawkins RA, Kim KT, et al. Use of thallium-201 SPECT to quantitate malignancy grade of gliomas. *J Neurosurg* 1989;71:342–346.

63. Baron GC, Lebrun-Grandie P, Collard P, et al. Noninvasive measurement of blood flow, oxygen consumption and glucose utilization in the same brain regions in man by positron emission tomography. *J Nucl Med* 1982;23:391–399.

64. Ingvar DH, Risberg J. Increase of regional cerebral blood flow during mental effort in normals and in patients with focal brain disorders. *Exp Brain Res* 1967;3:195–211.

65. Kety SS, Schmidt CF. The nitrous oxide method for quantitative determination of cerebral blood flow in man: theory, procedure and normal values. *J Clin Invest* 1948;27:476–483.

66. Mazziotta JC, Phelps ME, Carson RE, Kuhl DE. Tomographic mapping of human cerebral metabolism: auditory stimulation. *Neurology* 1982;32:921–937.

67. Phelps ME, Kuhl DE, Mazziotta JC. Metabolic mapping of the brain's response to visual stimulation: studies in humans. *Science* 1981;211:1445–1448.

68. Raichle ME, Grubb RL, Gado MH, et al. Correlation between regional cerebral blood flow and oxidative metabolism. *Arch Neurol* 1976;33:523–526.

69. Roland PE, Eriksson L, Stone-Elander S, Widen L. Does mental activity change the oxidative metabolism of the brain? *J Neurosci* 1987;7:2373–2389.

70. Mazziotta JC, Phelps ME, Carson RE, Kuhl DE. Tomographic mapping of human cerebral metabolism: sensory deprivation. *Ann Neurol* 1982;12:435–444.

71. Devous MD Sr, Stokely EM, Chehabi HH, Bonte FJ. Normal distribution of regional cerebral blood flow measured by dynamic single-photon emission tomography. *J Cereb Blood Flow Metab* 1986;6:95–104.

72. Gur RC, Gur RE, Obrist WD, et al. Age and regional cerebral blood flow at rest and during cognitive activity. *Arch Gen Psychiatry* 1987;44:617–621.

73. Hagstadius S, Risberg J. Regional cerebral blood flow characteristics and variations with age in resting normal subjects. *Brain Cogn* 1989;10:28–43.

74. Kuhl DE, Metter EJ, Riege WH, Phelps ME. Effects of human aging on patterns of local cerebral glucose utilization determined by the ^{18}F fluorodeoxyglucose method. *J Cereb Blood Flow Metab* 1982;2:163–171.

75. Mathew RJ, Wilson WH, Tant SR. Determinants of resting regional cerebral blood flow in normal subjects. *Biol Psychiatry* 1986;21:907–914.

76. Rogers RL, Meyer JS, Mortel KF. After reaching retirement age physical activity sustains cerebral perfusion and cognition. *J Am Geriatr Soc* 1990;38:123–128.

77. Baxter LR, Mazziotta JC, Phelps ME, et al. Cerebral glucose metabolic rates in normal human females vs. normal males. *Psychiatry Res* 1987;21:237–245.

78. Daniel DG, Mathew RJ, Wilson WH. Sex roles and regional cerebral blood flow. *Psychiatry Res* 1988;27:55–64.

79. Gur RC, Gur RE, Obrist WD, et al. Sex and handedness differences in cerebral blood flow during rest and cognitive activity. *Science* 1982;217:659–661.

80. Rodriguez G, Warkentin S, Risberg J, Rosadini G. Sex differences in regional cerebral blood flow. *J Cereb Blood Flow Metab* 1988;8:783–789.

81. Bonte FJ, Devous MD Sr, Reisch JS. The effect of acetazolamide on regional cerebral blood flow in normal human subjects as measured by single photon emission computed tomography. *Invest Radiol* 1988;23:564–568.

82. Rogg J, Rutigliano M, Yonas H, et al. The acetazolamide challenge: imaging techniques designed to evaluate cerebral blood flow reserve. *AJNR* 1989;10:803–810.

83. Sullivan HG, Kingsbury TB, Morgan ME, et al. The rCBF response to diamox in normal subjects and cerebrovascular disease patients. *J Neurosurg* 1987;67:525–534.

84. Vorstrup S, Brun B, Lassen NA. Evaluation of the cerebral vasodilatory capacity by the acetazolamide test before EC-IC bypass surgery in patients with occlusion of the internal carotid artery. *Stroke* 1986;17:1291–1298.

85. Mathew RJ, Barr DL, Weinman ML. Caffeine and cerebral blood flow. *Br J Psychiatry* 1983;143:604–608.

86. Rush AJ, Cain JW, Raese J, Stewart RS, et al. The neurobiological bases for psychiatric disorders. In: RN Rosenberg, ed. *Comprehensive neurology.* New York: Raven Press, 1991;555–603.

87. Petersen SE, Fox PT, Posner MI, et al. Positron emission tomographic studies of the cortical anatomy of single-word processing. *Nature* 1988;331:585–589.

88. Fox PT, Mintun MA, Raichle ME, et al. Mapping human visual cortex with positron emission tomography. *Nature* 1986;323:806–809.

89. Matsuda H, Tsuji S, Shuke N, et al. A quantitative approach to technetium-99m hexamethylpropylene amino oxime. *Eur J Nucl Med* 1992;19(3):195–200.

90. Matsuda H, Tsuji S, Shuke N, et al. Noninvasive measurements of regional cerebral blood flow using technetinum-99m hexamethylpropylene amine oxime. *Eur J Nucl Med* 1993;20(5):391–401.

91. Nussbaum RH. The linear no-threshold dose-effect relation: is it relevant to radiation protection regulation? *Med Phys* 1998;25:291–299.

92. Bond VP, Wielopolski L, Shani G. Current misinterpretations of the linear no-threshold hypothesis. *Health Phys* 1996;70:877–882.

93. Fry RJ, Grosovsky A, Hanawalt PC, et al. The impact of biology on risk assessment—workshop of the National Research Council's Board on Radiation Effects Research. July 21–22, 1997, National Academy of Sciences, Washington, DC. *Radiat Res* 1998;150:695–705.

94. Cohen BL. Test of the linear-no threshold theory of radiation carcinogenesis for inhaled radon decay products. *Health Phys* 1995;68:157–174.

95. Jaworowski Z. Beneficial effects of radiation and regulatory policy. *Aust Phys Eng Sci Med* 1997;20:125–138.

96. Little MP, Muirhead CR. Curvature in the cancer mortality dose response in Japanese atomic bomb survivors: absence of evidence of threshold. *Int J Radiat Biol* 1998;74:471–480.

97. Ron E. Ionizing radiation and cancer risk: evidence from epidemiology. *Radiat Res* 1998;150:S30–S41.

98. Pollycove M. Nonlinearity of radiation health effects. *Environ Health Perspect* 1998;106(suppl 1):363–368.

99. Mossman KL, Goldman M, Masse F, et al. Radiation risk in perspective: Health Physics Society position statement. *Health Phys Soc Newsl* 1996;24:2–3.

100. Ernst M, Freed ME, Zametkin AJ. Health hazards of radiation exposure in the context of brain imaging research: special consideration for children. *J Nucl Med* 1998;39:689–698.

101. Pollycove M. The issue of the decade: hormesis. *Eur J Nucl Med* 1995;22:399–401.

102. Bogen KT, Layton DW. Risk management for plausibly hormetic environmental carcinogens: the case of radon. *Hum Exp Toxicol* 1998;17:463–467.

103. Azzam EI, de Toledo SM, Raaphorst GP, Mitchel RE. Low-dose ionizing radiation decreases the frequency of neoplastic transformation to a level below the spontaneous rate in C3H 10T1/2 cells. *Radiat Res* 1996;146:369–373.

Functional Cerebral SPECT and PET Imaging, Third Edition,
edited by R.L. Van Heertum and R.S. Tikofsky,
Lippincott Williams & Wilkins, Philadelphia © 2000.

CHAPTER 2

PET Physics and Instrumentation

Peter D. Esser

POSITRON RADIATION PHYSICS

Brain scan images showing the physiologic and functional distribution of positron tracers are currently acquired at almost 400 clinical positron emission tomography (PET) imaging centers throughout the world. At these facilities, coincidence-imaging scanners detect collinear pairs of photons emitted from annihilation sites where positrons, also known as a positive electrons or β^+ particles, have united with electrons. Radioactive tracers tagged with neutron-deficient short-lived isotopes such as ^{11}C, ^{15}O, and ^{18}F emit the positrons. In this chapter we review the basic physics of positron decay and discuss the fundamentals of PET instrumentation. Additional details can be found in recent publications by Bendrie and Townsend (1) and others (2,3).

The pharmaceutical preparation of positron imaging agents begins at a cyclotron facility on site or nearby where an isotope target is bombarded with a beam of protons (hydrogen nuclei stripped of electrons). The most commonly administered β^+ radionuclide is ^{18}F, which is used for the production of [^{18}F]-2-deoxy-2-fluoro-D-glucose, or ^{18}FDG (4). This isotope is generated when ^{18}O-enriched water is employed as a target for high-energy protons. The reaction occurring during bombardment is summarized as $^{18}O(p,n)^{18}F$ or $^{18}O + p \Rightarrow {}^{18}F + n$. In a similar manner, radioactive ^{15}O is produced from an enriched ^{15}N target in the reaction $^{15}N(p,n)^{15}O$. In the above examples and other cyclotron reactions used to generate PET radioisotopes, the combination of neutrons and protons in the target is initially stable (e.g., ^{18}O with 8 protons and 10 neutrons). But during irradiation a new, unstable isotope with an unfavorable neutron-to-proton ratio is created when an extra proton is introduction into the target nucleus, increasing the atomic number from Z to Z + 1.

The unstable nuclei return to a more stable configuration by two competing processes that readjust the neutron-to-proton ratio. In the electron-capture decay mode, an orbital electron is captured by the nucleus and, in a transformation, the charge on a proton is neutralized, thereby generating a neutron. However, no useful gamma rays for imaging purposes are produced. In the alternative process, a proton loses its charge by the release of a β^+ particle, which is unstable in the presence of electrons. Fortunately, β^+ emission is the primary decay path for important biomolecular markers such as ^{11}C, ^{15}O, and ^{18}F. In addition, the relatively short half-lives of these isotopes, ranging from 2–110 min, are within the acceptable time range for emission imaging. The longer half-life of ^{18}F also has the advantage of allowing the imaging facility to use a cyclotron pharmacy with a delivery time of up to several hours; for comparison, ^{15}O requires an on-site pharmacy because of its very short half-life (2 min). Typical time parameters associated with the production of ^{18}F, labeling of ^{18}FDG, and patient scanning are shown in Table 2.1. Clinical scanning protocols for ^{18}FDG and ^{15}O are illustrated in Fig. 2.1.

For all positron-emitting radionuclides, a proton in the nucleus undergoes the transformation as follows:

Proton → neutron + positron (β^+) + neutrino (v)

In this decay process, a positron is emitted from the nucleus with a unit of charge while the number of nucleons remains constant. In term of energetics, the nucleus moves from an unstable energy state to a more stable level, as described by the general *nuclear* mass-energy balance equation:

$$ {}^A_Z X' = {}_{Z-1}^{A} Y' + \beta^+ + v + E_\gamma + Q $$

where X' is the parent's nuclear mass and Y' is the daughter's nuclear mass. Q is the total kinetic energy of the decay products and is different for each β^+-emitting isotope. In addition, gamma rays, with a total energy of E_γ, may be emitted after β^+ decay if the residual nucleus is left in an excited level above the ground state.

P. D. Esser: Department of Radiology, Columbia Presbyterian Medical Center, New York, New York 10032.

TABLE 2.1. *Typical time parameters associated with the production of* ^{18}F, *labeling of FDG, and patient scanning*

Production, QA and scan	
Cyclotron bombardment of ^{18}O target	60–120 min
Synthesis of FDG	60 min
Prerelease quality control (chromatography and half-life)	20 min
Measure dose	1 min
Delivery to site	1 min–3 hr
Measure dose and inject	3 min
Uptake in patient	30–60 min
Patient scan	24 min
Postrelease quality control of FDG	
Pyrogenicity	60 min
Sterility	2 weeks
Decay of 18F	
^{18}F half-life	109.8 min
β^+ lifetime in tissue	$\approx 10^{-11}$ sec
Positronimun half-life	$\approx 10^{-10}$ sec
Time of flight	$\approx 10^{-9}$ sec
Coincidence window	12×10^{-9} sec
Detector response	
Decay constant	
BGO	300×10^{-9} sec
NaI	230×10^{-9} sec
Max. trues count rate	
Ring	$\approx 5 \times 10^6$ cps
Camera	$\approx 2 \times 10^4$

In the decay process described above, a positron and a neutrino particle are simultaneously emitted. The positron carries a unit of positive charge from the nucleus, has the same mass as an electron, and also shares energy and momentum with the neutrino, which has no charge and seemingly no mass. Thus, while the total released energy, Q, from the transition is constant, the positron's energy varies in a probabilistic manner and does not have a unique value like that of an alpha particle. The presence of the neutrino explains the reproducible, continuous β^+ energy curve, with a maximum equal to Q, that is observed for β^+ decay of a particular nuclide (Fig. 2.2).

Another important feature of β^+ decay is the 1.022 MeV minimum energy necessary for this reaction to occur, since the atom (nucleus plus atomic electrons) loses the energy equivalent of two electron masses: a positron and an electron. The positron is released from the nucleus, reducing the atomic number by 1, and there is a corresponding reduction of the orbital configuration by one electron. Since the energy of the electron mass is 0.511 MeV, the total energy lost in the transition will be at least 1.022 MeV, with excess energy from the reaction distributed between the emitted neutrino and positron, as described above. To a good approximation, the *atomic* mass-energy balance equation is

$$^A_Z X = _{Z-1}^A Y + 2\beta^- + E_\gamma + Q$$

where X and Y are the neutral atomic masses of the parent and daughter, respectively.

Energetic positrons released in β^+ decay excite and ionize matter in a similar manner to electrons. Only below 100 keV are small differences observed in the average linear rate of energy loss (i.e., stopping power). Typically, the average single-collision energy loss by a fast beta particle in water is near 75 eV, while the most probable energy loss is close to 22 eV. (Note that the first ionization potential for water is only 12.6 eV.) Consistent with these losses, an 800-keV β and its secondary electrons produces on average of 32,000 ion pairs and a smaller number of excited molecules (5). In addition, as an energetic β particle moves through matter, it can be deflected by the electric field of a nucleus and emit photon radiation known as *bremsstrahlung* radiation. However, in the body, the radiation losses are negligible below 10 MeV for the PET isotopes—the radiation yield is only 0.35% for 1 MeV positrons in water. Bremsstrahlung varies with Z^2 and, as a consequence, low atomic-weight materials such as Lucite are used for β shielding instead of high-density metals such as lead, which emit considerably more radiation (at 1 MeV, 3% for positrons and 5% for electrons). In general, at the same energy, the radiative yield from positrons is slightly less than that from electrons. Also, the rate of total energy loss in water, including both collision and radiative energies, increases with decreasing energy (24.8 MeV cm^{-1} at 10 keV vs. 1.82 MeV cm^{-1} at 1 MeV) and is maximum near 110 eV.

When the initial kinetic energy of a positron has been almost lost, the probability of an annihilation reaction with an electron becomes very high. In this encounter, a positron and electron unite and disappear while transforming the energy equivalent of their masses into electromagnetic radiation. Since both energy and momentum must be conserved in the reaction, two photons of annihilation radiation are most often emitted. Each photon has 511 keV of energy and moves in the opposite direction, 180 degrees, of its partner. Often the positron is not completely at rest but has a small residual momentum at the time of annihilation. This produces a small change in the observed collinearity, 180 ± 0.25 degrees, and a small fluctuation, approximately +/− 5 eV, in the measured photon energy (6). The deviations in photon direction are an important limitation on scanner resolution.

Figure 2.3 traces the path of 4 positrons emitted from a point source in tissue. As shown, the positrons move erratically through the medium before undergoing annihilation and their total path length is significantly longer than the direct distance to their point of origin. The total distance along a positron's paths, regardless of direction, is the *range* of the particle. Since these paths are erratic with large deviations from the original trajectories, average range values are used for β particles (Table 2.2). The maximum *depth of penetration* as determined from experimental data is important for shielding calculations and is also given in Table 2.2.

While positrons deposit their energy over a very small distances (2.4 mm for ^{18}F), the 0.511-MeV annihilation radiation has sufficient energy to travel a much longer distance, 7.6 cm, before attenuation reduces their number by half. In

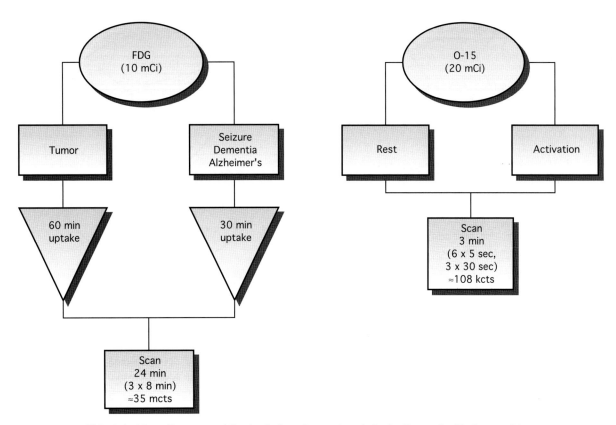

FIG. 2.1. Flow diagrams of the brain-imaging protocols typically used with ring gantries.

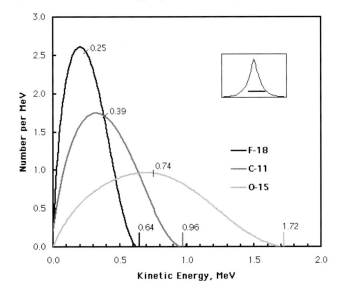

Positron Energy Spectra of $^{11}C, ^{15}O$ and ^{18}F

FIG. 2.2. Positron energy spectra for the most commonly used positron emission tomography (PET) isotopes for brain scanning. The average and maximum energies are indicated. The graph insert (relative intensity vs. distance) illustrates the two-dimensional distribution of positrons from a point source. The shape of the curve reflects the continuous distribution of β energies and is a contributing factor to reduced image resolution of PET systems. (Spectra based on data generated by WG Cross, N Freedman. A short atlas of beta-ray spectra. *Phys Med Biol* 1983;28:1251–1260.)

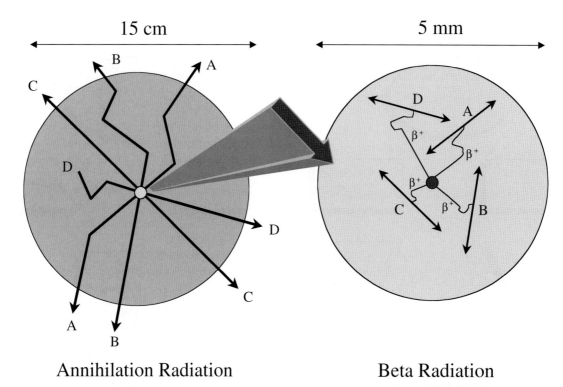

FIG. 2.3. Interactions of 511-keV annihilation photons (γ) and positrons (β^+) in soft tissue. The events (**A–D**) are approximated for positrons emitted from ^{18}F. Note the difference in scale between the left side, showing photons, and the zoomed right side, showing positrons.

comparison, the half-value layer for the 140-keV gamma rays of ^{99m}Tc is 4.6 cm. As a consequence, during a PET brain scan, a considerable portion of the internally emitted photons will pass out through the patient to the scanner's photon detectors. Compton scatter and photoelectric absorption are also important and are illustrated in Fig. 2.3.

The absorbed radiation dose to the patient is an important consideration for all radionuclide-scanning procedures. Energy is transferred to tissue by ionizing events from both positrons and annihilation radiation. The average positron energy (roughly two-fifths of the maximum energy) of ^{18}F and ^{15}O differs by a factor of approximately 3, but both deposit their energy over a relatively small distance compared to 511-keV photons (Table 2.2). The radiation doses for brain-imaging radiopharaceuticals are given in Table 2.3,

which for comparison also includes single-photon radiopharmaceuticals. While the biodistribution is different between agents, the radiation doses from PET pharmaceuticals are comparable to doses from single-photon-emission computed tomography (SPECT) agents.

PET imaging centers follow the standard radiation protection protocols used in nuclear medicine. However, PET technologists often have higher radiation exposure than workers doing similar tasks in single-photon studies (7,8). In addition, pharmacists in cyclotron facilities have even higher exposure rates, especially to their hands. The radiation dose to radiation workers in PET facilities can be reduced considerably by careful, rapid handling of the radioactive pharmaceutics using tongs, syringe shields, and lead barriers. Radiation exposure from patients to staff members is pri-

TABLE 2.2. *Physical properties of ^{18}F, ^{11}C, and ^{15}O*

| | | | | | Positrons | | | Resolution factor | |
Isotope	Half-life (min)	Photon energy (MeV)	Maximum energy (MeV)	Average energy (MeV)	Penetration depth in H$_2$O (mm)	Range in H$_2$O (mm)	Range in air (m)	FWHM† (mm)	FWTM† (mm)
^{18}F	109.77	0.511*	0.635	0.250	2.27	2.42	2.01	0.22	1.09
^{11}C	20.385	0.511	0.96	0.386	3.91	4.17	3.46	0.28	1.86
^{15}O	2.038	0.511	1.72	0.735	6.62	8.4	6.97	1.1	5.3
					6.72 lucite	0.05 lead			

* HVL for 0.511 MeV: concrete 3.4 cm; water 7.6 cm; lead 0.4 cm; exposure rate, γ, 0.6 mR/mCi-hr at 1 min.
† Data from CTI, Knoxville, TN: based on Derenzo SE, Procedeedings of the 5TH Annual Conference on Positron Annihilation except ^{15}O, which are estimates.

TABLE 2.3. *Estimates of radiation dose for brain-imaging radiopharmaceuticals (rad/mCl and rad for typical administered dose)*

Modality	^{18}FDG PET		^{15}O H$_2$O PET		^{99m}Tc ECD SPECT		^{99m}Tc HMPAO SPECT		^{201}Tl SPECT		^{123}Xe* SPECT	
dose in mCi	1	10	1	30	1	20	1	20	1	3	1	30
Brain	0.070	0.70	0.0049	0.15	0.0020	0.040	0.025	0.50	0.22	0.66	0.0025	0.075
Heart wall	0.22	2.2	0.0082	0.25	0.0065	0.13	0.014	0.28	1.0	3.0	0.0026	0.078
Kidneys	0.074	0.74	0.0072	0.22	0.029	0.58	0.13	2.60	1.7	5.1	0.0025	0.075
Ovaries	0.063	0.63	0.0013	0.04	0.029	0.58	0.026	0.52	0.37	1.1	0.0026	0.078
Red marrow	0.048	0.48	0.0033	0.10	0.0090	0.18	0.013	0.26	0.20	0.60	0.0031	0.093
Spleen	0.14	1.4	0.0058	0.17	0.0073	0.15	0.015	0.30	0.65	2.0	0.0025	0.075
Testes	0.048	0.48	0.0025	0.08	0.013	0.26	0.0084	0.17	0.73	2.2	0.0024	0.072
Thyroid	0.039	0.39	0.0063	0.19	0.0048	0.10	0.10	2.00	0.23	0.69	0.0025	0.075
Urinary bladder wall	0.70	7.0	0.0008	0.02	0.27	5.40	0.026	0.52	0.19	0.57	0.0026	0.078
Effective dose equivalent (rem)	0.11	1.1	0.0042	0.13	0.042	0.84	0.051	1.0	0.60	1.8	0.0028	0.084

* 5 min rebreathing.

Source: Stabin MG, Stubbs JB, Toohey RE. *Radiation dose for radiopharmaceuticals,* rev 4/30/96. Oak Ridge, TN: Radiation Internal Dose Information Center, Oak Ridge Institute for Science and Education, 1996.

marily from photons and not positrons. However, syringe preparation and patient injection can contribute a significant dose to the hands from both β and photon radiation and, with a possible positron range in air of up to 7 m, some eye exposure. These considerations are especially important for ^{15}O studies, since the maximum energy of the positrons is 1.72 MeV and the administered activity is usually 30 mCi or higher. (Research studies may require repetitive doses of 40–60 mCi.) In addition, to allow sufficient time to inject a patient with O^{15} after assaying the dose, the 2-min half-life necessitates that the measured activity in the dose calibrator should be 30–50% higher than the desired administered dose. Tungsten and acrylic syringe shields can reduce the radiation exposure of the hands. The University of Chicago (9), for example, has reported a factor of 5 reduction in the exposure rate from ^{15}O by using a 6-mm-thick acrylic syringe shield.

POSITRON TOMOGRAPHY PHYSICS

In the previous section, we discussed the physics of positron decay; now we continue by examining the methodology for detection and processing the 180-degree, dual-photon emission that is characteristic of decaying positrons. For simultaneous spatial positioning and registering two 511-keV photons, multidetector configurations and coincidence electronics are necessary, in contrast to simpler single-photon imaging cameras that can function with a single detector. The diagnostic potential of positron emitters for tumor imaging was first proposed by Wrenn et al. (10) in 1951 and was soon followed by Brownell and Sweet's (11) development of a dual-probe rectilinear scanner for the detection of positrons. In addition, the early history of nuclear medicine also included the pioneering work of Anger (12,13), who

configured dual single-crystal gamma cameras for positron imaging. The first ring system for brain scanning had 32 detectors and was developed at Brookhaven National Laboratory (14). Systems have continued to evolve into a variety of modern configurations, as shown in Fig. 2.4.

Contemporary commercial PET systems utilize thousands of small BGO (Bi$_4$Ge$_3$O$_{12}$) crystals in a ring configuration (e.g., 18,432, 4 × 4.4 × 30 mm, crystals in the HR+ scanner) or two to six larger single crystals of NaI. In Fig. 2.4, systems A, B, C, and F are optimized for PET imaging while the other two geometries, D and E, are multipurpose single-photon gamma cameras with additional coincidence circuitry. Since camera systems D and E are optimized for single-photon acquisition, their thin NaI crystals have significantly smaller gamma-ray capture efficiency than dedicated PET systems with thicker detectors. In addition, the count-rate capability of hybrid PET/SPECT camera is currently two orders of magnitude (Table 2.1) less than that of dedicated PET systems. In the future, new scintillator crystals such as lutetium oxyorthosilicate (LSO) may have a large impact on the performance of dedicated and hybrid systems. While the following discussion emphasizes the BGO ring-detectors system, the concepts are also applicable to NaI coincidence cameras.

The basic objective of PET image acquisition is to generate images with pixel values that are proportional to tracer concentration in the interior of the patient and that change linearly with concentration. In PET scanners, detecting photons and determining the coincidence photons' paths achieves this goal, as illustrated with the 16-detector PET system in Fig. 2.5. Images A and C show an off-center small source of activity, while B and D show a brain scan using a transaxial slice from a PET scan. As drawn in the illustration, two of the detectors are linked as they respond almost simul-

A) Partial Rings
- BGO

B) Rings with Septa
- BGO

C) Rings, no Septa
- BGO

D) 2 Heads - NaI

E) 3 Heads - NaI

F) 6 Heads - NaI

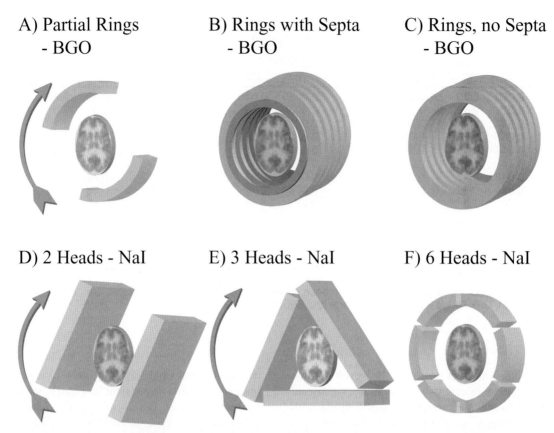

FIG. 2.4. Detector configuration of PET systems. Arrows indicate rotating systems. Two types of detector systems are shown. **A–C**: Multicrystal BGO ring systems. **D–F**: Multiheaded systems that use large rectangular NaI crystals for positioning scintillation events. **B** and **C**: The same system with the septa in position for two-dimensional imaging and removed for three-dimensional acquisition.

taneously to a coincidence emission from the tracer (the upper row of images). However, the finite size of the detectors (e.g., $6.75 \times 6.75 \times 20$ mm in the CTI EXACT scanner) limits the system's ability to precisely determine the location of the decayed positron except within a rectangular region or "tube" linking the detectors. During the data-acquisition interval, the joint response of the detector pair is proportional to the sum of the tracer concentration within the intersected region of the source. Figure 2.5A and B illustrates only one set of coupled detectors, but many other combinations are possible, as partially shown by the additional lines—*lines of response* (LORs)—joining detectors in Fig. 2.5C and D. The total number of LORs increases rapidly with the number of detectors; for the simple system shown, there are 120 possibilities, and for a single plane in a commercial scanner, there are close to 80,000 (depending on the number of detectors in the ring).

An ideal scanner would have very small field-of-view detector crystals with high light yield and rapid response, electronics that could instantaneously identify a coincidence, and shielding that would eliminate all scattered radiation. Current state-of-the-art scanners optimize the combination of BGO (or NaI) detectors, photomultiplier tubes, and high-speed electronics to achieve optimal performance. The coin-

cidence-resolving window between detectors is typically 12 nsec and the energy window for BGO detectors is several hundred keV. As a result of these types of instrumentation limitations, a significant percent of false coincidences are recorded as valid events. Figure 2.6 illustrates the various types of responses that occur in PET detector systems. Each photon event recorded by a detector is a *single,* and the processing logic for single events in a modern ring system is shown in Fig. 2.7. The authentic coincidences along a LOR are known as *trues.* There are, in addition, two types of events that contribute to coincidence misinformation: (a) one or both of the annihilation emissions from an positron decay in the patient are scattered and subsequently recorded with a LOR that indicates an incorrect location of the event (*scatter*) and (b) two unrelated events that occur so close together in time, less than 12 nsec, that the electronics registers them as a genuine coincidence along a LOR (*randoms*). Corrections for randoms are made with data recorded in a delayed coincidence window that measures the number of chance coincidences (Fig. 2.7). Approximately 97% of singles are eliminated by the coincidence window.

The count-rate performance curves of a HR + (CTI) ring-gantry system are shown in Fig. 2.8, based on measurements of activity in a standard phantom. Since ring systems can be

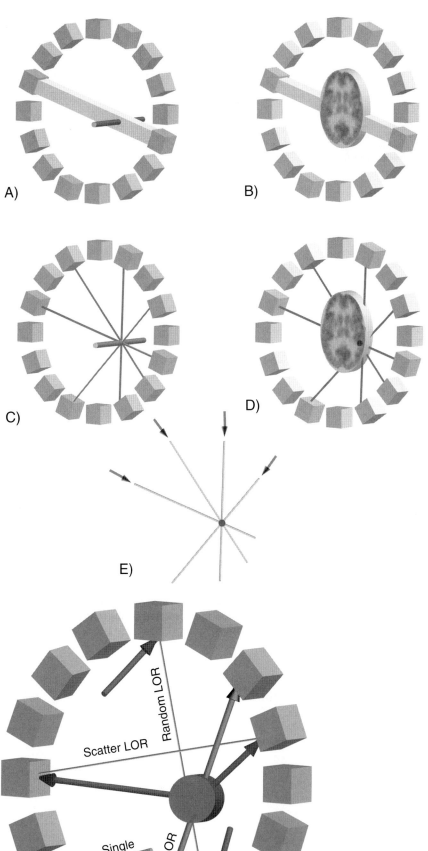

FIG. 2.5. Lines of response (LORs) for a 16-detector coincidence system. **A** and **B**: A single "tube" of response. **C** and **D**: Four LORs. **E**: The LORs are back-projected to reconstruct the original source of emission.

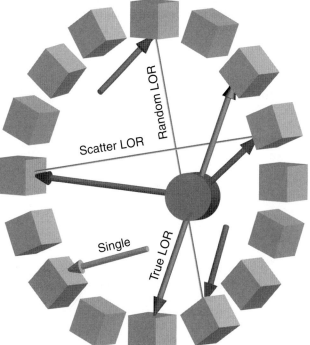

FIG. 2.6. LORs for true, random, and scattered events. Seven single events are shown. Of the three unrelated singles, two occur within the 12-nsec coincidence window and are recorded as a random LOR. In addition, a true and scatter LOR are shown.

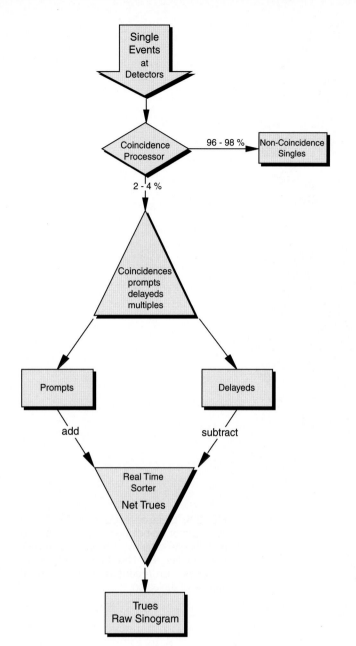

FIG. 2.7. Processing logic for single events in a ring gantry system (based on CTI PET systems). Prompt events occur when the coincidence processor determines that two detectors have registered two photons within the coincidence time window and delayed events occur in a similar manner within a delayed window. Randoms that occur within the coincidence window are corrected by the measured events in the delayed window.

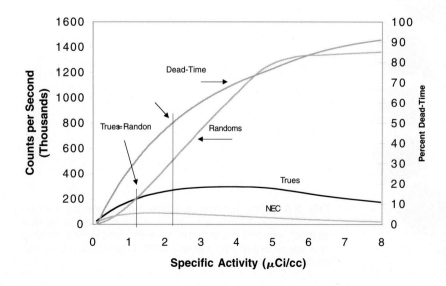

FIG. 2.8. Count rate vs. activity curve for an HR+ scanner in two-dimensional imaging mode (septa in place between detector rings). Curves were acquired during the decay of ^{18}F in a standard 20-cm-diameter phantom.

calibrated with a source of known activity, the ordinate is μCi/ml. In addition, the ratio of trues to randoms varies as a function of specific activity in the phantom, with the increase in randoms theoretically proportional to the square of activity. Above 1.2 μCi/ml the randoms start to predominate and continue to increase, while the trues show only small gains; in this region, a small increase in trues will occur at the expense of a large increase in random noise. The noise effective count rate (NEC) is often used to determine the optimum activity for imaging:

$$NEC = \frac{signal}{noise} = \frac{trues^2}{\sqrt{trues + 2 \cdot randoms + scatter}}$$

The curve for the NEC is also plotted in Fig. 2.8 and has a broad plateau region between 1 and 2 μCi/ml.

As indicated above, when a source of activity is scanned in a PET system, the detector electronics counts the number of events along each of the 80,000 or more LORs of each ring. Modern ring systems utilize a modified two-dimensional acquisition mode with rings also seeing events from five or more adjacent rings on either side. In full three-dimensional mode (with the septa retracted, Fig. 2.4C), events

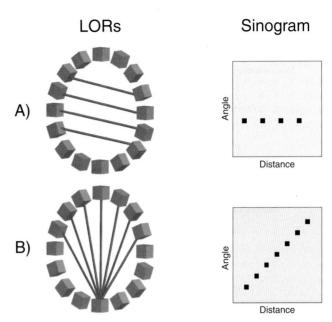

FIG. 2.10. Sinograms from parallel LORs and a LORs originating from a single detector.

can be detected between all rings and the number of LORs is correspondingly much greater. The coordinate system to locate each LOR (in two dimensions) is shown in Fig. 2.9. Each LOR is identified by a unique combination of distance s and angle ϕ and can be plotted as a discrete point on a graph. Figure 2.9A illustrates a single LOR between two detectors with the coordinates plotted in Fig. 2.9B. In Fig. 2.9C, a single source (Fig. 2.5) is shown, and the many LORs through the activity are graphed in Fig. 2.9D. The plotted curve has a sinusoidal shape; in general, the graphs of LORs are correspondingly known as *sinograms*. The intensity of each point on a sinogram corresponds to the number of events recorded for the LOR.

Two special cases of sinograms are shown in Fig. 2.10: for parallel LORs, angle ϕ will be constant, as shown in Fig. 2.10A; for a single detector, Fig. 2.10B, the field of view is determined by the other detectors with linking LORs, and the sinogram curve will be a diagonal line. Similar lines can be seen in "raw" sinogram curves before smoothing and attenuation corrections are applied. Figure 2.9E was acquired with rotating Ge-68 rod sources that expose the detectors to a uniform source of activity with no object in the gantry (a blank scan). Slight variations in detector sensitivity are easy to observe in this type of display. Finally, Fig. 2.9F shows a raw data set for an [18]FDG brain scan. After processing and reconstruction (Fig. 2.5E), the data is remapped into the standard x and y Cartesian coordinates for viewing.

Many steps are required in the data acquisition and processing to generate a final quantitative image. A simplified flow diagram is shown in Fig. 2.11. It is important to note that ring-gantry systems perform an on-the-fly randoms cor-

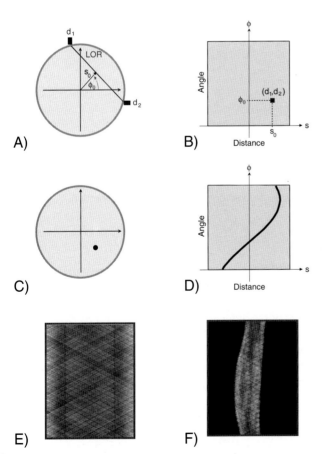

FIG. 2.9. The coordinate system for identifying LORs (**A**). Illustrative sinograms are shown (**B** and **D**). Actual data from a blank scan and a brain scan are also shown (**E** and **F**).

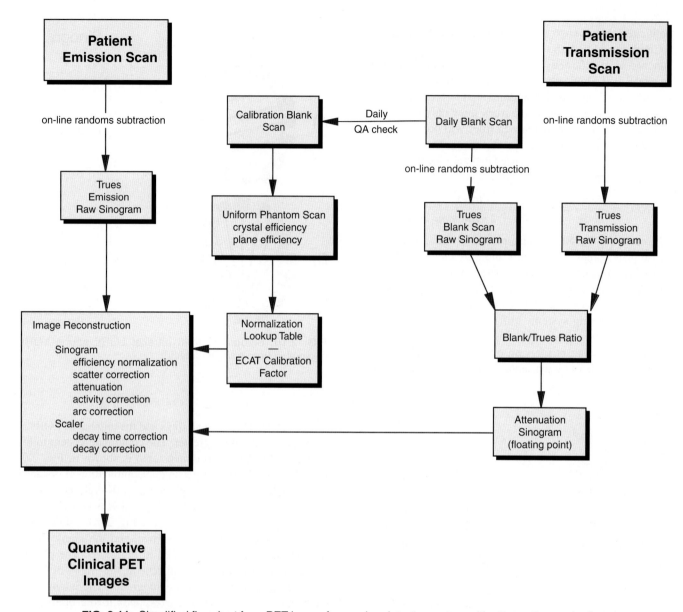

FIG. 2.11. Simplified flowchart for a PET image from a ring detector system with attenuation correction.

rection as well as correcting for dead time and scatter. For the most accurate quantitative results, one of the most important corrections to the acquired PET image is attenuation correction based on a transmission scan with a ^{68}Ge or ^{137}Cs source. For positron images, very accurate corrections can be made to the transmission scan, since the attenuation correction is a function of the total tissue thickness along each LOR ($e^{-\mu \cdot thickness}$) and is independent of the location of the decay.

Fig. 2.12 shows a comparison of attenuation corrections generated for a PET and a SPECT brain scan. For the PET image, the intensity is reduced by approximately 50% in the center of the brain as compared to 66% for SPECT. In addition, algorithms that theoretically estimate and correct the attenuation in the brain for 511-keV photons can generate almost identical images to data corrected with a transmission scan.

Raw Data

¹⁸F-FDG

Corrected Data

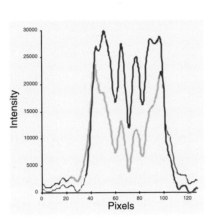

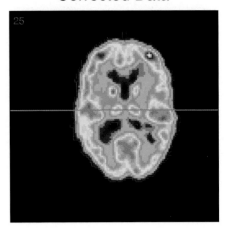

^{99m}TC-HMPAO

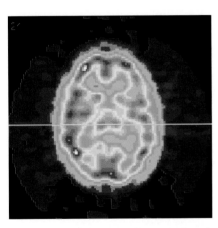

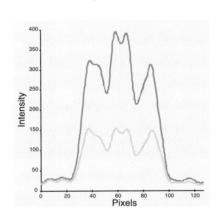

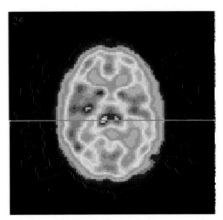

FIG. 2.12. Corrected and uncorrected images from PET and SPECT brain scans illustrating the importance of attenuation correction. The center illustrations are line-profile curves through the FDG and HMPAO brain images.

REFERENCES

1. Bendrie B, Townsend DW, eds. *The theory and practice of 3D PET.* Kluwer Academic Publishers, 1998.

2. Townsend DW, Defrise M. *Image reconstruction methods in positron tomography.* Lectures given in the academic training program of CERN, RD/904-2000-juin. Geneva 1993.

3. Welch MJ, Seigel BA (guest editors). The coming of age of PET (part 1). *Sem Nucl Med* 1998;28:247–267.

4. Reivich M, Kuhl D, Wolf A, et al. Measurement of local cerebral glucose metabolism in man with ¹⁸F-2-deoxy-2-fluoro-D-glucose. *Acta Neurol Scand Suppl* 1977;64:190–191.

5. Turner JE, Hamm RN, Souleyrette ML et al. Calculation for β dosimetry using Monte Carlo code (OREC) for electron transport in water. *Health Phys* 1988;55:741–749.

6. Anderson DW. *Absorption of ionizing radiation.* Baltimore, MD: University Park Press, 1984.

7. Chiesa C, De Sanctis V, Schiavini M, et al. Radiation dose to technicians per nuclear medicine procedure: comparison between technetium-99m, gallium-67, and iodine-131 radiotracers and fluorine-18 fluorodeoxyglucose. *Eur J Nucl Med* 1997;24:1380–1389.

8. Personal correspondence with James E. Carey and data from Vince McCormik, University of Michigan Medical Center, Ann Arbor MI 48109-0028.

9. Brown TF, Yasillo NJ. Radiation safety considerations for PET centers. *J Nucl Med Technol* 1997;25:98–102.

10. Wrenn FR, Good ML and Handler P. The use of positron emitting radioisotopes for the localization of brain tumors, *Science* 1951;1123:525–527.

11. Brownell GL, Sweet WH. Localization of brain tumors with positron emitters. *Nucleonics* 1953;11:40.

12. Anger HO. Scintillation camera. *Rev Sci Instr* 1958;29:27–33.

13. Anger HO, Rosenthal DJ. Scintillation camera and positron camera. *Medical radioisotope scanning.* Vienna: 1959:59–82.

14. Rankowitz S, Robertson JS, Higginbotham WA, et al. Positron scanner for locating brain tumors, *IRE Int Conv Rec* 1962;9:49–56.

Functional Cerebral SPECT and PET Imaging, Third Edition,
edited by R.L.Van Heertum and R.S. Tikofsky,
Lippincott Williams & Wilkins, Philadelphia © 2000.

CHAPTER 3

Normal and Correlative Anatomy

Charles R. Noback, David L. Daniels, Leighton P. Mark, Robert S. Hellman,
Ronald S. Tikofsky, and Ronald L. Van Heertum

The frontal, temporal, parietal, and occipital lobes are seen on the lateral view of the brain (Fig. 3.1). The central sulcus (fissure of Rolando) separates the frontal from parietal lobes. The Sylvian fissure divides the frontal from temporal and parietal lobes. There is no clear demarcation dividing the parietal from the occipital lobe. Functionally, the anterior portions of the frontal lobes are concerned with memory and emotional control, while the posterior portions are involved with the initiation and voluntary control of motor activity. The temporal lobe is involved with auditory function, and on the left side language comprehension. The parietal lobe is involved with the appreciation and interpretation of sensory input relating to form, shape, and weight. The occipital lobe is involved with primary visual function. The cerebellum is primarily involved with overall coordination of movement, including gait and balance. It is important to note that the two cerebral hemispheres do not have perfectly symmetric gross and microscopic anatomy, nor do they provide equivalent cognitive functions.

SAGITTAL VIEW OF THE BRAIN

The two hemispheres are interconnected by a large band of nerve fibers, the corpus callosum. The limbic (fifth) lobe, consisting of the cortex and associated structures superior to

C. R. Noback: Department of Anatomy and Cell Biology, Columbia University College of Physicians and Surgeons, New York, New York 10032.

D. L. Daniels, L. P. Mark, and R. S. Hellman: Department of Radiology, Medical College of Wisconsin, Milwaukee, Wisconsin 53226.

R. S. Tikofsky: Department of Radiology, Columbia University College of Physicians and Surgeons, Harlem Hospital Center, New York, New York, 10037.

R. L. Van Heertum: Department of Radiology, Columbia University College of Physicians and Surgeons, New York, New York 10032.

the corpus callosum, is involved in emotions, drives, and behavioral expression (Fig. 3.2).

The brain stem is involved in the control of respiration and cardiovascular activity. In addition, the major sensorimotor pathways pass through the brain stem to and from the cortex. The cerebellum, as noted above, is involved with motor coordination, gait, and balance.

THE VENTRICULAR SYSTEM

The ventricular system (Fig. 3.3) and subarachnoid space surrounding the brain are filled with cerebrospinal fluid (CSF). The fluid is formed by the choroid plexus in each ventricle. The CSF flows from the lateral ventricles through the interventricular foramen of Monro to the third ventricle, and then through the cerebral aqueduct and the fourth ventricle to the subarachnoid space. The system provides a fluid cushion upon which the brain "floats," protected from physical injury.

VASCULAR DISTRIBUTION

The arterial blood supply to the brain is derived from two major sources, i.e., the paired internal carotid (ICAs) and vertebral arteries (Fig. 3.4). The vertebral arteries join to form the basilar artery, which in turn usually terminates by dividing into the posterior cerebral arteries (PCAs). Branches of the PCAs supply blood to the brain stem, cerebellum, occipital lobes, and inferior portion of the temporal lobes. The ICAs usually terminate by dividing into anterior cerebral arteries (ACAs) and middle cerebral arteries (MCAs). The anterior and posterior circulations connect via the circle of Willis, an arterial ring found at the base of the brain.

As seen in the lateral view, the MCA extends laterally from the sylvian fissure to supply regions of the frontal, temporal, parietal, and occipital lobes (Fig. 3.5). However, the ACA provides the major arterial supply to the medial surface of the brain, in particular the superior surface of the corpus

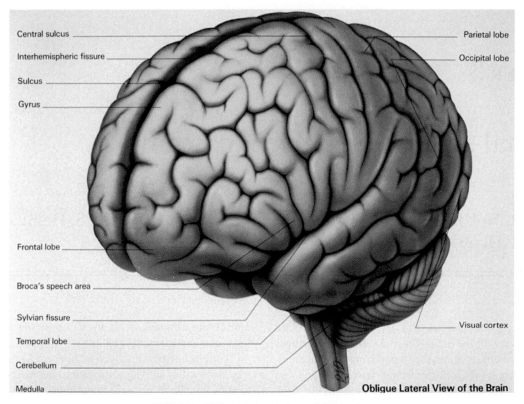

Central sulcus
Interhemispheric fissure
Sulcus
Gyrus
Frontal lobe
Broca's speech area
Sylvian fissure
Temporal lobe
Cerebellum
Medulla

Parietal lobe
Occipital lobe
Visual cortex

Oblique Lateral View of the Brain

FIG. 3.1. Oblique lateral view of the brain.

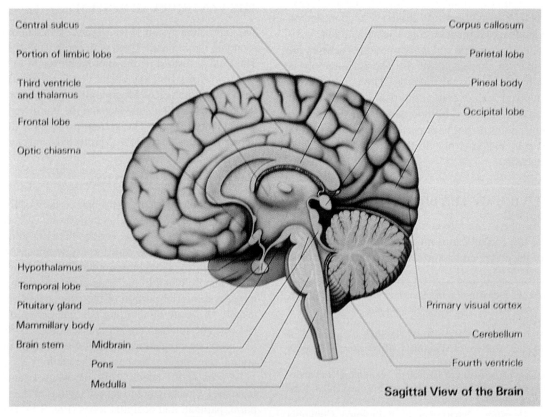

Central sulcus
Portion of limbic lobe
Third ventricle and thalamus
Frontal lobe
Optic chiasma
Hypothalamus
Temporal lobe
Pituitary gland
Mammillary body
Brain stem   Midbrain
             Pons
             Medulla

Corpus callosum
Parietal lobe
Pineal body
Occipital lobe
Primary visual cortex
Cerebellum
Fourth ventricle

Sagittal View of the Brain

FIG. 3.2. Sagittal view of the brain.

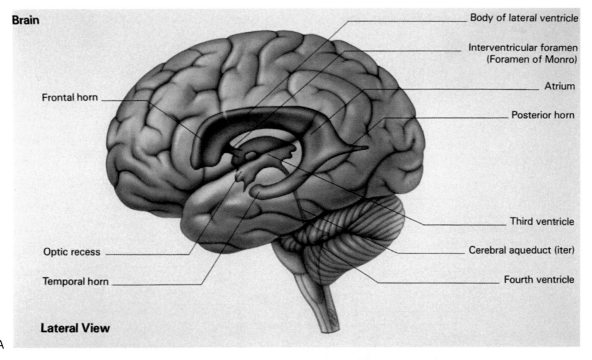

Brain

Frontal horn

Optic recess

Temporal horn

Lateral View

Body of lateral ventricle

Interventricular foramen
(Foramen of Monro)

Atrium

Posterior horn

Third ventricle

Cerebral aqueduct (iter)

Fourth ventricle

A

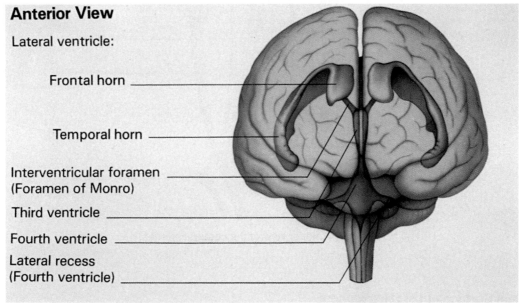

Anterior View

Lateral ventricle:

Frontal horn

Temporal horn

Interventricular foramen
(Foramen of Monro)

Third ventricle

Fourth ventricle

Lateral recess
(Fourth ventricle)

B

FIG. 3.3. Lateral **(A)** and anterior **(B)** views of the ventricles.

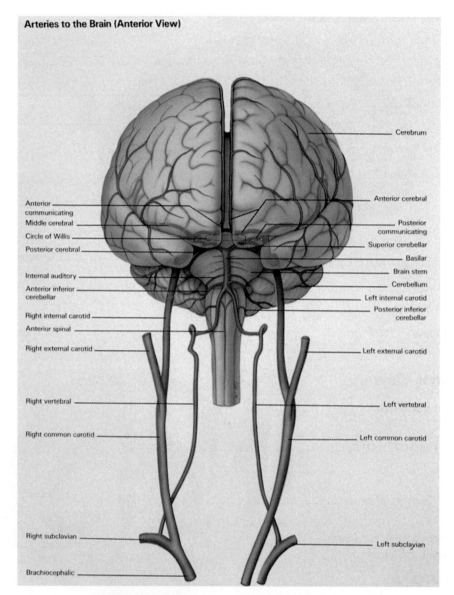

FIG. 3.4. Anterior view of the cerebral arteries.

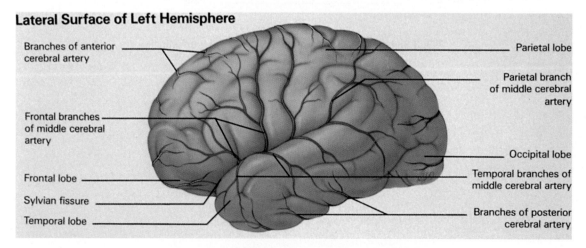

FIG. 3.5. Lateral surface of the left hemisphere.

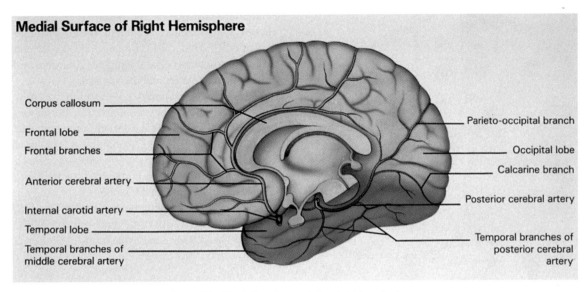

FIG. 3.6. Medial surface of the right hemisphere.

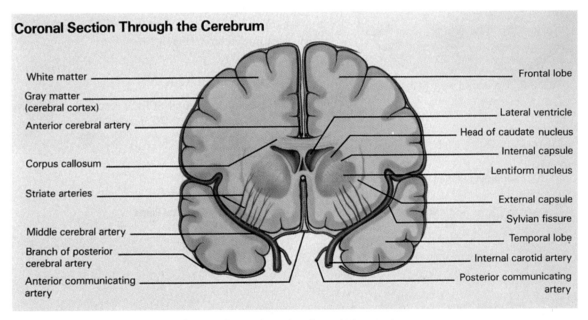

FIG. 3.7. Coronal section through the cerebrum.

callosum with branches reaching to the frontal and parietal lobes (Fig. 3.6). The PCA extends posteriorly and supplies the medial and posterior aspects of the temporal and occipital lobes.

On the coronal view, the MCAs are seen to extend between the temporal and parietal lobes (Fig. 3.7). Their deep branches—striate arteries—supply the corpus striatum of the basal ganglia and the internal capsules.

TRANSAXIAL VIEW OF THE BRAIN

The anterior and posterior limbs of the internal capsule are involved in motor activity. The caudate and putamen, structures

making up part of the basal ganglia are involved in fine motor coordination. The thalamus is a major structure for the perception of many types of sensory stimuli. It sends projections to the primary sensory/motor areas of the cerebral hemispheres (Fig. 3.8).

CORRELATIVE ANATOMY

Cerebral single-photon-emission computed tomography (SPECT) studies are displayed in transaxial, coronal, and sagittal planes (Fig. 3.9) adjacent to the corresponding magnetic resonance images (MRIs).

The major structures of the cerebrum such as the frontal, temporal, parietal, and occipital lobes are identified. The

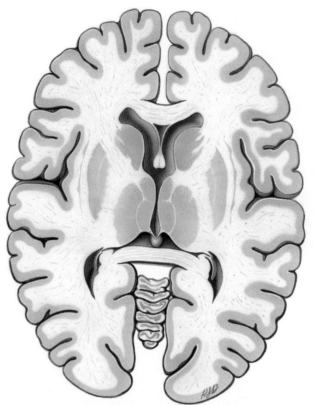

FIG. 3.8. Transaxial view of the brain.

cerebellar hemispheres and basal ganglia are also shown. However, the spatial resolution of SPECT images is less than that of MRI. Thus, SPECT images do not demonstrate the different structures of basal ganglia, brain stem, and the edge between white matter and the ventricles.

SPECT images should not be used to show detailed anatomy, although they demonstrate the major anatomic landmarks. SPECT imaging—when correlated with anatomic studies such as MRI and CT (computed tomography)—may be useful in delineating some pathologic processes using multiple planes. More importantly, in some disease states, changes in blood flow and metabolism may only be appreciated with SPECT imaging but not with CT or MRI. Figures 3.10, 3.11, and 3.12 illustrate representative SPECT images for single head (IMP) and triple head (HMPAU) adjacent to corresponding MRI images.

TRANSAXIAL PLANE

The transaxial cerebral SPECT sections are displayed in the same format as the MRI images. The sections begin inferiorly in the cerebellum and continue superiorly through the entire cerebrum (Fig. 3.10).

CORONAL PLANE

The coronal cerebral SPECT sections are displayed in the same format as the MRI images. The sections begin anteri-

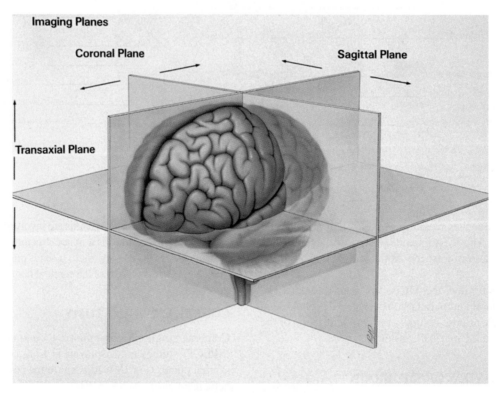

FIG. 3.9. Imaging planes.

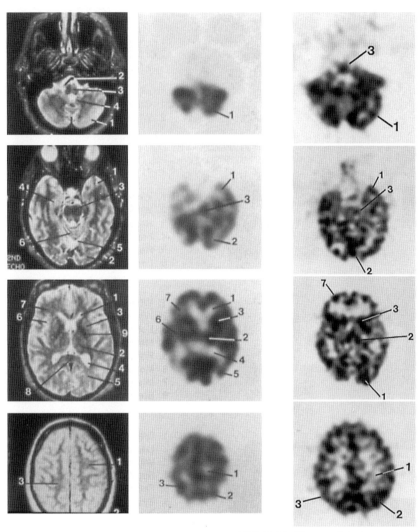

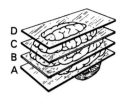

A. 1. Cerebellar hemisphere
   2. Vertebral artery
   3. Medulla oblongata
   4. Cerebellar tonsil

B. 1. Temporal lobe
   2. Occipital lobe
   3. Upper brain stem
   4. Temporal horn
   5. Tentorial notch
   6. Cerebellar vermis

C. 1. Frontal horn
   2. Thalamus
   3. Basal ganglia—lentiform nucleus
   4. Occipital horn
   5. Occipital lobe
   6. White matter
   7. Frontal lobe
   8. Splenium of corpus callosum
   9. Internal capsule

D. 1. White matter
   2. Gray matter
   3. Parietal lobe

FIG. 3.10. Transaxial plane.

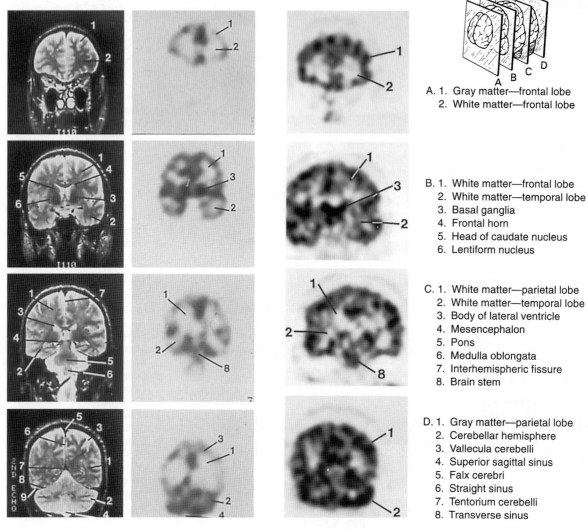

FIG. 3.11. Coronal plane.

A. 1. Gray matter—frontal lobe
2. White matter—frontal lobe

B. 1. White matter—frontal lobe
2. White matter—temporal lobe
3. Basal ganglia
4. Frontal horn
5. Head of caudate nucleus
6. Lentiform nucleus

C. 1. White matter—parietal lobe
2. White matter—temporal lobe
3. Body of lateral ventricle
4. Mesencephalon
5. Pons
6. Medulla oblongata
7. Interhemispheric fissure
8. Brain stem

D. 1. Gray matter—parietal lobe
2. Cerebellar hemisphere
3. Vallecula cerebelli
4. Superior sagittal sinus
5. Falx cerebri
6. Straight sinus
7. Tentorium cerebelli
8. Transverse sinus

orly in the frontal lobes and continue posteriorly through the entire brain (Fig. 3.11).

SAGITTAL PLANE

The sagittal cerebral SPECT sections are displayed in the same format as the MRI images. The images extend from the right side of the brain to the midline (Fig. 3.12).

HELPFUL HINTS

The examples that follow are designed to provide an overview of the general characteristics observed in normal and pathological regional cerebral blood flow/SPECT brain images. They serve as a general point of reference for comparison with the case presentations in the chapters that follow.

Normal Tracer Uptake

Typically, there is symmetric distribution of tracer uptake in both hemispheres. The basal ganglia, occipital cortex, and cerebellum will often appear darker than other regions.

Ventricles will not be as sharply defined as with CT or MRI because the tracer is not taken up by the ventricles or white matter surrounding the ventricles. When imaging is performed with multidetector systems it is possible to distinguish the heads of the caudate nuclei, the body of the caudate, and other lenticular structures. In addition, the thalamus can also be visualized in the transaxial images (Fig. 3.13).

Absent Tracer Uptake

Absent tracer uptake implies that tracer uptake is not present in a zone extending from deep within the brain through the cortical rim. These regions of absent uptake often have the appearance of a bite or wedge taken out of the brain. This type of finding is associated with a region of infarction seen on CT or MRI (Fig. 3.14). Areas of absent tracer uptake may also be observed in case of trauma and surgical resection.

Reduced but not Absent Tracer Uptake

Regions of reduced but not absent tracer uptake usually appear "less intense" than do the surrounding cortical regions

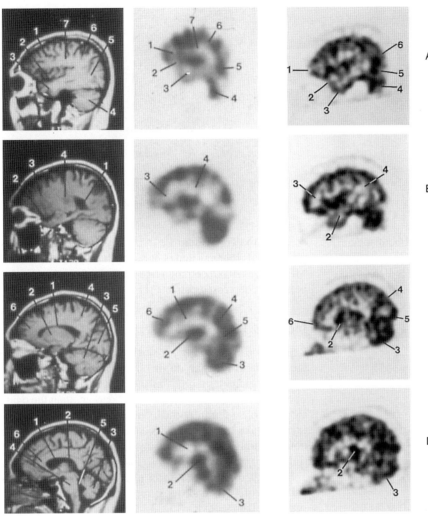
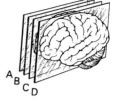

A. 1. Frontal lobe
   2. Sylvian fissure
   3. Temporal lobe
   4. Cerebellum
   5. Occipital lobe
   6. Parietal lobe
   7. White matter

B. 1. Atrium of lateral ventricle
   2. White matter—temporal lobe
   3. White matter—frontal lobe
   4. White matter—parietal lobe

C. 1. Lateral ventricle
   2. Basal ganglia
   3. Cerebellum
   4. Parietal lobe
   5. Occipital lobe
   6. Frontal lobe

D. 1. Lateral ventricle
   2. Thalamus
   3. Cerebellum
   4. Brain stem
   5. Fourth ventricle
   6. Corpus callosum

FIG. 3.12. Sagittal plane.

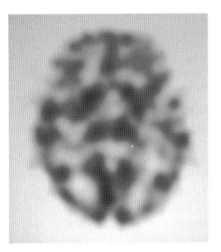

FIG. 3.13. Normal distribution.

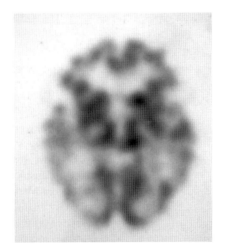

FIG. 3.14. Reduced tracer uptake.

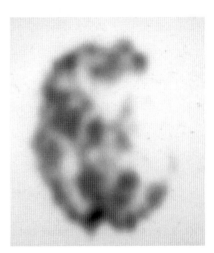

FIG. 3.15. Absent tracer uptake.

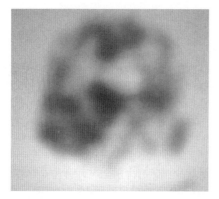

FIG. 3.16. Increased tracer uptake.

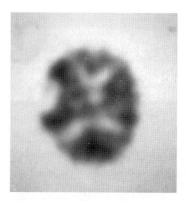

FIG. 3.18. Compressed cortex.

and corresponding regions of the contralateral hemisphere. They also will appear "thin" or "less intense" in comparison to equivalent regions seen in normal studies. It is also useful to compare regions thought to show reduced but not absent tracer uptake with the basal ganglia, occipital cortex, and

cerebellum. This finding is typically associated with the presence of ischemia and is not necessarily evident in CT or MRI images. It is a common finding in the dementia and may be seen in depressed patients (Fig. 3.15).

Increased Tracer Uptake

Regions of increased tracer uptake usually appear to have greater intensity" than do the surrounding cortical regions and corresponding regions of the contralateral hemisphere. They will also appear "thicker" and "darker" than the equivalent regions seen in normal studies. Findings of increased tracer uptake have been associated with one of two conditions: regions of hypermetabolism such as seizure activity (Fig. 3.16) or luxury perfusion (Fig. 3.17 A and B).

Findings of increased tracer uptake have been associated with one of two conditions: regions of hypermetabolism, such as seizure activity (Fig. 3.11), or luxury perfusion (Fig. 3.17 A and B).

Distortion of the Cortical Surface

Regions of "misshapen" or "distorted" cortical rim are often seen when there is an accumulation of extraaxial fluid or blood following trauma, and when there is an extraaxial mass. The extent of distortion is related to the amount of fluid accumulation and the size of the mass (Fig. 3.18).

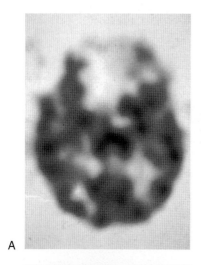

A

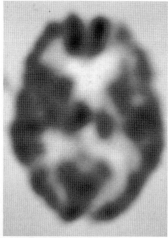

B

FIG. 3.17. Absent tracer uptake before luxury perfusion **(A)** and after the onset of luxury perfusion **(B).**

Examples of Normal Images

Figures 3.1 through 3.7 are examples of normal images obtained using SPECT, PET, and coincidence PET systems. For those who would examine a greater sampling of normal SPECT images using currently available tracers and imaging systems, we suggest accessing the normal database created under the auspices of the Brain Imaging Council of the Society of Nuclear Medicine. Information on the database can be obtained by visiting one of two Web pages. The sites can be accessed at: http://www.snm.org/about/new_councils_1.html or the brain imaging Web page: http://brainscans.med.yale.edu.

Normal Volunteer

CONTRIBUTORS:

Robert S. Hellman, M.D.,
Ronald S. Tikofsky, Ph.D.
Institution: Department of Radiology,
Section of Nuclear Medicine,
Medical College of Wisconsin

IMAGING ACQUISITION DATA:

Camera: GE Neurocam   **Dose:** 20 mCi
Tracer: ^{99m}Tc ECD

This 65-year-old healthy man volunteered to serve as a normal control.

Transverse-plane ^{99m}Tc-ECD SPECT images (Case Fig. 3.1) obtained at 10 and 75 min and 5 hr postinjection show uniform radiotracer uptake throughout the cerebral cortex, cerebellum (not shown in the figure), basal ganglia, and thalamus. Only minimal degradation of radiotracer uptake is seen between the 10- and 75-min postinjection acquisitions. However, there is significant reduction of radiotracer uptake in the cerebral cortex seen in the images acquired 5 hr postinjection except for the occipital regions and thalamus. The basal ganglia also reduced activity as to images acquired to images acquired at 10 and 75 min postinjection.

Teaching Points:

These examples illustrate that it is essential, in interpreting SPECT brain images, to take into account changes in radiotracer deposition as a function of time between injection and study acquisition. Delay in acquiring images may result in interpreting the SPECT study as shown at 5 hr as abnormal. This is especially the case with older patients.

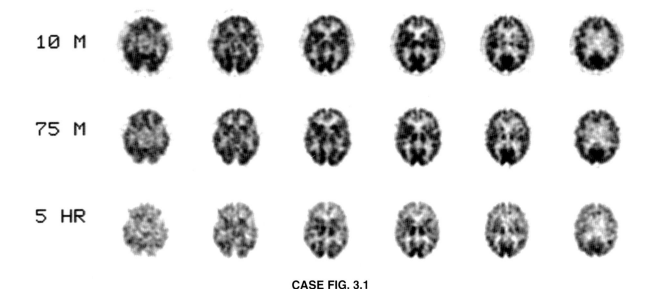

CASE FIG. 3.1

Normal Volunteer

CONTRIBUTOR:	IMAGING ACQUISITION DATA:	
Mansanori Ichise, M.D.	**Camera:** Picker PRISM 3000	**Collimator:** Ultra-high-resolution fan beam
Institution: Mount Sinai Hospital, Toronto, Canada	**Tracer:** 99mTc ECD	**Dose:** 20 mCi

This 22-year-old man (student) volunteered to serve as a normal control.

Findings of other imaging studies were normal.

Transverse-plane 99mTc-ECD SPECT images (Case Fig. 3.2) show uniform radiotracer uptake throughout the cerebral cortex, cerebellum, basal ganglia, and thalamus.

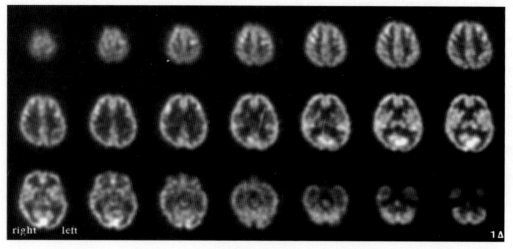

CASE FIG. 3.2

Normal Volunteer

CONTRIBUTOR:	IMAGING ACQUISITION DATA:	
Mansanori Ichise, M.D.	**Camera:** Picker PRISM 3000	**Collimator:** Ultra-high-resolution fan beam
Institution: Mount Sinai Hospital, Toronto, Canada	**Tracer:** 99mTc ECD	**Dose:** 20 mCi

This 53-year-old woman is a schoolteacher volunteer who served as a normal control.

Findings of other imaging studies were normal.

Transverse-plane 99mTc-ECD SPECT images (Case Fig. 3.3) show uniform radiotracer uptake throughout the cerebral cortex, cerebellum (not shown in the figure), basal ganglia, and thalamus.

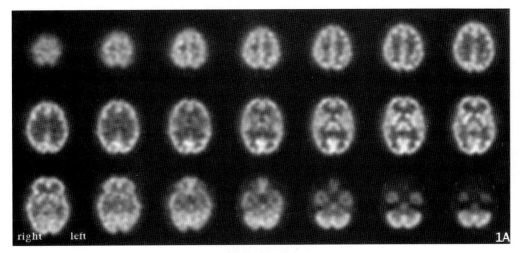

CASE FIG. 3.3

Normal Volunteer

CONTRIBUTOR:	**IMAGING ACQUISITION DATA:**	
Mansanori Ichise, M.D.	**Camera:** Picker PRISM 3000	**Collimator:** Ultra-high-resolution fan beam
Institution: Mount Sinai Hospital, Toronto, Canada	**Tracer:** ^{99m}Tc ECD	**Dose:** 20 mCi

This 96-year-old healthy woman volunteer served as a normal control.

Findings of other imaging studies were normal.

^{99m}Tc-ECD SPECT images in the transverse, coronal, and sagittal planes (Case Fig. 3.4A–C) show uniform radiotracer uptake throughout the cerebral cortex, cerebellum, basal ganglia, and thalamus.

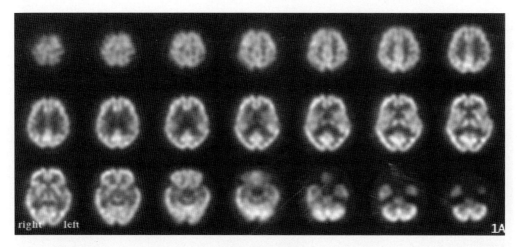

CASE FIG. 3.4A

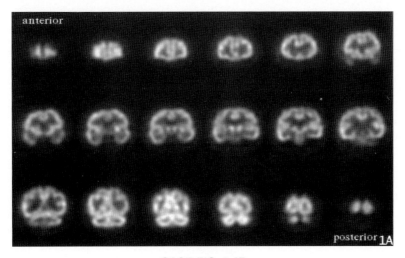

CASE FIG. 3.4B

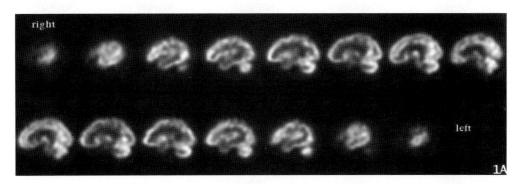

CASE FIG. 3.4C

Normal Volunteer

CONTRIBUTOR:

Michael M. Graham, Ph.D., M.D.

Institution: Department of Radiology,
Division of Nuclear Medicine,
University of Washington School
of Medicine

IMAGING ACQUISITION DATA:

Camera: GE Advance Scanner   **Dose:** 10 mCi
Tracer: ¹⁸FDG

This 40-year-old man served as a normal control.

PET images in the transverse plane reconstructed with filtered back projection (Case Fig. 3.5A and B), and iterative reconstruction (Case Fig. 3.5C and D).

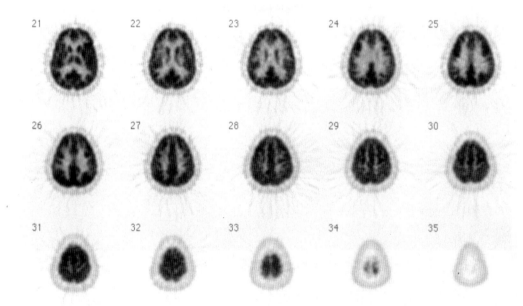

CASE FIG. 3.5A

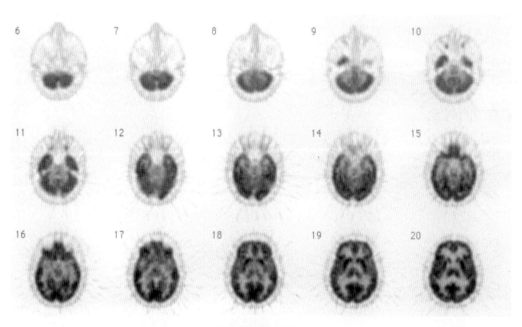

CASE FIG. 3.5B

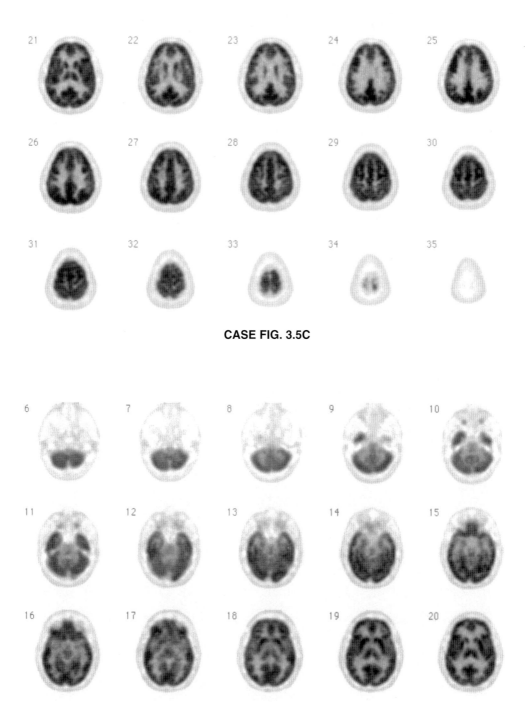

CASE FIG. 3.5C

CASE FIG. 3.5D

Normal Volunteer

CONTRIBUTORS:	IMAGING ACQUISITION DATA:	
James M. Mountz, M.D., Ph.D.,	**Camera:** ADAC MCD Vertex Plus	**Collimator:** None
Michael V. Yester, Ph.D.	**Tracer:** [18]FDG	**Dose:** 5 mCi Attenuation correction performed after a CS-transmission scan was acquired
Institution: The University of Alabama at Birmingham Medical Center		

This 35-year-old woman served as a normal volunteer.

[18]FDG ([F[18]] fluorodeoxyglucose) PET coincidence images in the transverse plane (Case Fig. 3.6). These images are typical of those that can be routinely achieved using coincidence imaging after injection of 5 mCi of [18]FDG and imaging with a dual-head camera without collimators.

Teaching Points:

Increased regional delivery of [18]FDG and new cameras and computers now permit the routine use of the metabolic tracer [18]FDG for nuclear medicine studies.

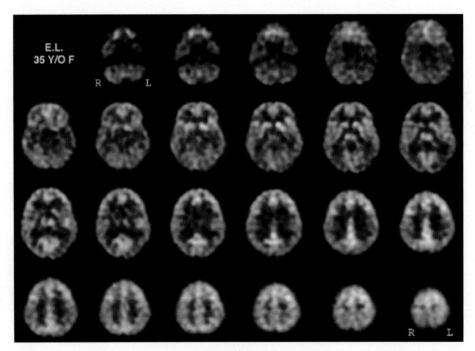

CASE FIG. 3.6

Normal Volunteer

CONTRIBUTORS:	IMAGING ACQUISITION DATA:

CONTRIBUTORS:

Martin P. Sandler, M.D.,

Dominique Delbeke, M.D., Ph.D.

Institution: Department of Radiology,
Vanderbilt University Medical
Center

IMAGING ACQUISITION DATA:

Cameras: Siemens ECAT 933 & Elscint
Varicam

Tracer: [18]FDG

Collimator: Slit Collilmator (Varicam)

Dose: 10 mCi

This 30-year-old woman who complained of headache.

[18]FDG PET image in the transverse plane (Fig. 3.7A) and an [18]FDG coincidence image obtained with dual-head camera (Fig. 3.7B) equipped with a 5/8-in. NaI (T1) crystal.

Teaching Points:

These images permit a comparison of image quality obtained by dual-head coincidence imaging vs. those obtained with a dedicated PET scanner.

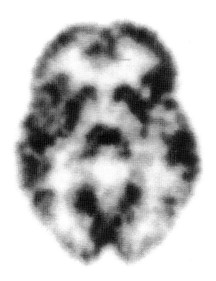

CASE FIG. 3.7A

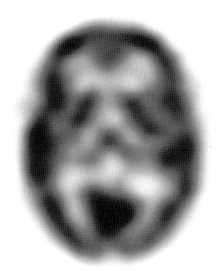

CASE FIG. 3.7B

Functional Cerebral SPECT and PET Imaging, Third Edition,
edited by R.L.Van Heertum and R.S. Tikofsky,
Lippincott Williams & Wilkins, New York © 2000.

CHAPTER 4

Functional Anatomy and SPECT Imaging

H. Branch Coslett

Interest in the anatomic underpinnings of behavior has a venerable history, dating at least to the ancient Greeks. In the fifth century B.C., for example, Hippocrates of Croton argued that the brain was the organ of intellect, whereas the heart was the organ of the senses. In the second century, Galen was the first to claim that cognition resided in the substance of the brain rather than the ventricles.

Perhaps the first modern attempt to localize behaviors to specific brain structures is found in the work of the phrenologist Franz Joseph Gall, who in the late 19th and early 20th centuries espoused the theory that mental faculties were localized in "centers" in the brain. Unfortunately, Gall is primarily remembered at this point not for his belief that definable brain regions were implicated in specific behaviors, but for his additional incorrect assertion that, because the brain's form shapes the overlying skull, the status of an individual's cognitive and behavioral capacities could be inferred by measuring the external contours of the skull.

Although they were ultimately discredited, the teachings of the phrenologists are clearly relevant to contemporary accounts of brain-behavior relationships in that these teachings exerted a significant influence on the French and German physicians of the mid-19th century, such as Paul Broca and Carl Wernicke, whose seminal contributions constitute the beginnings of the contemporary doctrine of the localization of cerebral functions. After hearing Aubertin, a student of Gall, describe the significance of the frontal lobes in speech, Broca (1) investigated a series of patients with "aphemia" (only later designated *aphasia*) and subsequently determined that the left frontal lobe is critical for speech. Additional observations by Hughlings Jackson (2), Bastian (3), and Wernicke (4) supporting the consistent association between sites of brain injury and specific behavioral disorders quickly

followed. Indeed, the exploration of brain-behavior relationships, to which single-photon-emission computed tomography (SPECT) brain imaging has made important contributions in recent years, continues to be a major subject of research in modern cognitive neuroscience.

This chapter provides a brief overview of insights on the functional anatomy of the human brain afforded by investigations conducted over the last 130 years. The *ablation paradigm*—that is, the investigation of the behavioral consequences of focal brain injury such as stroke or intracerebral hemorrhage—has been the richest source of information regarding the functional anatomy of the cerebral cortex. It should be noted, however, that a number of other lines of investigation—including brain stimulation in humans and animals, electrophysiological recordings in animals, manipulation of neurochemical systems in animals and, more recently, "activation" studies using SPECT positron emission tomography (PET) and magnetic resonance imaging (MRI) scans—have also contributed substantially to this body of knowledge.

Prior to a consideration of the behavioral disorders associated with dysfunction of different brain regions, it is important to note that the likelihood that brain dysfunction will result in the "classical" pattern of behavioral disturbance is influenced by a number of factors. The *age* at which the pathologic process is initiated, for example, may be critical to the outcome; thus, while the association between language dysfunction and left-hemispheric perisylvian dysfunction in right-handers has been repeatedly demonstrated since the time of Broca, a number of investigators have demonstrated that left-hemispheric insult—even including left hemispherectomy (5)—may cause minimal language dysfunction when the insult occurs prior to the age of 6. Similarly, the *nature* of the underlying pathologic process may play an important role in modulating the behavioral consequences of brain dysfunction; behavioral disturbances associated with right (nondominant) parietal lobe dysfunction may appear

---

H. Branch Coslett: Department of Neurology, Temple University School of Medicine Philadelphia, Pennsylvania 19140.

quite different in patients with brain tumors, for example, as opposed to those with stroke. Additional factors that may substantially influence the behavioral consequences of brain dysfunction include the time since insult, the rate of evolution of the pathologic process, depth and surface area of the lesion, and, of course, premorbid factors such as handedness and presence of previous neurologic or psychiatric disorders.

Because the present volume provides an excellent account of the utility of SPECT brain imaging in defining the functional anatomy of behavioral disorders, we have elected to describe the functional anatomy of the cerebral cortex with respect to specific brain regions (e.g., the temporal lobe) rather than, for example, describing the localization of specific behavioral disorders such as amnesia or aphasia. We have opted to present what we believe to be the most "typical" or consistent pattern of localization of function. In light of the complexity of the psychological processes underlying human behavior, we wish to make clear that many clinical syndromes may be associated with lesions in different brain regions.

FRONTAL LOBES

Describing the scope and characteristics of human cognition, the eminent Russian neuropsychologist A. Luria (6) wrote: "Man not only reacts passively to incoming information, but creates *intentions,* forms *plans* and *programs* of his actions, inspects their performance, and *regulates* his behavior so that it conforms to these plans and programs; finally, he *ver-*

ifies his conscious activity, comparing the effects of his actions with the original intentions and correcting many mistakes he has made" (pp. 78–79).

In fact, as shown below, it is the frontal lobe that provides the substrate for much of what Luria believed to be the essence of creative, synthetic, and goal-directed human behavior.

Perhaps the most striking evolutionary alteration in human brain structure has been the dramatic enlargement of the frontal lobe; the human frontal lobe makes up approximately 50% of brain volume and is characterized by both anatomic and functional diversity. The anatomic diversity is illustrated, for example, by the fact that the influential human neuroanatomist Brodmann identified 11 distinct cytoarchitectonic regions in the frontal lobe (Figs. 4.1 and 4.2).

In light of the size and complexity of this portion of the brain, it is perhaps not surprising that many different patterns of impairment may be observed as a consequence of frontal lobe lesions. Thus, despite the fact that clinicians frequently refer to a "frontal lobe syndrome," there is no single constellation of symptoms and signs characterizing frontal lobe lesions. Rather, the specific behavioral disturbance associated with frontal lobe pathology is to a large extent a function of the site of damage within the frontal lobe. Thus, although a seemingly bewildering array of behavioral deficits have been observed in association with frontal lobe dysfunction, a number of clinicoanatomic correlations have been established. For present purposes, one may distinguish four distinct functional regions of the frontal lobe, damage to which

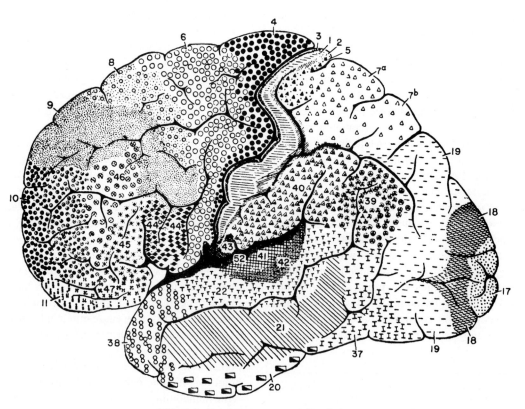

FIG. 4.1. Brodmann map—lateral view.

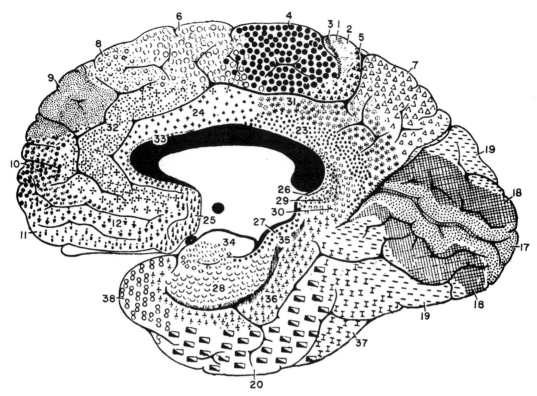

FIG. 4.2. Brodmann map—medial view.

typically is associated with different patterns of behavioral deficits.

The first of the functional regions, the *motor cortex,* extends from the sylvian fissure laterally to the medial surface of the frontal lobes and encompasses the precentral gyrus or "primary" motor cortex (Brodmann area 4) as well as the "premotor" cortex, comprised of the posterior portions of the three horizontally aligned frontal gyri (Brodmann area 6). These cortical regions are, of course, critical for fine motor activity; the majority of the axons of the corticospinal tract arise from neurons in these regions. As the primary behavioral consequences of damage to the motor cortex—that is, motor deficits ranging from clumsiness with mild weakness to hemiparesis—are well known, these regions are not considered further.

The balance of the frontal cortices, often designated the "prefrontal" cortex, includes three regions that are, at least in part, functionally distinct. These include the *orbitofrontal* cortex on the undersurface of the frontal lobe, the *dorsolateral* frontal cortices on the lateral surface of the frontal lobes (including at least portions of Brodmann areas 8–10 and 44–47), and the *medial* cortex of the frontal lobe (including parts of Brodmann areas 8–10 and 24). These three regions are discussed separately below.

Orbitofrontal Cortex

Dysfunction of the orbitofrontal cortex is typically associated with profound changes in personality characterized by emotional instability and unpredictability; damage to these structures is thought to be, at least in large part, responsible for symptoms and signs such as a "pseudobulbar affect," which is characterized by inappropriate expressions of emotion, and the closely related phenomenon of *Witzelsucht.* Interestingly, "intelligence," at least as assessed by standard tests of cognitive ability, may be normal.

The consequences of bilateral orbitofrontal lesions may be illustrated by the following accounts of two patients with damage to the orbitofrontal cortex.

Patient E.V.R.

Eslinger and Damasio (7) described a patient, E.V.R., who exhibited dramatic changes in behavior after resection of an orbitofrontal meningioma as well as substantial portions of the bilateral orbitofrontal cortex. By age 32, E.V.R. was married and had two children; he was a church elder and the comptroller of an accounting firm. At about this time, however, he began to exhibit changes in personality, marital difficulties, and an inability to discharge his professional responsibilities. These difficulties worsened over the course of the next several years, leading to his suspension from his job. When he reached age 35, a large orbitofrontal meningioma, which was compressing the anterior frontal lobes, was diagnosed and resected.

After the resection, E.V.R.'s problems apparently continued unabated. Once he was able to resume work, he returned to accounting for a short time before going into business with a man of dubious moral character. Against the advice of friends and family, he invested his entire savings in a venture that failed, forcing him to declare bankruptcy. He subsequently took and lost a number of jobs ranging from accountant to warehouse laborer. Within 2 years of his operation, his wife left him and filed for divorce. E.V.R. remarried within a month of his divorce and divorced again 2 years later. Interestingly, an extensive inpatient psychiatric evaluation revealed him to be of above normal intelligence with "no evidence of organic brain syndrome or frontal dysfunction" (7).

Evaluation at the University of Iowa several years later demonstrated that E.V.R. performed well on many conventional measures of intelligence and memory. For example, he obtained a verbal IQ of 129 (97th percentile) and a performance IQ of 135 (99th percentile) as well as a Weschler Memory Scale Score of 143 (well above average).

Patient C.C.

The behavior of C.C., one of our patients, also illustrates the consequences of dysfunction of the orbitofrontal cortex. C.C. was a seemingly happy and well-adjusted young girl until the age of approximately 15, when family and teachers noted that she had become increasingly "difficult" and unpredictable. Although her behavior was initially attributed to an adolescent adjustment reaction, if deteriorated, over the course of several years, to the point where she displayed "sociopathic" and on occasion violent behavior, ultimately leading to her suspension from school. At the age of 17, she complained of increasingly severe generalized headaches; medical evaluation at that point revealed a large (8×8 cm) meningioma arising from the right sphenoid wing and extending superiorly into the posterior portion of the orbitofrontal cortex and basal forebrain; the tumor and surrounding edema distorted most of the orbitofrontal cortex bilaterally as well as portions of the mesial frontal lobes.

Following resection of the tumor and small amounts of surrounding basal forebrain, a dramatic change in C.C.'s behavior was observed. Her irritability, aggressiveness, and unpredictability disappeared and the previously observed warm and affectionate relationships with family and friends resurfaced. Thus, according to her mother, C.C.'s personality reverted to what it had been in childhood.

C.C. did not, however, return to her premorbid state in all respects; she continues to exhibit a prominent and disabling deficit often associated with lesions of the posterior portions of the orbitofrontal cortex and basal forebrain—amnesia (see later).

These two cases, as well as those of previously reported patients (8), attest to the role of the orbitofrontal cortex in the mediation of complex social behavior as well as memory.

Medial Frontal Cortex

The mesial frontal cortex receives projections from the limbic system and has extensive reciprocal projections with the polymodal sensory association cortex as well as cortical regions mediating motor planning. Thus, as emphasized by Mesulam (9), the medial frontal cortex (and cingulate gyri in particular) may play an important role in the integration of limbic information that pertains to motivational significance and emotional valence; such information combines with sensory input and other data about past experience and current needs to generate plans of action. In other words, the medial frontal cortex may be critical for generating and initiating behavior that serves to modulate current and anticipated needs and goals.

This hypothesis is consistent with observations regarding the effects of brain lesions in humans. For example, bilateral lesions of the medial frontal lobes produce the syndrome of akinetic mutism; patients with this disorder may be awake and apparently alert yet fail to interact with the examiner or with their environment more generally; when spoken to, these patients may not respond, and when asked to execute a movement, they typically produce no response. Observation of the patients often reveals that the movements made by a normal resting individual (e.g., eye-blinking and grooming movements) are markedly reduced.

Patients with medial frontal lesions typically adopt a quite passive attitude toward their environment, exhibiting little initiative. Laplane et al. (10), for example, reported a patient with destruction of portions of the bilateral medial frontal cortex who, despite a lack of food for 24 hrs, never complained of hunger or initiated any action to obtain food. When finally provided with a meal tray, she expressed no surprise or relief but ate in her usual fashion. Interestingly, when provided a second meal a short while later, she expressed no consternation but consumed the meal just as she had the first.

Finally, a striking flatness of affect or emotional expression is a frequent consequence of medial frontal damage. These patients typically appear neither happy nor sad but are seemingly indifferent to the emotional valence and content of social interactions.

Unilateral lesions of the mesial frontal cortex typically produce similar but far less dramatic deficits. Damage to the left medial frontal region is associated with an akinesia of speech—that is, "transcortical motor aphasia"—which is characterized by a marked reduction in the length and frequency of utterances but a relative preservation of the ability to repeat.

Patient M.S.

The behavioral deficits associated with lesions of the medial frontal cortex are illustrated by the account of patient M.S. He was a high-ranking executive until the age of 60, when he was noted by business colleagues to be less "energetic" and motivated. Although the quality of his work remained exemplary, he failed to complete his usual tasks despite working the same schedule. At approximately the same time, his wife noted that he became less affectionate; he exhibited less and less interest in his friends and hobbies and spent increasing amounts of leisure time "just sitting." During the ensuing 2 years, the symptoms became more pronounced. After being encouraged to take early retirement, he finally sought medical attention.

Neurologic examination revealed M.S. to be alert and oriented, with excellent mathematical and analytical skills. His memory appeared normal. Two striking abnormalities were observed, however. First, although cooperative and responsive, M.S. virtually never initiated interactions with his wife or the examiner. He sat passively in a wheelchair, exhibiting little affect and rare spontaneous movements. He exhibited normal strength and only mild rigidity. When asked to walk, however, he stood but appeared to be rooted to the floor. When sufficient force was exerted to displace his center of gravity, he recovered his balance and, seemingly without effort, walked a few steps. While sitting, he was able to demonstrate stepping movements with both legs.

Second, M.S. manifested a dramatic delay in responding. When greeted, for example, he invariably provided an appropriate (if bland) salutation, but he required up to 30 sec to respond. Similar delays were noted in response to commands to execute movements. He required as long as a minute to generate a (usually correct) response to a simple problem. Although spontaneous speech was markedly diminished, he exhibited no impairment in accuracy of naming, reading, writing, or comprehension. M.S. was frequently incontinent of urine; he stated that he sensed when his bladder was full and could inhibit evacuation but was indifferent to the incontinence.

A SPECT scan showed a substantial reduction in blood flow in the medial frontal cortex and anterior temporal lobes bilaterally.

Dorsolateral Frontal Lobes

Although recent investigations in nonhuman primates (11) have demonstrated the dorsolateral frontal cortex (cortex surrounding the arcuate and principal sulci) to be implicated in a variety of motor, sensory, and even visual functions, investigations of patients with lesions of the dorsolateral frontal lobes suggest that the primary consequence of dysfunction in this region is an impairment in planning, problem solving, abstract reasoning, and high-level cognitive abilities more generally.

Patients with bilateral dorsolateral frontal lesions frequently exhibit a lack of flexibility in their thinking and planning and appear rigid and perseverative. Many but not all patients with these lesions exhibit deficits on standard intelligence tests (e.g., the Weschler Adult Intelligence Scale—Revised or Raven's Progressive Matrices); other patients, often with less extensive lesions, may appear to family and friends to be less insightful, innovative, or analytical in their thinking but do not demonstrate clear-cut cognitive abnormalities.

As noted above with respect to other frontal lobe regions,

unilateral lesions of the dorsolateral frontal cortex often produce substantially less prominent symptoms and signs of cognitive dysfunction. Lesions of the left (that is, dominant) dorsolateral frontal cortex, for example, are typically associated with language deficits, whereas lesions of the right dorsolateral frontal lobe are often associated with an impairment in the expression of emotion in conjunction with a relatively preserved ability to apprehend the emotional significance of affect expressed in speech or facial expressions (12).

The severity of the language deficit associated with left dorsolateral frontal lobe damage varies widely. Extensive lesions that disrupt the posterior portion of the left dorsolateral frontal lobe (e.g., Brodmann areas 44 and 45, or Broca's area) as well as portions of the motor cortex and insular cortex typically produce the syndrome of Broca's aphasia, characterized by nonfluent, halting, "telegraphic" speech. In contrast, lesions *restricted* to the dorsolateral frontal lobe are typically not associated with a severe aphasia but manifest as an impairment in verbal fluency and sometimes subtle impairment in the ability to adequately express oneself (13). Thus, Mohr et al. (14) have demonstrated that lesions restricted to Broca's area, for example, are not associated with Broca's aphasia.

PARIETAL LOBES

For the sake of convenience, the parietal lobes may be divided into three distinct regions, the *primary sensory cortices* (Brodmann areas 1–3), the *inferior parietal lobule* (Brodmann areas 39 and 40), and the *superior parietal lobule* (Brodmann areas 5 and 7).

Lesions restricted to the primary sensory cortex of the postcentral gyrus are infrequent. These lesions may be asymptomatic or may be associated with relatively minor and restricted primary sensory deficits, such as a reduction or alteration in the perception of light touch. In light of their rarity and the relatively straightforward nature of the associated deficits, these impairments are not discussed further.

Inferior Parietal Lobule

Lesions of the inferior parietal lobule, in contrast, are commonly observed in infarctions in the territory of the middle cerebral artery (MCA) in association with damage to either the frontal and/or parietal lobes, or, in the case of an embolus, the posterior portion of the superior division of the MCA.

The behavioral deficits associated with unilateral lesions of the inferior parietal lobules differ markedly as a function of the side of the lesion. Dysfunction of the left inferior parietal lobule is typically associated with a deficit in speech comprehension, often in the presence of preserved repetition (that is, transcortical sensory aphasia). Additionally, at least since Dejerine's (15) classic description over 100 years ago of alexia with agraphia, damage to the dominant inferior parietal lobule has been associated with impairments in reading and writing.

Other cognitive deficits typically associated with damage to the left inferior parietal lobule include an impairment in the ability to perform calculations and right/left confusion. When encountered in conjunction with finger agnosia and agraphia (an impairment in writing), acalculia and right/left orientation are designated *Gerstmann's syndrome,* a constellation of deficits claimed by many investigators to be associated with dysfunction of the dominant angular gyrus.

Lesions of the right inferior parietal lobule are frequently associated with two behavior deficits. The first is the neglect syndrome, a striking and disabling disorder characterized by a failure to report, orient to, or respond to salient stimuli presented in the side opposite a brain lesion that is not attributable to a primary sensory deficit (e.g., hemianopia) or weakness (16). Although observed in conjunction with lesions in a number of cortical (e.g., dorsolateral frontal, dominant inferior parietal lobule) and subcortical (e.g., thalamus) structures, the neglect syndrome is most frequently encountered in association with dysfunction of the nondominant inferior parietal lobule.

Patients with neglect may fail to groom or dress the neglected side of their body; for some patients with this syndrome, the neglect of their extremities is so severe that they fail to recognize their arms as their own; thus patients who have felt their neglected extremity with their "good" arm may complain that another person has climbed into their bed. Interestingly, the sensory and motor performance of patients with neglect may be influenced by factors such as the location with respect to their bodies where testing occurs; these patients may, for example, exhibit greater "strength" when power is assessed with the hand placed on the *ipsilesional* compared with the contralesional side of the body.

The second deficit frequently associated with lesions of the nondominant inferior parietal lobule is an impairment in the ability to understand affect, whether expressed in speech or by means of facial expressions. At least in part as a consequence of this deficit, these patients are often judged by family members and friends to be emotionally flat and indifferent.

Focal structural lesions of the bilateral inferior parietal lobules are relatively rare but are associated with dramatic behavioral deficits such as simultanagnosia, a condition in which patients "see" only one object at a time despite the fact that they have normal visual acuity and visual fields. We have recently reported a patient with this striking disorder (17).

Patient B.P.

B.P., a 67-year-old woman, had suffered a small infarct of the left inferior parietal lobe as well as a larger right inferior parietal infarct. The patient's major complaint was that her environment appeared fragmented; although she saw individual items clearly, they appeared to be isolated, and she could not discern any meaningful relationship among them. She stated, for example, that she could find her way about within her home (in which she had lived for 25 years) with her eyes closed, but she became confused with her eyes open. On one occasion, for example, she attempted to find her way to her bedroom by using a large lamp as a landmark; while walking toward the lamp, she fell over her dining room table. Although she enjoyed listening to the radio, television programs bewildered her because she could only "see" one person or object at a time and therefore could not determine who was speaking or being spoken to. She reported watching a movie in which, after hearing a heated argument, she noted to her surprise and consternation that the character she had been watching was suddenly sent reeling across the room, apparently as a consequence of a punch thrown by a character she had never seen. Although she was able to read single words effortlessly, she stopped reading because the "competing words" confused her. She was unable to write, as she was able to see only a single letter; thus, in creating a letter, she saw only the tip of the pencil and the letter under construction and "lost" the previously constructed letters.

Neurologic examination at that time revealed her to be alert and oriented. Cranial nerve examination revealed normal visual fields to confrontation and normal ocular movements; strength, reflexes, sensation, and coordination were normal. Examination of higher nervous system functions revealed no general intellectual impairment. The patient performed well on tests of abstract reasoning. She demonstrated no impairment in the production or recognition of gesture. No hemisensory neglect or extinction of auditory, tactile, or visual stimuli was noted. She exhibited a profound dressing impairment; B.P. was unable to put on a single item of clothing without assistance.

The most frequent clinical setting in which bilateral inferior parietal dysfunction is encountered is in the context of dementing illnesses such as Alzheimer's disease. Although the full spectrum of behavioral disorders observed in these patients varies widely, presumably as a function of the extent of dysfunction in other brain regions such as the temporal and frontal lobes, some patients with dementing illness appear to present with dysfunction at least relatively restricted to the inferior parietal lobules. The behavioral deficits exhibited by these patients are similar in many crucial respects to those demonstrated by patients with structural abnormalities in the same regions. The following case report illustrates the pattern of deficits typically encountered in these patients.

Patient R.C.

R.C. is a 60 year-old right-handed man who, at age 55, first noted difficulty locating tools on his cluttered workbench. At approximately the same time, he also noted difficulties in reading text, which he attributed to "getting lost" on the page. Over the ensuing 5 years, his difficulties in reading and locating objects embedded in an array slowly progressed. At the time of the evaluation reported here, for example, he stated that he could not visually locate items in the refrigerator but identified them by palpation. Over the course of the last 2 years, he began to notice difficulties recognizing some objects, particularly large ones. He experienced less trouble with small objects and, for example, routinely assisted his wife by threading her needles.

He denied tripping over or bumping into stationary objects and drove a car without incident until shortly before the time of the present evaluation. He had only recently become forgetful; he has not noted problems with names, language, or simple calculations.

Neurologic examination revealed that he was able to reach to visualized targets accurately with either hand but performed poorly, especially with the left hand, when asked to point to a target after closing his eyes.

Visual acuity was 20/25 ou with correction, and ocular movements were normal except for a modest reduction in upgaze. Visual field examination to confrontation revealed that he detected finger movements in both visual fields quickly and accurately.

Magnetic resonance imaging (MRI) revealed mild generalized atrophy; SPECT demonstrated markedly diminished perfusion of the inferior parietal and lateral occipital regions with normal perfusion of primary visual cortex. Consistent with the asymmetric visual field deficit, the perfusion defect was worse in the right hemisphere.

Superior Parietal Lobules

The association cortex of the superior parietal lobules (Brodmann areas 5 and 7) appears to be critical for integration of multiple sensory and motor inputs for the body and external space. The postero superior parietal lobule receives dense projections from the visual association cortex; experiments in monkeys suggest that this cortical region is critical for the "where" component of the visual system—that is, the representation of peri- and extrapersonal space. This contention is supported by Gordon Holmes' (18) elegant investigations of the behavioral consequences of penetrating missile injuries of the superior parietal lobules. Holmes described patients with bilateral superior parietal damage who, although able to identify and describe visually presented objects normally, were unable to reach to grasp the visualized object, a phenomenon termed *optic ataxia.* Similarly, these patients were able to identify their cots, for example, but were utterly unable to walk to them; while attempting to reach the cot, the patient would walk into chairs and even walls.

The anterior portion of the superior parietal lobule (Brodmann area 5) appears, in contrast, to represent high-level, multimodal sensory information including a representation of the body in three-dimensional space. We have observed patients with ischemic infarction restricted to Brodmann area 5 on the left who, in spite of apparently normal sensory thresholds to pain, temperature, and light touch, were unable to name from touch objects placed in the right hand. The same objects were accurately named when placed in the left hand, demonstrating that the impaired performance with the right hand was not attributable to a language deficit.

The clinical deficits associated with dysfunction of the superior parietal lobule are illustrated by the following case history.

Patient G.W.

G.W., a 63-year-old right-handed woman, was in good health until approximately 6 years prior to our evaluation, when she began to have difficulty driving. She was involved in five accidents over the course of approximately 1 year, all of which she attributed to an inability to determine the spatial relationships between her car and other cars or objects. Over the ensuing years, she experienced increasing difficulty in navigating through familiar areas such as her town and even her house; despite having clearly seen and identified objects around her, she tended to bump into things on either side of her. She also began to have difficulty sitting down in chairs and positioning herself to lie in bed. Early in the course of her illness, for example, she attempted to take her seat in a restaurant, only to miss the chair and find herself sprawled on the floor.

A second problem of which G.W. was aware was an inability to localize sounds. While crossing a street, for example, she was unable to determine if the sound of a horn honking emanated from a car to her left or her right. Similarly, it was noted that she often turned in the wrong direction when greeted by someone who was out of her line of vision.

G.W. experienced no difficulties recognizing people or objects. She also denied problems with language or memory and stated that she continued to enjoy reading, although she admitted to losing her place on the page when reading text. She experienced no difficulties in tasks such as locating a magazine on a crowded desk or eating from a tray. Despite her problems, the patient was able to continue working until approximately 18 months prior to the time of testing.

Neurologic examination performed 6 years after the onset of symptoms revealed mild rigidity of all extremities that was more pronounced on the left. No spasticity or weakness was noted, but the left arm was often held in an awkward manner, with adduction of the upper arm and flexion of the elbow, causing her left hand to rest on or below her chin. Occasional myoclonic jerks were observed, the vast majority of which involved the left arm. With eyes open, she accurately touched the examiner's finger with either hand; when instructed to touch the examiner's finger after closing her eyes, however, she appeared to grope aimlessly while stating that the finger had "disappeared." Similarly, she was unable, with eyes closed, to touch her free hand to her stationary, extended hand. She was slower with the left hand on both tasks. With eyes open or closed, she was able to point to named proximal body parts such as her elbow, chest, or knee.

Perhaps the most striking abnormality on the neurologic examination was the patient's inability to position herself in space. When instructed to lie down on her bed with her head on the pillow, she sat on the edge of the bed and, over the course of approximately 10 min, made many futile attempts (some of which caused her to almost fall off the bed) to orient her body in the desired fashion. During this time, she was consistently able to articulate her objective, point to the pillow, and provide a description of the action that would permit her to achieve that end. Unlike R.C., G.W. was not simultanagnosic. She was able to interpret complex scenes when shown a series of line drawings and pictures. She quickly and accurately identified the contents of the scenes but made occasional errors in identifying the spatial relationships between the objects or individuals in the scenes.

Magnetic resonance imaging revealed focal atrophy in the superior parietal lobules bilaterally.

TEMPORAL LOBES

Four major functional systems may be identified in the temporal lobe. The superior temporal gyrus contains the primary (Brodmann areas 41 and 42) as well as secondary (Brodmann area 22) auditory cortex, which is critical for the conscious perception and interpretation of sound. Although unilateral lesions restricted to these structures appear to produce little functional deficit, bilateral disruption of these structures may be associated with syndromes ranging from cortical deafness, a quite rare disorder characterized by the loss or substantial reduction in the ability to detect sound, to auditory agnosia and pure word deafness. Auditory agnosia is characterized by the preserved ability to detect and discriminate sounds but an impaired ability to recognize them; patients with this disorder may, for example, "hear" a telephone ringing but cannot name or indicate the meaning of the sound. Patients with pure word deafness, in contrast, recognize nonverbal sounds but are unable to understand speech. For example, we reported a patient with this disorder who, after identifying a series of nonverbal sounds correctly, responded to a verbal request by saying "I know you are talking to me, but I can't understand a word you are saying." Pure word deafness is differentiated from aphasia by the preservation of all language skills (such as naming, reading, writing, and speech production) that are not dependent on auditory input.

The second functional system mediated at least in part by the temporal lobe is language. The posterior portion of the superior temporal gyrus, or Wernicke's area, appears to be critical for the comprehension of speech. Dysfunction in this region causes a receptive or Wernicke's aphasia characterized by an inability to understand speech and the fluent production of semantically impoverished speech that typically contains distorted or contextually inappropriate words ("paraphasic errors"). It should be noted that severe Wernicke's aphasia is typically associated with lesions that extend into the inferior parietal lobule or inferiorly into the middle temporal gyrus (Brodmann area 21).

The third distinct functional system supported by the temporal lobe is memory. Since the landmark investigations by Milner and colleagues (19) of the patient H.M. in the 1950s, it has been clear that the limbic structures of the mesiobasal temporal lobe, in particular the hippocampi and surrounding cortex, are critical for memory. Since undergoing ablations of the bilateral anterior temporal lobe (including amygdala and hippocampus) for the treatment of intractable epilepsy, H.M. has exhibited a profound and utterly disabling inability to acquire new information (that is, H.M. exhibits an "anterograde amnesia"). Although able to recall information about events prior to the operations, H.M. has failed to learn such basic information as the name of present-day politicians, athletes, and celebrities; when asked the ages of his children, he provides ages appropriate to the time of the operation.

We recently evaluated a patient (R.H.) with bilateral infarctions of the mesiobasal temporal lobes whose behavior is quite similar to that of H.M. Although he possesses an IQ of 129 and performs normally on a variety of tests of facial recognition, he fails to recognize people whom he has met on approximately 40 occasions. Similarly, he cannot find his way from the front door of the building to our laboratory, although he has visited over 50 times. A self-described football fan, R.H. names Johnny Unitas (who retired in 1974) as his favorite active player and cannot name a single current player.

The fourth functional system supported by the temporal lobes is the "what" component of the visual system, for which the inferior temporal cortex is critical. In contrast to the "where" processing stream supported by the superior parietal lobule, the "what" system appears to be critical for object identification. Lesions of the bilateral inferior temporal lobe (and, occasionally, the unilateral left) may produce the clinical syndrome of "visual object agnosia," characterized by an inability to recognize visually presented objects that is not attributable to low-level visual deficits. Although there is substantial variability in this poorly defined clinical syndrome, at least some patients with this disorder may be unable to name or match to sample visually presented objects or pictures despite normal visual fields and acuity. The preserved ability to name the same objects from palpation demonstrates that the impairment is not simply attributable to language or general cognitive deficits.

More recent investigations suggest that the inferior temporal cortex may be important not only for the visual aspects of object identification but also for supporting the general body of knowledge about objects and concepts that constitute the semantic system. A number of patients with lesions of the inferior temporal cortex have been described who exhibit selective impairment in specific categories of knowledge; patients have been reported who had a relatively selective impairment in the recognition and knowledge of animals but who had preserved information on a variety of other domains, such as nonliving things. Once again, we recently evaluated a patient whose performance is relevant in this context.

Patient D.M.

D.M. is a 56-year-old right-handed professional who presented for evaluation of slowly progressive forgetfulness and difficulty reading. Although able to work full time for several years after the onset of symptoms, he frequently complained that he was "overwhelmed" by his professional responsibilities and simply could not keep up with his work.

The patient's wife and colleagues also noted a deterioration in his performance. One of the striking observations made by his wife was that he appeared to have lost knowledge about a variety of subjects; one subject about which he became increasingly confused, for example, was animals. When asked by his wife to name a squirrel running across his lawn, for example, he stated that it was "a deer, but awfully small"; additionally, when questioned about the attributes of common animals with which he had been familiar, he frequently responded incorrectly. It should be noted that in spite of his gradual loss of information (or "semantic knowledge"), D.M.'s personality and behavior remained largely unchanged. He was aware of his cognitive deficits and pursued a vigorous course of remediation, to no avail.

When examined in our laboratory, the neurologic examination was normal except for a mild dementia. D.M.'s IQ was 86, a score that certainly represents a decline from his premorbid level of function. Memory was mildly impaired. Extensive testing of visual processing demonstrated normal visual acuity and visual fields. He did, however, exhibit an impairment in the recognition of at least some types of objects. For example, D.M. was able to name line drawings of tools and furniture substantially better than he was able to name drawings of animals and kitchen utensils.

His knowledge of the world was tested in a variety of ways. On the "Pyramids and Palm Trees" test, in which the subject is shown a picture (e.g., a pyramid) and must select which one of two other pictures (e.g., palm tree or pine tree) is most closely related or associated, D.M. performed significantly worse than controls, indicating a loss of stored information.

One of the most striking aspects of his performance was a preservation of information pertaining to "abstract" compared with "concrete" words. In this context, the abstract/concrete dimension refers to the extent to which the referent of a word can be experienced by the senses; thus concrete words include apple, table, and bunion, whereas abstract words include destiny, thought, and passion. Unlike normal controls and the vast majority of patients with brain lesions, D.M. performed *better* on a variety of tasks with abstract as opposed to concrete words.

SPECT scan demonstrated decreased blood flow to the anterior portions of the inferior temporal and occipitotemproal gyri; this decrease was greater on the left than on the right.

OCCIPITAL LOBES

The occipital lobes, which include the primary and secondary visual cortex, are critical for the conscious processing of visual stimuli. Lesions of the occipital lobe typically cause a homonymous visual field deficit that may range in severity from mild (e.g., color desaturation) to a complete loss of vision in the affected portion of the visual field contralateral to the affected hemisphere. Large, bilateral lesions of the occipital lobes may cause the syndrome of "cortical blindness," in which patients fail to detect visual stimuli. Occasionally, patients with acquired blindness secondary to cortical pathology or dysfunction elsewhere in the visual system explicity deny their visual loss; this condition is termed Anton's syndrome.

Although investigations in human brains have delineated only a relatively small number of visual areas defined on cytoarchitectonic grounds (e.g., Brodmann areas 17–19), recent investigations in monkeys have identified at least 20 distinct cortical regions differing in function. Evidence consistent with such a differentiation in visual cortex in humans comes from observations of the effects of brain lesions in humans. Achromatopsia, or the acquired inability to discriminate color, for example, has been consistently observed in association with lesions of the inferior surface of the occipital lobe, in particular the lingual and fusiform gyri. Unilateral inferior occipital lesions may produce achromatopsia only in the contralateral visual field, whereas bilateral lesions produce a complete loss of ability to discriminate color. Similarly, recent PET studies have defined a lateral temporooccipital lesion that may be important for the appreciation of motion, which may be analogous to are MT in monkeys, which mediates, at least in part, the perception of movement.

As illustrated by the previous brief discussions of the behavioral consequences of brain dysfunction, progress in understanding brain-behavior relationships has been substantial. The tentative nature of the previous discussion and the presence of obvious gaps in the current knowledge base demonstrate compellingly, however, that a great deal remains to be learned. In light of the achievements of the last decade and the accelerating rate of technological advancement, we believe that functional brain imaging techniques such as SPECT will continue to provide critical insights into the functional anatomy of complex human behaviors.

REFERENCES

1. Broca P. Sur la faculté du langage articule. *Bull Soc Anthropol Paris* 1865;6:337–393.
2. Jackson H. On the affections of speech from disease of the brain. *Brain* 1878;1:304–330.
3. Bastian HC. On the various forms of loss of speech in cerebral disease. *Br Foreign Medico Surg Rev* 1869;43:470–492.
4. Wernicke C. *Des aphasische Symptomenkomplex.* Breslau: Cohn and Weigart, 1874.
5. Dennis M, Whitaker HA. Language acquisition following hemidecortication: linguistic superiority of the left over the right hemisphere. *Brain Lang* 1976;3:404–433.
6. Luria A. *The working brain.* London: Allan Lane, Penguin Press, 1973.
7. Eslinger PJ, Damasio AR. Severe disturbance of higher cognition after bilateral frontal lobe ablation: patient EVR. *Neurology* 1985;35:1731–1741.

8. Brickner RM. *The intellectual functions of the frontal lobes: study based upon observation of a man after partial bilateral frontal lobectomy.* New York: Macmillan, 1936.

9. Mesulam M-M. A cortical network for directed attention and unilateral neglect. *Ann Neurol* 1980;10:309–325.

10. Laplane D, Degos JD, Baulac M, Gray F. Bilateral infarction of the anterior cingulate gyri and of the fornices. *J Neurol Sci* 1981;51:289–300.

11. Goldman-Rakic PS. Topography of cognition: parallel distributed networks in primate association cortex. *Annu Rev Neurosci* 1988;11:137–156.

12. Ross E. The aprosodias. *Arch Neurol* 1981;38:561–569.

13. Coslett HB, Bowers D, Verfaellie M, Heilman KM. Phonological amnesia. *Arch Neurol* 1991;48:949–955.

14. Mohr JP, Pessin MS, Finkelstein S, et al. Broca aphasia: pathologic and clinical. *Neurology* 1978;28:311–324.

15. Dejerine J. Sur un cas de cecite verbale avec agraphie, suivi d'autopsie. *Mem Soc Biol* 1891;3:197–201.

16. Heilman KM, Watson RT, Valenstein E. Neglect and related disorders. In: Heilman KM, Valenstein E, eds. *Clinical neuropsychology.* New York: Oxford University Press, 1985.

17. Coslett HB, Saffran EM. Simultanagnosia: to see but not two see. *Brain* 1991;114:1082–1107.

18. Holmes G. Disturbances of vision by cerebral lesions. *Bri J Ophthalmol* 1918;2:353–384.

19. Milner B. Amnesia following operation on the temporal lobes. In: Whitty CWM, Zangwill OL, eds. *Amnesia.* London: Butterworth, 1966.

SECTION II

Clinical Disease States

Functional Cerebral SPECT and PET Imaging, Third Edition,
edited by R.L.Van Heertum and R.S. Tikofsky,
Lippincott Williams & Wilkins, New York © 2000.

CHAPTER 5

Cerebrovascular Diseases

Ronald L. Van Heertum, Alan B. Rubens, and H. Branch Coslett

Cerebral infarctions can be divided into two major groups: hemorrhagic infarctions, which make up about 25% of all infarctions, and ischemic infarctions, which constitute approximately 75%. Ischemic infarcts may, in turn, be divided into two major groups on the basis of the presumed pathophysiologic mechanism; embolic infarctions are thought to be caused by substances in the arterial circulation lodging in the lumen of the carotid, vertebral, or intracranial arteries and thereby disrupting the blood flow to structures irrigated by that vessel. Most emboli originate from intraarterial atheromatous plaque, often from bifurcation of the internal and external carotid arteries. Alternatively, emboli may originate in the heart, typically from mural thrombi or heart valve vegetations; recent investigations have also emphasized that emboli may arise in the systemic circulation and reach the brain by means of a right-to-left shunt in the heart ("paradoxical" emboli). Thrombotic infarctions, in contrast, are attributable to a reduction or obliteration of the arterial lumen caused by the accumulation of atheromatous plaque or fibrin-containing debris.

Although it is frequently difficult or even impossible to distinguish between ischemic and embolic infarctions on the basis of clinical considerations alone, most neurologists believe that the sudden onset of maximal deficit in the absence of prodromal symptoms is suggestive of an embolus.

Intracerebral hemorrhages are usually but certainly not invariably encountered in patients with hypertension. "Hypertensive" hemorrhages tend to occur deep in the brain, arising in the thalamus, basal ganglia, or internal capsule.

The clinical deficit associated with intracerebral hemorrhage usually differs from that of ischemic stroke in that, following an abrupt onset of symptoms, the patient's signs and general level of consciousness often worsen substantially over the course of hours.

PATHOPHYSIOLOGY OF STROKE

In all instances of cerebrovascular disease (CVD), there is interference with the normal flow of blood to the brain. Brain metabolism is dependent on an adequate supply of oxygenated blood. It is known that in normals there is a close linkage between blood flow and metabolism. Autoregulation and vasodilatory reserve permit minor modifications of flow to be matched to metabolic demand. However, if there is a significant alteration of blood flow to the brain, as in the case of a progressive stroke, then there is an onset of neurologic deficit due to the reduction or interruption of the blood supply to vessels subserving the regions of the brain producing the deficit. Thus, the deficit occurs because the blood flow to the brain has dropped to a point where increasing oxygen extraction can no longer sustain normal metabolic activity.

When blood flow exceeds the metabolic demand of the tissue involved, as in the case of cerebral infarction, "luxury perfusion" will often occur. This phenomenon can occur in the acute phase, 3–7 days after onset, where normal cerebrovascular autoregulation fails, or in the period 14–21 days after onset, where it is the result of capillary hyperplasia. Therefore, when imaging with hexamethylpropyleneamineoxine (HMPAO), which will frequently be confounded by luxury perfusion, it is necessary to be aware of the time the single-photon-emission computed tomography (SPECT) study is performed relative to onset of symptoms (1). This phenomenon will not be seen to the same degree on scans obtained with IMP or ethyl cisteinate dimer (ECD) (2) or with positron emission tomography (PET) scans using the ^{15}O-labeled H_2O oxygen methods (3).

R. L. Van Heertum: Department of Radiology, Columbia University College of Physicians and Surgeons, New York, New York 10032.

A. B. Rubens: Department of Neurology, University of Arizona College of Medicine, Tucson, Arizona 85724.

H. Branch Coslett: Department of Neurology, Temple University School of Medicine, Philadelphia, Pennsylvania 19140.

SPECT is of considerable clinical value in stroke because it provides a three-dimensional representation of perfusion that is neither invasive nor expensive. It delivers low doses of radiation, is widely available, and uses conventional nuclear medicine equipment. In CBV, SPECT and PET are useful in patients with a spectrum of disorders ranging from transient ischemic attacks (TIAs) (4) to completed stroke (5–9).

In acute cerebral infarction, SPECT and PET imaging demonstrates hypoperfusion in the early hours of onset, a period when computed tomography (CT) scans are usually still normal. In the acute period, used in conjunction with CT scans, SPECT is helpful in distinguishing between frank infarction, cortical diaschisis, and reversible ischemia (10,11). In patients with chronic symptoms and signs of CVD but a negative CT, a positive SPECT or PET study implicates cerebral ischemia and suggests the presence of a hemodynamically significant arterial stenosis or occlusion (12). SPECT also has a clinical application in monitoring ischemia associated with vasospasm following subarachnoid hemorrhage (13,14) and in assessing perilesional ischemia in intracerebral hemorrhage (15). This is of great importance in planning surgical management. SPECT and PET imaging therefore complements the information available from CT, magnetic resonance imaging (MRI), and cerebral angiography. By showing both brain perfusion and brain metabolism, these techniques have proven to be very useful in delineating the physiologic evolution of acute infarction and in identifying areas of viable but ischemic brain tissue surrounding chronic infarcts (16,17). The role of SPECT in planning therapy and predicting short-term prognosis in acute stroke has become more clearly defined (18,19). In addition, the role of SPECT and PET in determining prognosis and treatment in the chronic stage has also begun to show real growth (20).

FUNCTIONAL LOCALIZATION

Functional localization of strokes and of the reduction of blood flow to the cerebral hemisphere depends on which of the major arteries are involved and on the laterality of the stroke and the reduced flow.

Infarction of the Anterior Cerebral Artery (ACA)

Occlusion of the ACA produces deficits related to destruction of the medial frontoparietal area and the corpus callosum. Infarction or ischemia of the paracentral lobule results in weakness and sensory loss in the contralateral leg. There may be forced grasping and groping of the contralateral hand. When the infarction extends to the upper convexity, there may be proximal arm weakness. When the proximal deep branches supplying the anterior limb and genu of the internal capsule are involved, weakness of the contralateral face and hand are present. Urinary incontinence—and, to a lesser extent, fecal incontinence—may be found with a unilateral or bilateral stroke of the ACA. Unilateral occlusion of the left ACA results in language disturbance in which there

occurs marked reduction of spontaneous speech, sometimes to the point of muteness. Infarction of the corpus callosum may produce an interhemispheric disconnection syndrome with apraxia and agraphia of the left hand and an inability to name objects palpated with the left hand without the aid of vision. With bilateral infarction of the medial frontal lobe, there occurs a state of akinetic mutism in which there is unresponsiveness to the environment in the absence of alterations of the sensorimotor mechanism, or coma.

Infarction of the Left Middle Cerebral Artery (LMCA)

Total infarction in the territory of the LMCA produces global aphasia with right hemiparesis and right hemisensory loss, often with right hemianopia and poor conjugate gaze to the right in the acute state. Involvement of the superior division of the LMCA produces a frontocentral parietal infarct, with Broca's aphasia, hemiparesis, and apraxia of the unparalyzed left upper extremity. Broca's aphasia is characterized by relatively intact auditory comprehension, with severe reduction in the amount of grammatical complexity of speech. Involvement with the inferior division of the left middle cerebral artery produces temporal lobe infarction, with associated Wernicke's aphasia but without motor or sensory deficits. Right hemianopia—or, more commonly, a superior quadrantanopia—is sometimes found. Wernicke's aphasia is characterized by poor auditory comprehension and copious fluent speech that contains little meaning. Focal involvement of the left parietal lobe produces agraphia, alexia, and aphasia in which the ability to name objects is the major deficit.

Right Middle Cerebral Artery (RMCA)

Occlusion of the RMCA, in addition to producing left hemiparesis and hemisensory deficit, results in sensory neglect of the left visual space, difficulty in drawing and copying, left visual field deficit, and poor conjugate gaze to the right in the acute state. The area of the right hemisphere most apt to produce sensory neglect is the parietal lobe. Patients with severe sensory neglect may manifest anosognosia, a condition in which the patient denies the sensory motor deficit. Deep small lesions in the territory of the lenticulostriate arteries take the form of lacunar strokes that, because of the involvement of the internal capsule, produce varying degrees of hemiparesis of the contralateral side without major abnormalities of higher cortical function.

Posterior Cerebral Artery (PCA)

Occlusion of the left PCA results in infarction of the mesial occipital lobe and produces a right visual field defect, sometimes in association with alexia but without a concomitant writing disorder or aphasia. Involvement of the right PCA produces a left visual field defect, sometimes accompanied by posopagnosia, or the impaired ability to recognize familiar faces. Bilateral PCA lesions produce cortical blindness, often in association with severe memory disorder because of the involvement of branches of the inferior medial temporal lobe that supply the left and right hippocampi. When the penetrating branches of the PCA are involved, thalamic infarction may occur, with associated numbness or decreased sensibility of the opposite side of the body. Some patients with left thalamic strokes develop transient aphasia. Strokes may also involve the posterior fossa area, including the cerebellar hemispheres (Case 5.27).

EVALUATING CEREBROVASCULAR RESERVE

The evaluation of cerebrovascular reserve in patients with a history of transient ischemic attacks (TIA) who have negative CTs can be enhanced by using brain SPECT and PET (21–24). This can be accomplished by studying vascular reactivity using vasodilators, such as acetazolamide and inhaled carbon dioxide. A carbonic anhydrase inhibitor, acetazolamide acts to indirectly produce dilation of the cerebrovasculature by increasing CO_2 levels. In normal individuals, there is typically a uniform increase in regional cerebral blood flow (rCBF) associated with acetazolamide administration as compared to a baseline (nonacetazolamide scan). This technique will, therefore, increase the contrast between regions of adequate vascular reserve and those in which there is inadequate reserve. Regions of poor vascular reserve will not demonstrate the expected increase in rCBF associated with acetazolamide administration. In fact, postacetazolamide studies may reveal defects of reserve not evident on baseline scans. In general, it is recommended that if this procedure is being considered, the acetazolamide scan be performed first; if it is within normal range, a second baseline scan is not required. If an abnormality is found, a second study should be performed to determine if there are abnormalities present during unenhanced flow states.

REFERENCES

1. Hellman RS, Tikofsky RS. An overview of the contribution of regional cerebral blood flow studies in cerebrovascular disease: is there a role for single photon emission computed tomography? *Sem Nucl Med* 1990;20:303–324.
2. Moretti J, Defer G, Cinotti L, et al. "Luxury perfusion" with ^{99m}Tc-HMPAO and ^{123}I-IMP SPECT imaging during the subacute phase of stroke. *Eur J Nucl Med* 1990;16:17–22.
3. Marchal G, Beaudouin V, Rioux P, et al. Prolonged persistence of substantial volumes of potentially viable brain tissue after stroke: a correlative PET-CT study with voxel-based data analysis. *Stroke* 1996;27:599–606.
4. Bogousslavsky J, Delaloye-Bischof A, Regli F, Delaloye B. Prolonged hypoperfusion and early stroke after transient ischemic attack. *Stroke* 1990;21:40–46.
5. Smith FW, Donald RT, Morris AJ, et al. The study of regional cerebral blood flow in stroke patients using technetium 99m HMPAO. *Br J Radiol* 1988;61:358–361.
6. Holman BL, Hellman RS, Goldsmith SJ, et al. Biodistribution, dosimetry, and clinical evaluation of Tc-99m ethyl cysteinate dimer (ECD) in normal subjects and in patients with chronic cerebral infarction. *J Nucl Med* 1989;30:1018–1024.
7. Ell PJ, Hacknell JML, Jarrit PH, et al. A 99mTc radiotracer for the investigation of cerebral vascular disease. *Nucl Med Commun* 1985;6:437–431.
8. Duncan DB, Fink GR, Wirth M, et al. Heterogeneity of cerebral dynamics and metabolism in carotid artery disease. *J Nucl Med* 1996;37:429–432.
9. Tommasino C, Grana C, Lucignani G, et al. Regional cerebral metabolism of glucose in comatose and vegetative state patients. *J Neurosurg Anesthesiol* 1995;7:109–116.
10. Yeh S, Lui RS, Hu HH, et al. Brain SPECT imaging with 99m Tc-hexamethlpropyleneamine oxime in the early detection of cerebral infarction: comparison with transmission computed tomography. *Nucl Med Commun* 1986;7:873–878.
11. Feldmann M, Voth E, Dressler D, et al. 99m-Tc-Hexamethylpropylene amine oxime SPECT and x-ray CT in acute cerebral ischemia. *J Neurol* 1990;237:475–479.
12. Raynaud C, Rancurel G, Tzourio N, et al. SPECT analysis of recent cerebral infarction. *Stroke* 1989;20:192–204.
13. Hino A, Mizukawa N, Tenjin H, et al. Postoperative hemodynamic and metabolic changes in patients with subarachnoid hemorrhage. *Stroke* 1989;20:1504–1510.
14. Davis S, Andrews J, Lichtenstein M, et al. A single-photon emission computed tomography study of hypoperfusion after subarachnoid hemorrhage. *Stroke* 1990;21:252–259.
15. Mayer SA, Lignelli A, Fink ME, et al. Perilesional blood flow and edema formation in acute intracerebral hemorrhage: a SPECT study. *Stroke* 1998;29:1791–1798.
16. Defer G, Moretti J, Cesaro P, et al. Early and delayed SPECT using N-isopropyl p-iodoamphetamine iodine 123 in cerebral ischemia: a prognostic index for clinical recovery. *Arch Neurol* 1987;44:715–718.
17. Nakane H, Ibayashi S, Fujii K, et al. Cerebral blood flow and metabolism in patients with silent brain infarction: occult misery perfusion in the cerebral cortex. *J Neurol Neurosurg Psychiatry* 1998;65:317–321.
18. Mountz JM, Modell JG, Foster NL, et al. Prognostication of recovery following stroke using the comparison of CT and technetium-99m HMPAO SPECT. *J Nucl Med* 1990;31:61–66.
19. Hanson SK, Grotta JC, Rhoades HJ., et al. Value of single-photon emission computed tomography in acute stroke therapeutic trials. *Stroke* 1993;24:1322–1329.
20. Giubilei F, Lenzi GL, Di Piero V, et al. Predictive value of brain perfusion single-photon emission computed tomography in acute ischemic stroke. *Stroke* 1990;21:895–900.
21. Chollet F, Celsis P, Clanet M, et al. SPECT study of cerebral blood flow reactivity after acetazolamide in patients with transient ischemic attacks. *Stroke* 1989;20:458–464.
22. Burt RW, Witt RM, Cikrit DF, Carter J. Increased brain retention of Tc-99m HMPAO following acetazolamide administration. *Clin Nucl Med* 1991;16:568.
23. Burt RW, Witt RM, Cikrit DF, Reddy RV. Carotid artery disease: evaluation with acetazolamide-enhanced Tc-99m HMPAO SPECT. *Radiology* 1992;182:461–466.
24. Knop J, Thie A, Fuchs C, et al. Tc99m-HMPAO-SPECT with acetazolamide challenge to detect hemodynamic compromise in occlusive cerebrovascular disease. *Stroke* 1992;23:1733–1742.

CASE 5-1   **Clinical Diagnosis:**

Acute Infarction of the Right Middle Cerebral Artery

CONTRIBUTOR:	IMAGING DATA:	
Ronald L. Van Heertum, M.D.	**Camera:** SGE 3000 XCT	**Collimator:** Ultra-high-resolution, parallel-
Institution: St. Vincent's Hospital and	**Tracer:** ^{99m}Tc ECD	hole
Medical Center		**Dose:** 21.8 mCi

This 38-year-old man with documented sickle cell trait presented with an acute progressive left-sided weakness and a severe headache in the right temporal area. A duplex Doppler study, performed 24 hr after initial clinical presentation, revealed a thrombus in the right middle cerebral artery with extension into the distal right internal carotid artery.

The initial CT scan (Case Fig. 5.1A) showed some loss of definition in the deep gray and white matter in the right posterior frontal and anterior temporal lobes and calcification of the horizontal portion of the right middle cerebral artery. No definite mass lesion was noted.

The ethyl cisteinate dimer (ECD) SPECT, transaxial plane (Case Fig. 5.1B), revealed a large perfusion deficit in the right posterior frontal, anterior temporal, and basal ganglia regions.

A 10-day follow-up CT scan (Case Fig. 5.1C) revealed a large well-defined (hypodensity) area of infarction corresponding in size and location to the cerebral SPECT study.

Teaching Point:

Cerebral SPECT is complementary to CT and duplex Doppler in the evaluation of acute cerebral infarction.

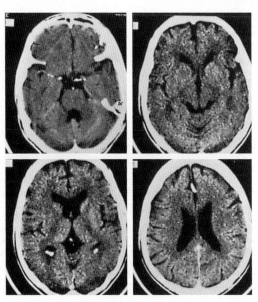

CASE FIG. 5.1A

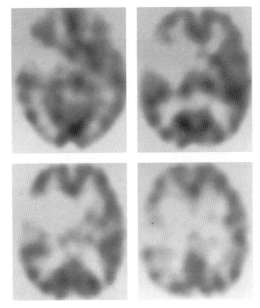

CASE FIG. 5.1B

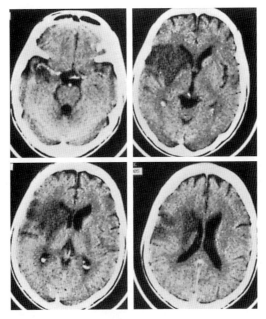

CASE FIG. 5.1C

Clinical Diagnosis:

Acute Infarction—Posterior Branch of the Left Middle Cerebral Artery

CONTRIBUTOR:	IMAGING DATA:	
Ronald L. Van Heertum, M.D.	**Camera:** GE Neurocam	**Collimator:** Ultra-high-resolution, parallel-hole
Institution: Columbia-Presbyterian Medical Center	**Tracer:** ^{99m}Tc HMPAO	**Dose:** 21.7 mCi

This 73-year-old man was admitted to the hospital for evaluation and treatment of a major depressive episode (bipolar disorder). During his hospital stay, the patient was started on a course of electroconvulsive therapy (ECT) treatments. Soon after his 11th ECT treatment, the patient was observed to be confused and was thought to have a combined receptive and expressive aphasia and a right hemiparesis. Both the aphasia and hemiparesis were noted to be transient in nature.

An initial CT scan revealed mild diffuse atrophy and was otherwise unremarkable. An HMPAO SPECT study in the coronal (Case Fig. 5.2A) and sagittal (Case Fig. 5.2B) planes revealed a wedge-shaped area of absent radiotracer activity in the posterosuperior aspect of the left parietal lobe that was felt to be compatible with an infarction in this region.

A follow-up CT scan 4 days later revealed a hypodensity in the same region as on the SPECT scan. The CT scan findings confirmed that the patient had sustained a left posterior branch occlusion, most likely secondary to a thromboembolus, possibly secondary to an atherosclerotic plaque.

Teaching Point:

In some cases, post-ECT sequelae may be difficult to distinguish from an underlying evolving stroke or ischemia. Cerebral SPECT may be very helpful in such cases, particularly when the CT or MRI study is equivocal or negative.

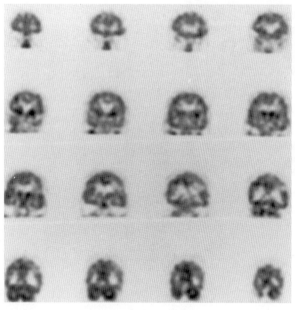

CASE FIG. 5.2A

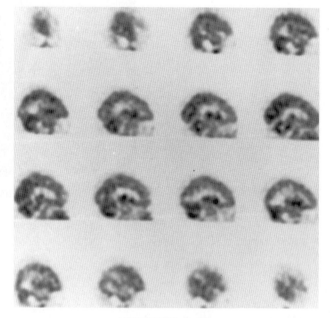

CASE FIG. 5.2B

Clinical Diagnosis:

Progressive Stroke of the Right Hemisphere

CONTRIBUTOR:	IMAGING DATA:	
Ronald L. Van Heertum, M.D.	**Camera:** GE 3000 XCT	**Collimator:** Ultra-high-resolution
Institution: St. Vincent's Hospital and Medical Center	**Tracer:** ^{99m}Tc HMPAO	**Dose:** 22.2 mCi

This 60-year-old woman with a known history of chronic hypertension and diabetes presented to the emergency room after having sustained a fall. Physical examination at that time revealed slurred speech, eyes deviated to the right, and a left hemiplegia.

An initial CT scan (Case Fig. 5.3A) revealed hypodensities in the white matter in the right hemisphere consistent with changes related to a subcortical arteriosclerotic encephalopathy. In addition, an area of infarction in the right occipital lobe was observed.

An HMPAO SPECT study (Case Fig. 5.3B) in the transaxial plane revealed focal absence of radiotracer activity in the right occipital lobe corresponding to the area of infarction noted on CT. Crossed cerebellar diaschisis with diminished radiotracer activity in the left cerebellar hemisphere was also noted. In addition, there was extensive decrease in radiotracer accumulation throughout the right cerebral hemisphere that was significantly greater than the area of abnormality noted on the CT scan. This latter finding was felt to be related to underlying carotid occlusive disease.

The patient's hospital course was relatively uneventful; however, at the time of discharge, the patient's left hemiplegia had not improved. Approximately 9 months after discharge from the hospital, the patient again presented to the emergency room. At that time, it was felt that she had sustained an extension of her prior stroke.

The CT scan (Case Fig. 5.3C) performed at the time of her second hospital admission revealed an extensive infarction involving the right occipital, temporal, parietal, and frontal lobes.

The follow-up HMPAO SPECT study (Fig. 5.3D) in the transaxial plane revealed an extensive area of absent radiotracer activity corresponding to the area of infarction noted on the CT scan.

Published with permission from Van Heertum RL, Pile-Spellman J, Miller SH, Bixon R. The Role of Brain SPECT Imaging in Cerebrovascular Disease. *Appl Radiol* 1993;22:35–44.

> ***Teaching Point:***
>
> This case is an excellent example of the potential role for cerebral SPECT in the assessment of acute stroke. The initial SPECT study revealed hypoperfusion throughout the right cerebral hemisphere, suggesting the possibility of a low hemodynamic due to occlusion of the right internal carotid artery. In such a situation, the patient is at an increased risk of developing an extension of the area of infarction if left untreated.

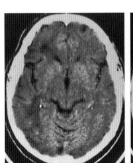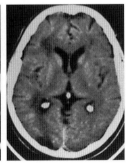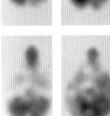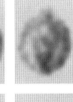

CASE FIG. 5.3A　　　　　　　　　　　**CASE FIG. 5.3B**

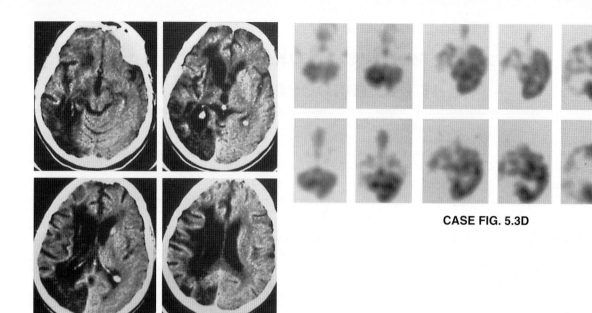

CASE FIG. 5.3C

CASE FIG. 5.3D

CASE 5-4

Clinical Diagnosis:
Massive Left Cerebrovascular Accident Secondary to Cocaine Abuse

CONTRIBUTORS:

Robert S. Hellman, M.D.,
Ronald S. Tikofsky, Ph.D.
Institution: Medical College of Wisconsin

IMAGING DATA:

Camera: GE Neurocam
Tracer: 99mTc HMPAO

Collimator: High-resolution, parallel-hole
Dose: 30 mCi

This 32-year-old man presented for evaluation 1 day after having collapsed while walking. At that time, his family reported that the patient was confused and unable to communicate or move his right side. At the time of presentation to the emergency room, a urine screen for cocaine was positive. Other risk factors, in addition to cocaine abuse, included a long-term history of smoking.

The initial CT scan (Case Fig. 5.4A) was unremarkable, with no evidence of mass effect, hemorrhage, or acute infarction.

The HMPAO SPECT study performed 1 day later (Case Fig. 5.4B) in the transaxial plane showed a large area of absent radiotracer uptake in the territory of the left middle cerebral artery, consistent with an area of infarction. A second, smaller area of absent radiotracer activity was also noted in the left posterior and superior parietal regions, suggesting an additional area of infarction. In addition, crossed cerebellar diaschisis with decreased radiotracer activity in the right cerebellar hemisphere was noted.

A follow-up HMPAO SPECT study 19 days later (Case Fig. 5.4C) in the transaxial plane revealed a dramatic increase in radiotracer accumulation at the two sites of previously noted diminished uptake, which was felt to be secondary to luxury perfusion. In addition, crossed cerebellar diaschisis was no longer evident.

A third HMPAO SPECT study performed approximately 6 months following the initial presentation (Case Fig. 5.4D) in the transaxial plane again revealed absent radiotracer activity in the left frontal, temporal, and parietal lobes along with crossed cerebellar diaschisis.

Teaching Points:

1. The HMPAO SPECT studies in this case illustrate one of the characteristic findings that may be seen in cocaine abuse, namely, cerebral infarction.

2. In addition, this case demonstrates the difficulties associated with luxury perfusion that may arise when initial studies are performed 3–5 days after ictus due to a loss of autoregulation. Similar patterns of increased radiotracer uptake may be seen with capillary hyperplasia (neovascularity) 14–21 days after ictus. When using 99mTc HMPAO, follow-up studies should be obtained at a time when luxury perfusion is not likely to be present, (i.e., 3–6 months after ictus).

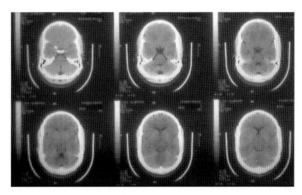

CASE FIG. 5.4A

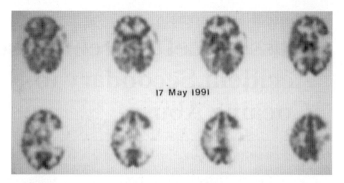

CASE FIG. 5.4B

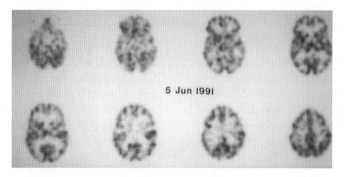

CASE FIG. 5.4C

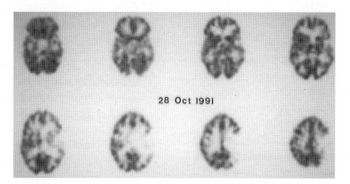

CASE FIG. 5.4D

Clinical Diagnosis:
Progressive Supranuclear Palsy

CONTRIBUTORS:	IMAGING DATA:	
Ronald L. Van Heertum, M.D.,	**PET Scanner:** Siemens XACT 47	**Attenuation Correction Method:**
Murray D. Becker, M.D.	**Tracer:** ^{18}FDG	Autoattenuation
Institution: New York Presbyterian Medical		**Dose:** 10.02 mCi
Center		

This 69-year-old man had a history of progressive supranuclear palsy, atypical Parkinson's disease, hypertension, and atrial fibrillation.

An MRI (Case Fig. 5.5A) revealed a resolving infarction of the territory of the right MCA.

Transverse-plane PET images (Case Fig. 5.5B) reveal a marked decrease in radiotracer activity in the region of the right frontal lobe and insular cortex. A slight decrease in radiotracer activity is also noted in the inferolateral aspect of the left frontal lobe in the region of encephalomalacia noted on the MRI. A marked decrease in radiotracer activity is present throughout the white matter, which is disproportionate to the size of the ventricles as seen in the MRI. This finding is indicative of diffuse white matter disease.

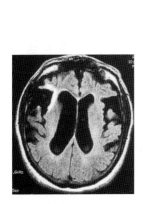

CASE FIG. 5.5A

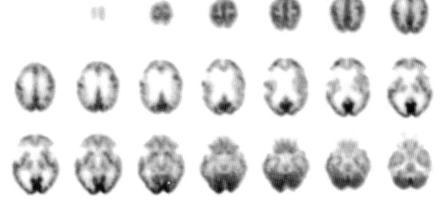

CASE FIG. 5.5B

CASE 5-6

Clinical Diagnosis:

Infarction of the Left Middle Cerebral Artery (MCA) Secondary to Embolic Disease

CONTRIBUTORS:	**IMAGING DATA:**	
Ronald S. Tikofsky, Ph.D., Roberta C. Locko, M.D. **Institution:** Columbia University, Harlem Hospital Affiliation	**PET Scanner:** Picker PRISM 3000 **Tracer:** ^{99m}Tc ECD	**Collimator:** LEUHR fan-beam **Dose:** 31.2 mCi

This 41-year-old man had an embolism of the left middle cerebral artery and subsequent right hemiplegia, sensory loss, and global aphasia.

A noncontrast CT reveals a left temporofrontal infarct in the territory of the left MCA. Old infarcts involving the left basal ganglia, anterior limb of the left internal capsule, and cerebellum are also visualized (Case Fig. 5.6A).

Transverse ECD brain SPECT images reveal an area of marked decrease of radiotracer activity in the region of the sensory motor cortex in the left hemisphere. There is also significantly reduced radiotracer activity in the left basal ganglia and absent radiotracer activity in the medial aspect of the left cerebellar hemisphere (Case Fig. 5.6B), consistent with the CT findings.

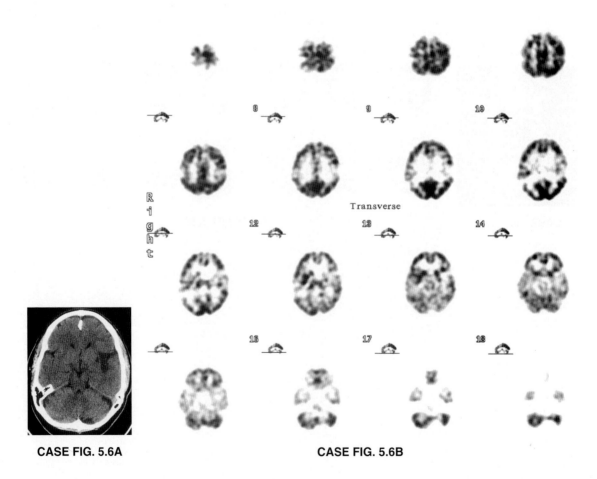

CASE FIG. 5.6A

CASE FIG. 5.6B

CASE 5-7   **Clinical Diagnosis:**

Infarction of the Left Middle Cerebral Artery

CONTRIBUTORS:	IMAGING DATA:	
James M. Mountz, M.D., Ph.D.,	**Camera:** PRISM 3000	**Collimator:** LEUHR parallel-hole
Elmer C. San Pedro, M.D.	**Tracer:** ^{99m}Tc HMPAO	**Dose:** 20 mCi
Institution: The University of Alabama at Birmingham Medical Center		

This 60-year-old man had an infarction of the left middle cerebral artery. He had neurocognitive symptoms associated with right posterior hemispheric deficits as well those resulting from the left middle cerebral artery infarct.

Case Figure 5.7 demonstrates absent radiotracer activity in the left hemisphere consistent with a left middle cerebral artery infarct. In addition, this figure illustrates cross-callosal diaschisis (*arrow*).

Teaching Points:

Cross-callosal diaschisis and diaschisis, in general, is an important component of the stroke process, which may in part help to explain mental deficits in very distant brain areas. Functional imaging with SPECT or PET may be useful in visualizing diaschisis.

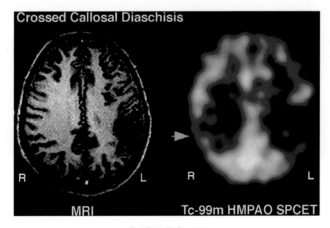

CASE FIG. 5.7

CASE 5-8　　　**Clinical Diagnosis:**

Infarction of the Left Middle Cerebral Artery (MCA)

CONTRIBUTORS:	IMAGING DATA:	
James M. Mountz, M.D., Ph.D.,	**Camera:** PRISM 3000	**Collimator:** LEUHR parallel-hole
Elmer C. San Pedro, M.D.	**Tracer:** ^{99m}Tc HMPAO/^{99m}Tc ECD/	**Dose:** 25 mCi/15 mCi/45 mCi
Institution: The University of Alabama at	^{99m}Tc HMPAO	
Birmingham Medical Center		

This 67-year-old man had an infarction of the left middle cerebral artery.

MRI (Case Fig. 5.8) reveals a 2-week-old LMCA infarction (**A,** *arrows*).

^{99m}Tc HMPAO brain SPECT scan (Case Fig. 5.8) demonstrates luxury perfusion at the site of infarction (**B,** *arrows*), a phenomenon that occurs during the subacute phase of stroke. A repeat set of SPECT scans were obtained 5 days later using a low-dose (15 mCi) ^{99m}Tc ECD protocol. These showed no perfusion in the region of the previously observed luxury perfusion (**C,** Case Fig. 5.8). On the same day, a second high-dose (45 mCi) ^{99m}Tc HMPAO scan was performed. This scan showed perfusion (**D,** Case Fig. 5.8) in the region of absent radiotracer activity demonstrated on the ECD scan.

Teaching Point:

These images demonstrate that ^{99m}Tc HMPAO much more frequently demonstrates luxury perfusion than ^{99m}Tc ECD.

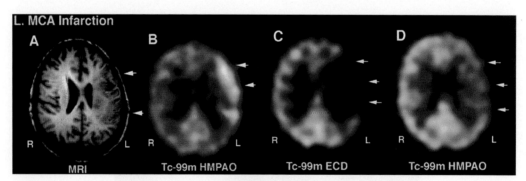

CASE FIG. 5.8

CASE 5-9

Clinical Diagnosis:

Antiphospholipid Antibody Syndrome

CONTRIBUTORS:	IMAGING DATA:	
Elmer C. San Pedro, M.D.,	**Camera:** PRISM 3000	**Collimator:** LEUHR parallel-hole
James M. Mountz, M.D., Ph.D.	**Tracer:** ^{99m}Tc HMPAO × 2	**Dose:** 25 mCi × 2
Institution: The University of Alabama at Birmingham Medical Center		

This 39-year-old woman had progressive left hemiparesis over the course of 2 weeks.

CT revealed an infarction of the RMCA (Case Fig. 5.9A).

An initial ^{99m}Tc HMPAO brain SPECT scan demonstrated "luxury perfusion" at the site of the right MCA infarction with associated decreased radiotracer activity in the right posterior region (Case Fig. 5.9B, left image). A repeat brain SPECT scan 2 weeks later revealed a region of absent perfusion in the mid-MCA territory on the right, and luxury perfusion in the posterior right MCA territory.

> **Teaching Point:**
>
> This case illustrates the various phases of luxury perfusion as demonstrated on the serial SPECT brain studies. The typical pattern is that of isoperfusion, hyperperfusion, isoperfusion, and hypoperfusion.

Image reproduced by permission from San Pedro EC, Mountz JM. CNS vasculitis in systemic lupus erythematosus complicated by antiphospholipid antibody snyndrome: temporal evaluation by repeated Tc-99m HMPAO SPECT. *Clin Nucl Med* 1998;23:709–710.

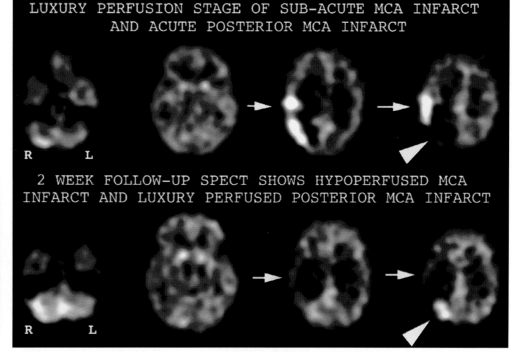

LUXURY PERFUSION STAGE OF SUB-ACUTE MCA INFARCT AND ACUTE POSTERIOR MCA INFARCT

2 WEEK FOLLOW-UP SPECT SHOWS HYPOPERFUSED MCA INFARCT AND LUXURY PERFUSED POSTERIOR MCA INFARCT

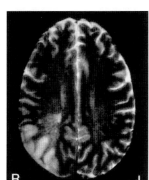

CASE FIG. 5.9A

CASE FIG. 5.9B

81

Clinical Diagnosis:

Acute Infarction of the Left Posterior Cerebral Artery

CONTRIBUTOR:	IMAGING DATA:	
Richard Rome, M.D.	**Camera:** Elscint Helix	**Collimator:** High-resolution
Institution: Huguley Memorial Medical Center	**Tracer:** [123]I IMP	**Dose:** 2.6 mCi

This 59-year-old man with a long-standing history of labile hypertension presented for evaluation following a sudden loss of vision involving the nasal and temporal fields in his right eye. The visual fields in his left eye remained intact.

A CT scan at the time of presentation was negative.

An HMPAO SPECT study (Case Fig. 5.10) in the transaxial plane revealed markedly decreased radiotracer activity in the left occipital lobe.

Teaching Point:

Cerebral SPECT can be very useful in differentiating acute infarction from other causes of acute presentation of visual field deficits. The SPECT study may be particularly helpful, particulary when CT and MRI are negative or equivocal.

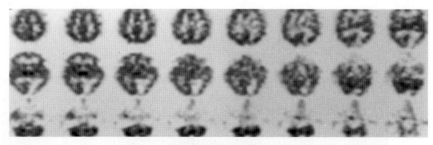

CASE FIG. 5.10

CASE 5-11

Clinical Diagnosis:
Bleed of the Left Middle Cerebral Artery

CONTRIBUTORS:	IMAGING DATA:	
Ronald S. Tikofsky, Ph.D.,	**PET Scanner:** Picker PRISM 3000	**Collimator:** LEUHR fan-beam
Roberta C. Locko, M.D.	**Tracer:** ^{99m}Tc ECD	**Dose:** 28.7 mCi
Institution: Columbia University, Harlem		
Hospital Affiliation		

This 77-year-old woman had a hemorrhage of the left middle cerebral artery, subsequent right hemiplegia, and aphasia.

An initial noncontrast CT revealed a left posterior temporal and parietooccipital hemorrhage probably extending into the left lateral ventricle. Follow-up CT showed retraction of the hemorrhage with encephalomacia (Case Fig. 5.11A).

Transverse ECD brain SPECT images reveal a large area of absent radiotracer activity in the left temporoparietal region extending deep to the thalamus and basal ganglia (Case Fig. 5.11B), consistent with the initial CT findings.

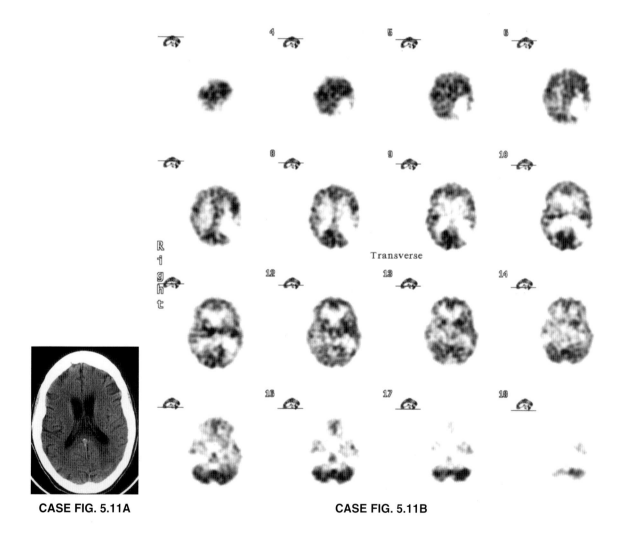

CASE FIG. 5.11A

CASE FIG. 5.11B

Clinical Diagnosis:

Infarction of the Right Anterior Cerebral Artery

CONTRIBUTORS:	IMAGING DATA:	
Robert S. Hellman, M.D.,	**Camera:** GE 400AC/T;STAR	**Collimator:** High-resolution
Ronald S. Tikofsky, Ph.D.	**Tracer:** [123]I IMP	**Dose:** 5.0 mCi
Institution: Medical College of Wisconsin		

This 69-year-old-man was referred for evaluation of progressive dementia, possibly of the Alzheimer's type.

A cerebral SPECT study (Case Fig. 5.12) in the transaxial **(A),** coronal **(B),** and sagittal **(C)** planes revealed decreased tracer uptake in the medial aspect of the right frontal lobe (*arrow*). This pattern is typical of an infarction of the anterior cerebral artery.

Teaching Point:

The pattern demonstrated in this case is quite different from the bilateral reduction of tracer uptake in the posterior temporoparietal lobe, which is typically associated with Alzheimer's disease. The pattern here is much more compatible with infarction as a cause of the patient's dementia.

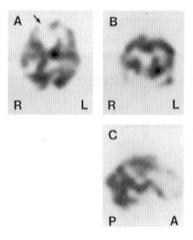

CASE FIG. 5.12

Clinical Diagnosis:

Acute Infarction of the Right Posterior Cerebral Artery

CONTRIBUTOR:	IMAGING DATA:	
Ronald L. Van Heertum, M.D.	**Camera:** GE 400 AC/T;STAR II	**Collimator:** High-resolution
Institution: Columbia-Presbyterian Medical Center	**Tracer:** ^{123}I IMP	**Dose:** 3.0 mCi

This 60-year-old woman was referred for evaluation of a single episode of occipital headache, loss of vision, and transient loss of consciousness.

The initial CT scan (Case Fig. 5.13A) revealed an osteoma projecting from the inner table of the left parietal bone. The study was otherwise unremarkable.

The cerebral SPECT study (Case Fig. 5.13B) in the transaxial **(A),** coronal **(B),** and sagittal **(C)** planes showed an area of absent tracer deposition in the right occipital lobe, with involvement of the visual cortex *(arrows.)* The adjacent posterior temporal lobe and posterior right thalamus were also involved.

A follow-up CT scan (Case Fig. 5.13C) revealed an evolving infarction of the right occipital lobe, with involvement of the right temporal lobe and thalamus corresponding to the deficit seen on the cerebral SPECT study.

The overall findings are quite typical of an acute infarction in the territory of the right posterior cerebral artery.

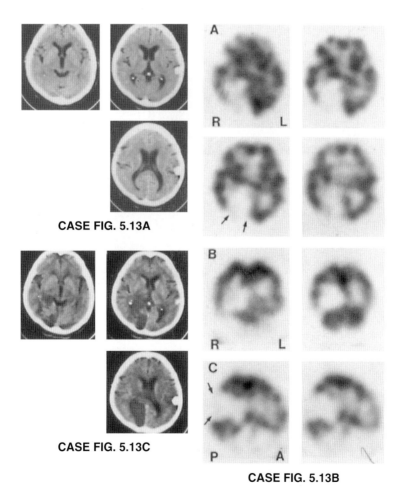

CASE FIG. 5.13A

CASE FIG. 5.13C

CASE FIG. 5.13B

85

CASE 5-14

Clinical Diagnosis:

Acute Infarction of the Right Posterior Cerebral Artery

CONTRIBUTORS:

Paul Hoffer, M.D.,
David Moon, M.D.
Institution: Yale University School of
Medicine

IMAGING DATA:

Camera: Picker PRISM 3000
Tracer: ^{99m}Tc HMPAO

Collimator: High-resolution, fan-beam
Dose: 20 mCi

This 69-year-old woman was referred for evaluation of the acute onset of a visual field deficit that developed immediately following a cerebral arteriogram.

An initial CT scan (Case Fig. 5.14A) demonstrated an area of infarction in the right posterior occipital lobe with adjacent white matter changes felt to be secondary to ischemia.

The HMPAO SPECT study (Case Fig. 5.14B) revealed absent radiotracer activity in the right occipital lobe, corresponding to the combined area of infarction and ischemia noted on CT. Inaddition, diminished radiotracer activity was noted in the right anterior temporal lobe.

Teaching Point:

Highly valuable information can be obtained by comparing the size of the deficit on SPECT with that on CT. In this case, the right occipital lobe deficit noted on the SPECT study corresponded to the combined areas of ischemia and infarction noted on CT. In addition, the SPECT study suggested that additional disease existed in the territory of the right middle cerebral artery distribution.

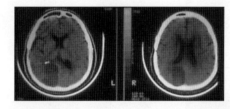

CASE FIG. 5.14A

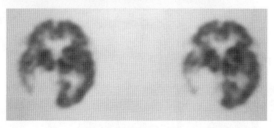

CASE FIG. 5.14B

Clinical Diagnosis:
Balint Syndrome

CONTRIBUTOR:	IMAGING DATA:	
Jean Luc Moretti, M.D.	**Camera:** GE 400AC	**Collimator:** LEAP
Institution: Hôpital Avicenne	**Tracer:** ^{123}I IMP	**Dose:** 10.0 mCi

This 77-year-old woman presented for evaluation of progressive symptoms of optic ataxia with altitudinal hemianopia and object agnosia. Physical examination revealed shrinking visual fields. The overall clinical findings were felt to be compatible with Balint's syndrome secondary to a posterior stroke.

The HMPAO SPECT study (**A** in Case Fig. 5.15) in the transaxial plane revealed bilateral decrease in radiotracer activity at 0 min post-IMP injection that remained un-changed on the follow-up SPECT study (**B** in Case Fig. 5.15), at 200 min post-IMP injection. The findings were felt to be compatible with bilateral occipital lobe infarctions.

Teaching Point:

This case and the previous four cases demonstrate the spectrum of SPECT findings in patients presenting with acute visual field abnormalities due to underlying occipital lobe lesions of a cerebrovascular etiology.

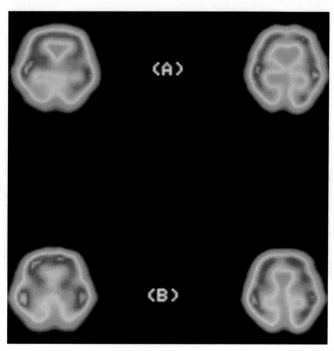

CASE FIG. 5.15

CASE 5-16　　　**Clinical Diagnosis:**

Occlusion of the Left Internal Carotid Artery

CONTRIBUTOR:	IMAGING DATA:	
Kazufumi Kimura, M.D.	**Camera:** SPECT 2000 H-40	**Collimator:** High-resolution
Institution: Osaka University Medical School	**Tracer:** ^{123}I IMP	**Dose:** 3.0 mCi

This patient had a known occlusion of the left internal carotid artery, with an infarction in the distribution of the left middle cerebral artery.

The cerebral SPECT study (Case Fig. 5.16) in the transaxial plane indicated an absence of tracer uptake throughout most of the left cerebral hemisphere. This tracer distribution pattern was consistent with an internal carotid artery occlusion.

Teaching Point:

A pattern of absent tracer activity throughout a hemisphere is generally indicative of internal carotid occlusive disease, as demonstrated in this case.

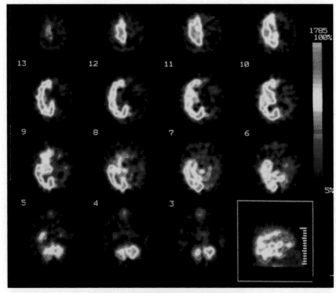

CASE FIG. 5.16

Clinical Diagnosis:
Hemodynamic Insufficiency Secondary to Nifedipine Therapy

CONTRIBUTOR:	IMAGING DATA:	
Jean Luc Moretti, M.D.	**Camera:** GE 400AC	**Collimator:** LEAP
Institution: Hôpital Avicenne	**Tracer:** ^{99m}Tc HMPAO	**Dose:** 20.0 mCi

This 77-year-old man with known arterial hypertension and gait disturbance was referred for evaluation of progressive cognitive impairment, dysarthria, and worsening of his gait disturbance. The patient's symptoms had commenced approximately 4 months previously, soon after he had been started on nifedipine.

An HMPAO SPECT study (**A** in Case Fig. 5.17) in the transaxial plane revealed a diffuse decrease in radiotracer activity in the frontal lobes as well as throughout the entire left hemisphere.

Following the SPECT study, the nifedipine treatment was stopped. Soon after discontinuing nifedipine, the patient began to show dramatic clinical improvement in his gait and reversal of his cognitive disturbances.

A follow-up HMPAO SPECT study (**B** in Case Fig. 5.17) in the transaxial plane revealed improved radiotracer activity in the frontal lobes. Some decrease is still seen in the left hemisphere, presumably due to underlying atherosclerotic disease.

Teaching Point:

Antihypertensive therapy may, on occasion, give rise to clinically significant cerebral hemodynamic insufficiency, particularly in cases with underlying clinically significant atheromatous vessels. In such cases, brain SPECT may be useful for identifying regional or more generalized changes in cerebral perfusion.

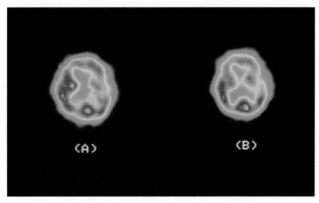

CASE FIG. 5.17

Clinical Diagnosis:
Recurrent Transient Ischemic Attacks

CONTRIBUTORS:	IMAGING DATA:	
Robert S. Hellman, M.D.,	**Camera:** GE Neurocam	**Collimator:** High-resolution
Ronald S. Tikofsky, Ph.D.	**Tracer:** ^{99m}Tc HMPAO	**Dose:** 30.4 mCi
Institution: Medical College of Wisconsin		

This 80-year-old woman was referred for evaluation of recurrent episodes of suspected transient ischemia manifested as vertigo attacks. At the time of referral, she had experienced a well-defined TIA while undergoing a cerebral arteriogram. During the episode, she developed a right hemiplegia and aphasia and became progressively more unresponsive. Her symptoms lasted for approximately 5 min, after which she slowly returned to her baseline neurologic status.

An MRA study revealed an aneurysm of the right internal carotid artery near the origin of the posterior communicating artery measuring approximately 12 mm in diameter. A cerebral arteriogram confirmed the presence of an aneurysm of the right internal carotid artery with evidence of plaque involving the origin of the right internal carotid artery. No hemodynamically significant lesion was seen on the left side; however, the study was abbreviated due to the patient developing symptoms of a TIA.

An HMPAO SPECT study (Case Fig. 5.18A) in the transaxial plane, which was performed soon after her TIA in the angiography suite, showed decreased radiotracer activity in the left temporal and posterior parietal lobes. In addition, an adjacent area of increased radiotracer activity was seen in the left anterior temporal lobe extending superior and posterior into the parietal lobe.

At 24 hr, a follow-up HMPAO SPECT study (Case Fig. 5.18B) in the transaxial plane revealed an overall improvement in radiotracer activity in the left temporal and posterior parietal lobes that correlated with the patient's improved neurologic status. A small deficit persisted in the left posterior temporal lobe.

Teaching Points:

Cerebral SPECT imaging is a highly sensitive technique for documenting regional perfusion abnormalities in patients experiencing a TIA. Perfusion deficits seen on SPECT scan will generally resolve within 24 to 48 hr following the TIA. Patients with persistent defects at 72 hr after TIA appear to be at greater risk for developing a progressive stroke and, therefore, should be evaluated for potential surgery on a more emergency basis.

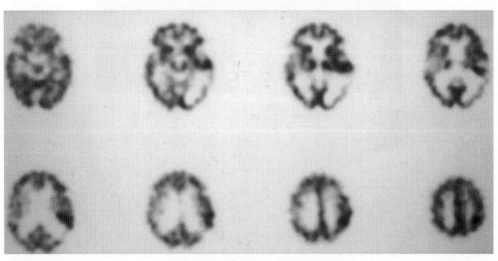

CASE FIG. 5.18A

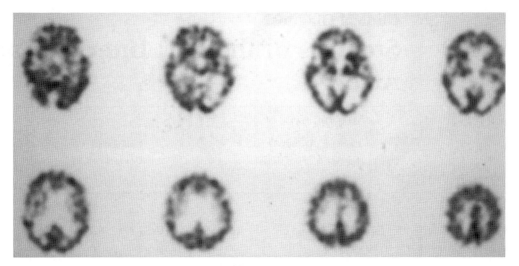

CASE FIG. 5.18B

CASE 5-19

Clinical Diagnosis:

Stenosis of the Left Internal Carotid Artery

CONTRIBUTORS:	IMAGING DATA:	
Paul Katz, M.D., Janet Lan, M.D. **Institution:** Montefiore Medical Center	**Camera:** Trionix-Triad **Tracer:** ^{99m}Tc HMPAO	**Collimator:** Ultra-high-resolution **Dose:** 20 mCi

This 70-year-old man was referred for further evaluation of monocular blindness (OS) secondary to an occlusion of the central retinal artery. The neurologic examination was otherwise within normal limits. There was no prior history of neurologic disease or symptoms; however, the patient did have a long-standing history of hypertension.

A CT scan (Case Fig. 5.19A and B) was normal. A cerebral arteriogram revealed a high-grade stenosis of the left internal carotid artery (Case Fig. 5.19C and D) with collateral flow from the right side via the anterior communicating artery.

An HMPAO SPECT (Fig. 5.19E) in the transaxial, sagittal, and coronal planes, was performed to assess the hemodynamic significance of the stenosis. The SPECT study revealed a normal symmetric pattern of radiotracer uptake indicative of an intact and adequate collateral circulation at rest.

Teaching Point:

Cerebral SPECT imaging can be a useful predictor of a competent intracranial collateral circulation pathway.

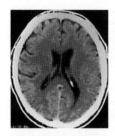 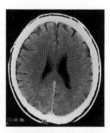

CASE FIG. 5.19A   **CASE FIG. 5.19B**

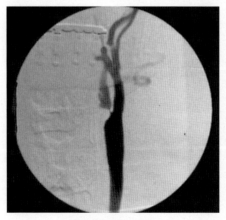 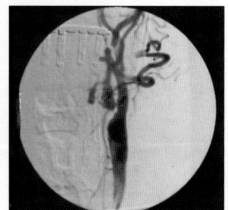

CASE FIG. 5.19C   **CASE FIG. 5.19D**

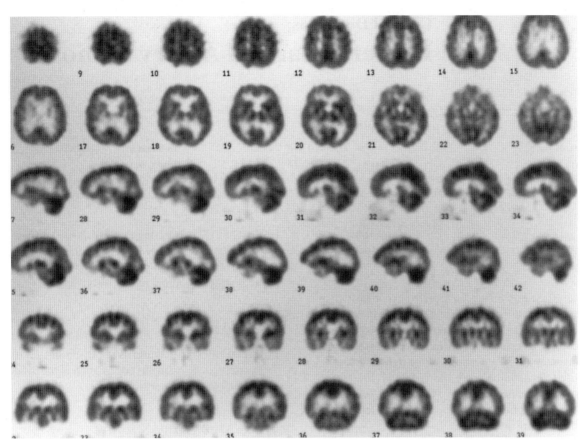

CASE FIG. 5.19E

Clinical Diagnosis:
Bilateral Carotid Artery Stenoses

CONTRIBUTORS:	IMAGING DATA:	
Paul Katz, M.D.,	**Camera:** Trionix-Triad	**Collimator:** Ultra-high-resolution
Janet Lan, M.D.	**Tracer:** ^{99m}Tc HMPAO	**Dose:** 20 mCi
Institution: Montefiore Medical Center		

This 58-year-old woman with known atherosclerotic aortoiliac disease was referred for evaluation of suspected bilateral carotid artery stenoses.

A CT scan (Case Fig. 5.20A–C) revealed hypodensities in the cortex of the left frontal lobe and the white matter of the left parietal lobe. Carotid arteriography confirmed the presence of complete occlusion of the left internal carotid artery and a moderate (70–80%) stenosis of the right internal carotid artery. In addition, there was collateral flow from the anterior communicating artery (Case Fig. 5.20D), with incomplete filling of the territories of the distal left anterior and middle cerebral arteries.

HMPAO SPECT (Case Fig. 5.20E) showed diffuse decrease radiotracer activity throughout the left hemisphere, most marked in the high parietal region, corresponding to the angiographic finding of decreased distal perfusion.

Teaching Point:

Cerebral SPECT imaging, as shown in this case, can be very useful in assessing hypoperfusion of the distal hemodynamic (watershed territory).

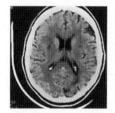 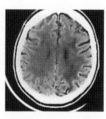 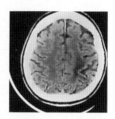

CASE FIG. 5.20A   **CASE FIG. 5.20B**   **CASE FIG. 5.20C**

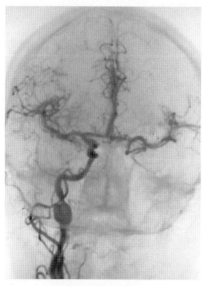

CASE FIG. 5.20D

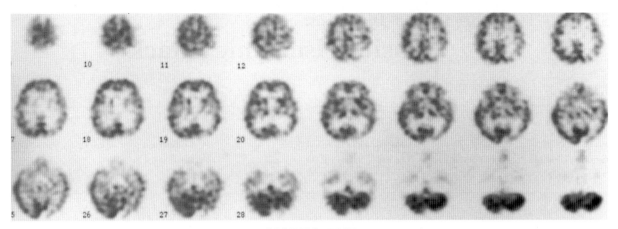

CASE FIG. 5.20E

Clinical Diagnosis:

Transient Ischemic Attack

CONTRIBUTOR:

Ronald L. Van Heertum, M.D.
Institution: Columbia-Presbyterian Medical
            Center

IMAGING DATA:

Camera: Picker PRISM 3000
Tracer: ^{99m}Tc HMPAO

Collimator: Ultra-high-resolution, fan-beam
Dose: 18.0 mCi

This 73-year-old man, with known long-standing insulin-dependent diabetes mellitus, was referred for evaluation of suspected TIAs. Specifically, the patient complained of three separate episodes of transient dizzy spells lasting approximately 30 to 40 min.

Duplex Doppler and MRI studies revealed bilateral severe (85%) stenoses of the internal carotid arteries (ICA).

An HMPAO SPECT study in the transaxial plane (Case Fig. 5.21A) and coronal plane (Case Fig. 5.21B) after intra-venous acetazolamide administration revealed diminished radiotracer activity throughout the right cerebral hemisphere consistent with a loss of cerebrovascular reserve in the region of the right ICA territory.

Teaching Point:

In cases with bilateral carotid stenoses, cerebral SPECT can be very useful for identifying which lesion is of greatest hemodynamic significance.

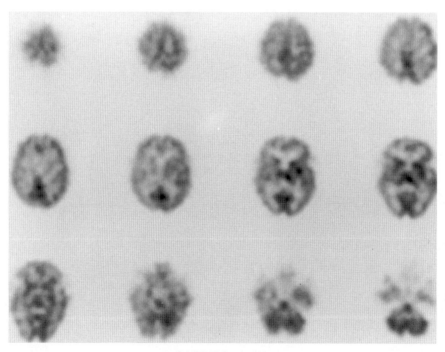

CASE FIG. 5.21A

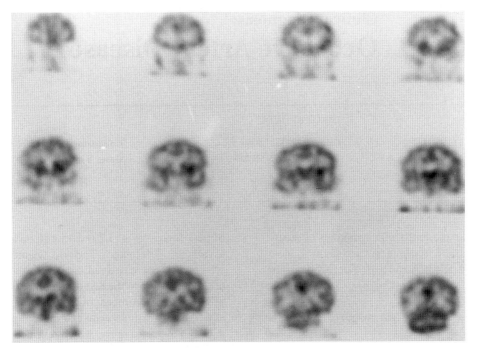

CASE FIG. 5.21B

Clinical Diagnosis:

Occlusive Artery Disease

CONTRIBUTORS:	IMAGING DATA:	
James M. Mountz, M.D., Ph.D.,	**Camera:** PRISM 3000	**Collimator:** LEUHR parallel-hole
Elmer C. San Pedro, M.D.	**Tracer:** ^{99m}Tc HMPAO	**Dose:** 8 mCi, 32 mCi
Institution: The University of Alabama at Birmingham Medical Center		

This 58-year-old man presented with symptoms of recurrent episodes of transient ischemia. He was know to have total occulsion of the left ICA and a 90% occlusion of the right ICA.

MRI revealed diffuse atrophy (right image) (Case Fig. 5.22).

HMPAO brain SPECT scanning was performed using a low-dose/high-dose protocol. The low-dose study was performed first, with 8 mCi of the tracer injected during the resting state study, followed by intravenous infusion of 1 g of acetazolamide (Diamox) and, after a 15-min delay, 32 mCi of the radiotracer. The baseline transverse-plane brain

SPECT images (Fig. 5.22) demonstrate a left-to-right asymmetry (left image). The post-Diamox brain SPECT scan reveals decreased radiotracer activity in the left ICA territory relative to the rest of the brain (Fig. 5.22, right SPECT image). A repeat of the this protocol was performed after the patient underwent external carotid–internal carotid (EC–IC) bypass surgery, which revealed no asymmetry during the Diamox state.

Teaching Point:

Acetazolamide challenge brain SPECT imaging can be very useful for assessing cerebrovascular reserve in patients with cerebral occlusive vascular disease.

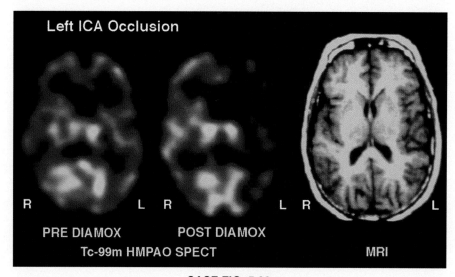

CASE FIG. 5.22

Clinical Diagnosis:
Chronic Perfusion Failure

CONTRIBUTOR:	IMAGING DATA:	
Ronald L. Van Heertum, M.D.	**PET Scanner:** Siemens XACT 47	**Attenuation Correction**
Institution: New York Presbyterian Medical Center	**Tracer:** [18]FDG	**Method:** Autoattenuation
		Dose: 9.9 mCi

This 60-year-old man had undergone a right internal carotid endarterectomy complicated by a intrasurgical stroke 3 years prior to the PET.

MRI revealed volume loss in the right cerebral hemisphere with extensive periventricular white matter changes (Fig. 5.23A).

Transverse, coronal, and sagittal plane FDG PET images (Case Fig. 5.23B,C,D) reveal a marked decrease in radiotracer activity in the central white matter of the right hemi-sphere compatible with extensive periventricular white matter disease. Focal decreased radiotracer uptake is also noted in the right posterior watershed region compatible with an area of infarction. In addition, there is generalized decreased radiotracer activity throughout the entire right cerebral hemisphere secondary to right-sided carotid occlusive disease. Associated decreased radiotracer activity is also noted in the right thalamus and basal ganglia; there is also decreased radiotracer activity in the left cerebellum, compatible with crossed cerebellar diaschisis.

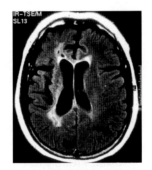

CASE FIG. 5.23A

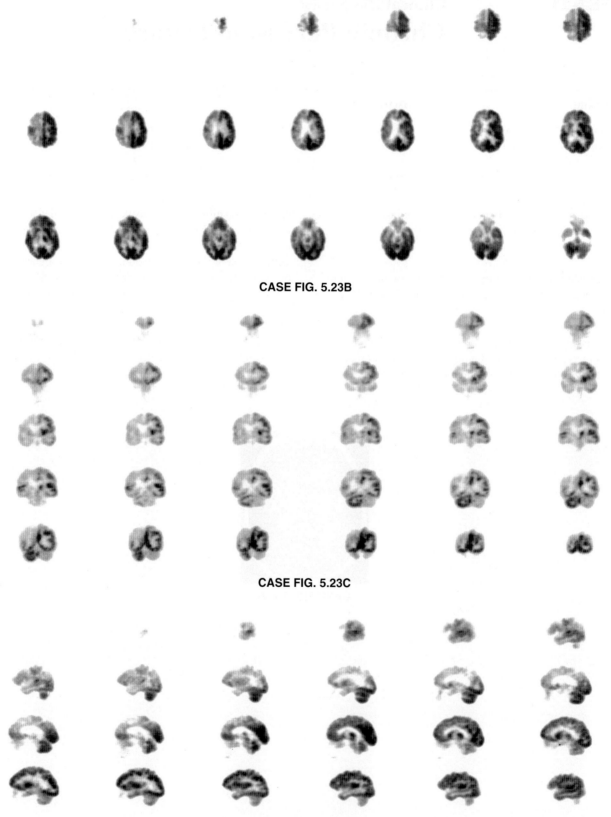

CASE FIG. 5.23B

CASE FIG. 5.23C

CASE FIG. 5.23D

Clinical Diagnosis:

Infarction in the Posterior Limb of the Internal Capsule

CONTRIBUTORS:

James M. Mountz, M.D., Ph.D.,
Elmer C. San Pedro, M.D.
Institution: The University of Alabama at
Birmingham Medical Center

IMAGING DATA:

Camera: PRISM 3000 XP
Tracer: ⁹⁹ᵐTc HMPAO

Collimator: LEUHR parallel-hole
Dose: 30mCi

This 47-year-old woman presented with sudden onset of left hemiparesis.

MRI reveals an infarction in the posterior limb of the right internal capsule and lentiform nucleus (*top left,* Case Figure 5-24).

A ⁹⁹ᵐTc HMPAO transverse-plane brain SPECT scan at the same levels as the MRI reveals an infarction in the posterior limb of the right internal capsule. The bottom row of Case Fig. 5.24 at a higher level reveals cortical diaschisis (*arrowheads*), while the MRI at this level is normal. A

Diamox (acetazolamide) brain SPECT reveals relative normalization of radiotracer activity in this cortical region.

Teaching Points:

1. This case illustrates that hypoperfusion due to distant diaschisis is evident as an indirect effect of axonal disruption and loss of normal cerebral activity that is not due to ischemia.

2. The lack of ischemia is confirmed by the Diamox brain SPECT, which reveals an increase in cerebral perfusion relative to the contralateral hemisphere.

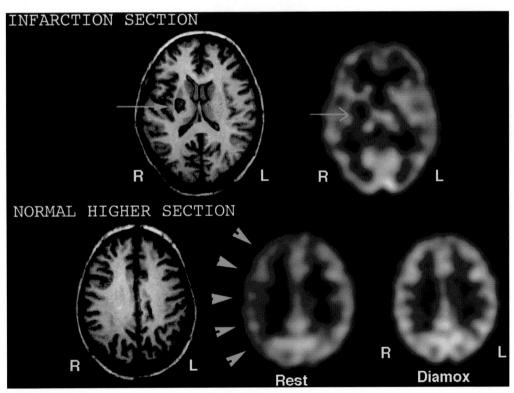

CASE FIG. 5.24

Clinical Diagnosis:

Left Thalamic Intracerebral Hemorrhage

CONTRIBUTORS:	IMAGING DATA:	
Robert S. Hellman, M.D.,	**Camera:** GE 400AC/T;STAR	**Collimator:** High-resolution
Ronald S. Tikofsky, Ph.D.	**Tracer:** ^{123}I IMP	**Dose:** 5.0 mCi
Institution: Medical College of Wisconsin		

This 45-year-old, right-handed woman had sustained a cerebrovascular accident of the left hemisphere 2 months before the cerebral SPECT study. At the time of the SPECT examination, she had a mild expressive/receptive aphasia and a moderate right hemiparesis in which the effect on the upper extremity was greater than that on the lower.

A CT scan (Case Fig. 5.25A) revealed a large hemorrhage involving the lateral aspect of the left thalamus and adjacent subcortical structures.

The cerebral SPECT study (Case Fig. 5.25B) in the transaxial plane demonstrated an absence of tracer uptake at the site of the hemorrhage (*arrow*). In addition, a larger zone of decreased tracer deposition, involving most of the left cerebral hemisphere (*arrowheads*), was observed. This findings was felt to be compatible with a larger area of associated ischemia.

Teaching Point:

This case is a good example of the complementary role of cerebral SPECT, when used in conjunction with CT and MRI, in the assessment of subcortical cerebrovascular disease.

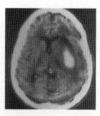

CASE FIG. 5.25A

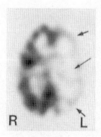 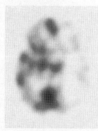 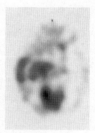

CASE FIG. 5.25B

CASE 5-26

Clinical Diagnosis:

Hypertensive Intracerebral Hemorrhage

CONTRIBUTORS:	IMAGING DATA:	
Robert S. Hellman, M.D.,	**Camera:** GE Neurocam	**Collimator:** High-resolution, parallel-hole
Ronald S. Tikofsky, Ph.D.	**Tracer:** ^{99m}Tc HMPAO	**Dose:** 30 mCi
Institution: Medical College of Wisconsin		

On the morning of admission, this 66-year-old woman, with a 30-year history of hypertension, began to experience a severe headache along with a transient syncopal episode. At the time of presentation to the hospital, the patient was noted to have a rapidly progressive left hemipheresis.

The initial CT scan (Case Fig. 5.26A) revealed a large right-sided intracerebral hematoma with extension into the right basal ganglia and associated midline shift to the left.

The HMPAO SPECT study (Case Fig. 5.26B) in the transaxial plane showed a a large deficit involving the right posterior frontal, temporal, and parietal lobes. The SPECT deficit was noted to be significantly larger than the area of hemorrhage noted on CT. In addition, decrease in left frontal radiotracer activity was noted.

A 2-month follow-up CT scan (Case Fig. 5.26C) revealed a hypodensity involving the deep right parietal and basal ganglia regions consistent with the residual of an evolving intracerebral bleed. A left basal ganglia hypodensity, secondary to a prior infarction, was also noted.

Teaching Point:

SPECT deficits associated with intracerebral hemorrhages may be significantly larger than the area of hemorrhage noted on CT scan. The larger deficit on SPECT is due to a penumbra zone surrounding the area of hemorrhage. This penumbra zone may be due to edema, selective neuronal loss, ischemia, or diaschisis.

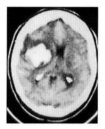

CASE FIG. 5.26A

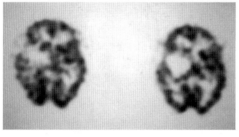

CASE FIG. 5.26B

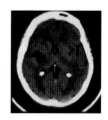

CASE FIG. 5.26C

Clinical Diagnosis:

Intracerebral Hemorrhage— Left Occipital Lobe

CONTRIBUTOR:	IMAGING DATA:	
Kazufumi Kimura, M.D.	**Camera:** SPECT 2000H-40 (Hitachi)	**Collimator:** High-resolution
Institution: Osaka University Medical School	**Tracer:** ^{123}I IMP	**Dose:** 3.0 mCi

This patient was referred for evaluation of a known intracerebral hemorrhage in the left occipital lobe.

The immediate cerebral SPECT study (Case Fig. 5.27A) in the transaxial and sagittal planes showed absent tracer deposition in the left occipital lobe (*arrows*).

The delayed study (Case Fig. 5.27B) revealed a smaller area of absent tracer deposition of tracer (*arrowhead*), suggesting the presence of a zone of ischemia surrounding the area of infarction.

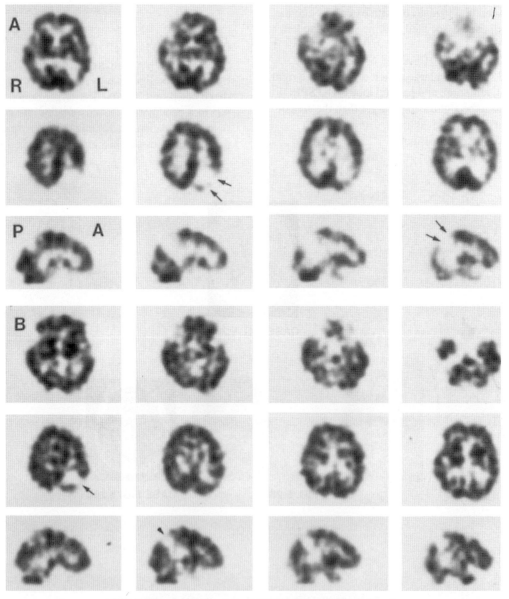

CASE FIG. 5.27A (top) **and CASE FIG. 5.27B** (bottom)

Clinical Diagnosis:
Left Putamenal Hemorrhage

CONTRIBUTORS:	IMAGING DATA:	
Ronald S. Tikofsky, Ph.D.,	**PET Scanner:** Picker PRISM 3000	**Collimator:** LEUHR fan-beam
Candido Quinones, M.D.	**Tracer:** ^{99m}Tc ECD	**Dose:** 30.1 mCi
Institution: Columbia University, Harlem		
Hospital Affiliation		

This 55-year-old woman with a history of hypertension had sustained a left putamenal hemorrhage accompanied by aphasia and right hemiparesis.

A noncontrast CT revealed a large putamenal hemorrhage (Case Fig. 5.28A).

Transverse ECD brain SPECT images reveal an area of absent tracer uptake in the left basal ganglia and thalamus (Case Fig. 5.28B). There is also a significant reduction of tracer activity in the left hemisphere, probably secondary to a disconnect (diaschisis). In addition, there is significant crossed cerebellar radiotracer activity. Temporal lobe cuts (Case Fig. 5.28C) show the effect of the hemorrhage on the medial aspects of the temporal lobe.

Teaching Points:

1. Hemorrhage to the deep structures (basal ganglia and thalamus) often produce significant perfusion deficits to the surrounding cortical regions.

2. Recognition of these perfusion deficits often provides a clearer understanding of the patient's clinical presentation.

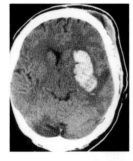

CASE FIG. 5.28A

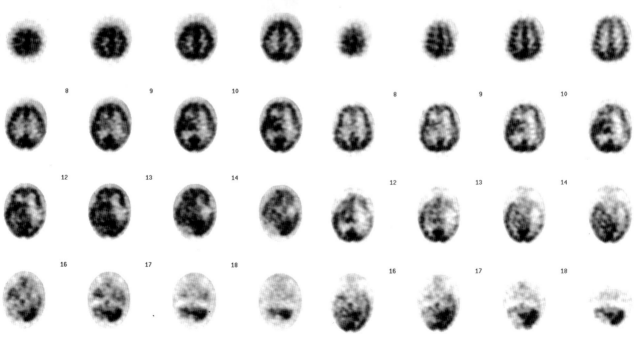

CASE FIG. 5.28B   CASE FIG. 5.28C

CASE 5-29

Clinical Diagnosis:

Subarachnoid Hemorrhage/Question of Vasospasm

CONTRIBUTORS:	IMAGING DATA:	
Rashid Fawwaz, M.D.,	**PET Scanner:** Picker PRISM 3000	**Attenuation:** LEUHR fan-beam
Karolyn R. Kerr, M.D.	**Tracer:** ^{99m}Tc ECD	**Dose:** 22 mCi
Institution: New York Presbyterian Medical Center		

This 62-year-old woman sustained a subarachnoid hemorrhage and possible vasospasm following clipping of an anterior communicating artery (ACA) aneurysm.

An CT scan (Case Fig. 5.29A) revealed a defect in both frontal lobes with fresh blood in the ventricles.

Transverse, coronal, and sagittal plane acetazolimde brain ECD SPECT images (Case Fig. 5.29B–D) were obtained 2 days postaneurysm surgery. The protocol involves the intravenous infusion of 1 g of Diamox 20 min prior to the injection of ECD, with imaging initiated 30 min post-ECD injection. ECD brain SPECT images reveal a large bilateral tracer perfusion defect in the frontal lobes (*right greater than left*) and cerebellum, consistent for the presence of vasospasm and known right-ACA aneurysm. There is also decreased global cerebral and cerebellar radiotracer activity.

Teaching Point:

Subarachnoid hemorrhage associated with intraventricular hemorrhage will be associated with moderate to severe global hypoperfusion.

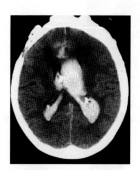

CASE FIG. 5.29A

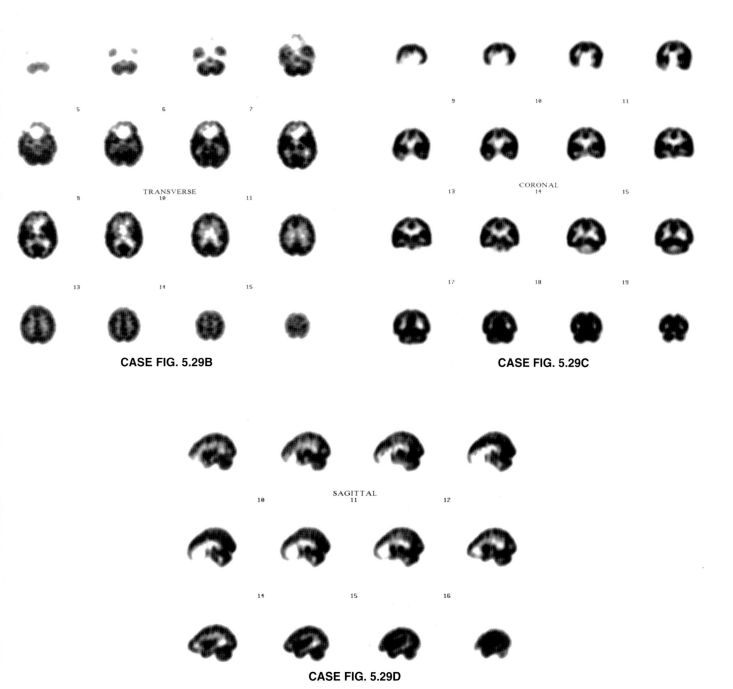

CASE FIG. 5.29B

TRANSVERSE

CASE FIG. 5.29C

CORONAL

SAGITTAL

CASE FIG. 5.29D

Clinical Diagnosis:
Subarachnoid Hemorrage

CONTRIBUTORS:

Rashid Fawwaz, M.D.,
Murray D. Becker, M.D.
Institution: New York Presbyterian Medical
Center

IMAGING DATA:

PET Scanner: Picker PRISM 3000
Tracer: ^{99m}Tc ECD

Collimator: LEUHR fan-beam
Dose: 22 mCi

This 44-year-old woman sustained a subarchnoid hemorrhage following clipping of an anterior communicating artery aneurysm.

An MRI (Case Fig. 5.30A) revealed a resolving infarction of the territory of the RMCA.

Transverse, coronal and sagittal plane acetazolimde brain ECD SPECT images (Case Fig. 5.30 B–D) were obtained 2 days post-aneurysm surgery. The protocol involves the intravenous infusion of 1 g of acetazolide 20 min prior to the injection of ECD, with imaging initiated 30 min post-ECD injection. ECD brain SPECT images reveal a large radiotracer perfusion defect in the left frontal lobe and associated decreased global cerebral and deceased radiocerebellar tracer activity.

Teaching Point:

Subarachnoid hemorrhage associated with intraventricular hemorrhage will be associated with moderate to severe global hypoperfusion.

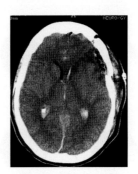

CASE FIG. 5.30A

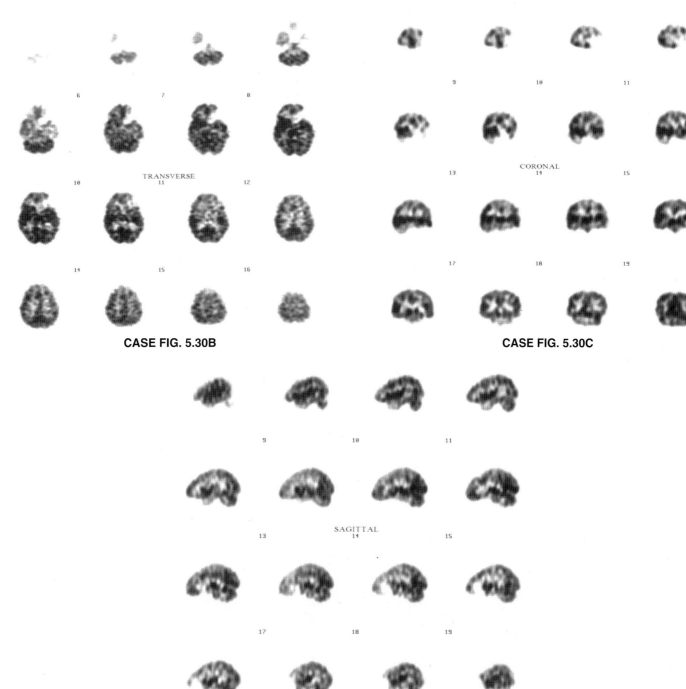

TRANSVERSE

CORONAL

CASE FIG. 5.30B

CASE FIG. 5.30C

SAGITTAL

CASE FIG. 5.30D

Clinical Diagnosis:
Vasospasm Secondary to Subarachnoid Hemorrhage

CONTRIBUTOR:	IMAGING DATA:	
David H. Lewis, M.D.	**PET Scanner:** Picker PRISM 3000	**Collimator:** High-resolution parallel-hole
Institution: Harborview Medical Center	**Tracer:** ^{99m}Tc ECD	**Dose:** 15 mCi × 2

This 39-year-old woman had a grade 4 subarachnoid hemorrhage and concomitant neurogenic cardiomyopathy.

Angiography revealed an aneurysm of the right posterior communicating artery, which was treated with endovascular coils. The right supraclinoid carotid and M-1 segment of the MCA showed severe vasospasm; this was treated with intraarterial papaverine, with significant improvement in luminal diameter of the vessels.

SPECT studies were performed before (Case Fig. 5.31) and after intraarterial papaverine infusion of the right internal carotid artery. Images show a severe perfusion defect in the posterior temporal and parietal cortex on the right in a posterior branch of the right MCA distribution. The defect had resolved on follow-up scan, after intervention, indicating restoration of blood flow to the ischemic region.

Teaching Points:

1. Brain SPECT is useful in monitoring cerebral ischemia due to cerebral vasospasm. It can aid neurosurgeons and neurologists in their management decisions regarding the need for aggressive medical, hemodynamic or interventional therapy.

2. Postintervention scans can also monitor response to therapy.

3. Unstable, critically ill patients are often difficult to assess clinically as regards new neurologic deficits. Clinical vasospasm in such patients may be underestimated because they are already quite impaired by the initial ictus.

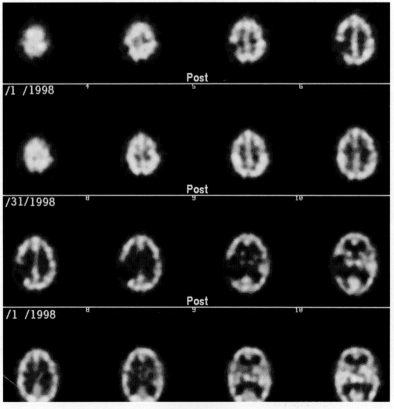

CASE FIG. 5.31

Clinical Diagnosis:

Subarachnoid Hemorrhage

CONTRIBUTOR:	IMAGING DATA:	
David H. Lewis, M.D.	**PET Scanner:** Picker PRISM 3000	**Collimator:** High-resolution parallel-hole
Institution: Harborview Medical Center	**Tracer:** ^{99m}Tc ECD	**Dose:** 25 mCi × 2

This 48-year-old woman had a grade 4 (Hunt and Hess score) subarachnoid hemorrhage caused by rupture of a posterior inferior cerebellar artery (PICA) aneurysm. The patient did not awaken following clipping of the PICA aneurysm.

A postoperative CT scan was suggestive of early right cerebellar hemisphere infarction. Angiography showed vasospasm of the vertebral and basilar arteries.

SPECT studies (Case Fig. 5.32) were performed before and a day after surgery. Transverse images reveal a new absolute perfusion defect (*arrows*) in the majority of the right cerebellar hemisphere as compared to the preoperative scan. The patient improved following decompressive occipital craniectomy to prevent brain stem herniation.

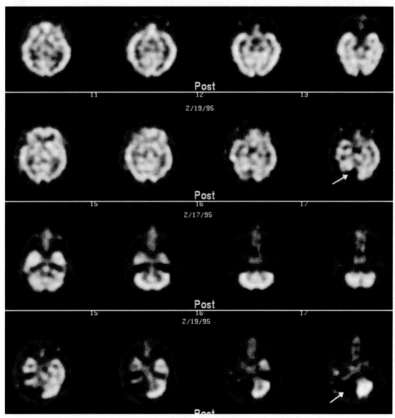

CASE FIG. 5.32

CASE 5-33

Clinical Diagnosis:
Subarachnoid Hemorrhage

CONTRIBUTOR:	IMAGING DATA:	
David H. Lewis, MD	**Scanner:** Picker PRISM 3000	**Collimator:** High-Resolution parallel hole
Institution: Harborview Medical Center	**Tracer:** ^{99m}Tc ECD	**Dose:** 25 mCi $\times$ 2

This is a 57-year-old woman who had a grade 5 subarachnoid hemorrhage (Hunt and Hess score) caused by a basilar tip aneurysm rupture with coils placed into the aneurysm.

Early signs of left cerebellar infarction were noted on CT. Angiography showed vasospasm of the vertebral arteries, and a thrombus in the left posterior cerebral artery (PCA) treated with intraarterial urokinase.

SPECT studies were performed prior to neuro-embolization of the aneurysm and again on the day after intervention (Case Fig. 5.33). Transverse ECD brain SPECT images reveal a new perfusion defect in the medial 2/3rds of the left cerebellar hemisphere. The patient subsequently expired

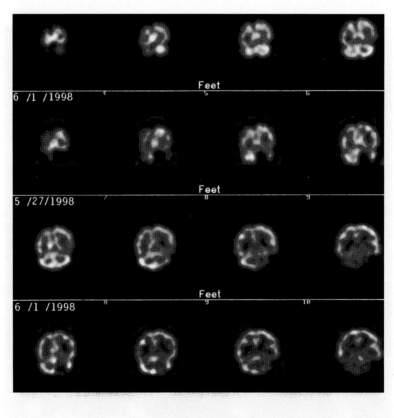

CASE FIG. 5.33

Clinical Diagnosis:
Moyamoya Disease

CONTRIBUTOR:	IMAGING DATA:	
Matthew Bloom, M.D.	**Camera:** Picker PRISM 3000	**Collimator:** Ultra-high-resolution
Institution: Columbia-Presbyterian Medical Center	**Tracer:** ^{99m}Tc HMPAO	**Dose:** 20.5 mCi

This 34-year-old woman presented for evaluation following the acute onset of a progressive left hemiplegia and dysarthria. The patient had experienced similar symptoms approximately 3 years prior to her current presentation. At that time, her symptoms were transient and were felt to be related to a TIA.

A CT scan (Case Fig. 5.34A and B) revealed a large area of infarction in the right basal ganglia and sulcal effacement in the right frontotemporal region.

A subsequent MRI scan confirmed the infarction of the right basal ganglia along with smaller areas of infarction in the right frontoparietal region. An MRA study (Case Fig. 5.34C) and a cerebral arteriogram revealed bilateral occlusions of the ICAs in a pattern compatible with moyamoya disease.

An HMPAO SPECT study (Case Fig. 5.34D) in the transaxial plane revealed a diffuse decrease in radiotracer activity throughout the right cerebral hemisphere.

A follow-up HMPAO study after intravenous acetazolamide (Case Fig. 34E) in the transaxial plane revealed a more marked decrease in radiotracer activity in the right cerebral hemisphere as well as significant decrease in tracer uptake in the left hemisphere. The overall findings are consistent with a significant bilateral loss of cerebrovascular reserve.

Teaching Point:

Acetazolamide-enhanced cerebral SPECT imaging is very useful for identifying which areas of the brain are most hemodynamically impaired, as demonstrated in this case with bilateral carotid occlusive disease.

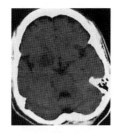 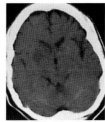

CASE FIG. 5.34A   CASE FIG. 5.34B

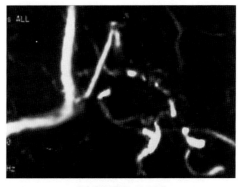

CASE FIG. 5.34C

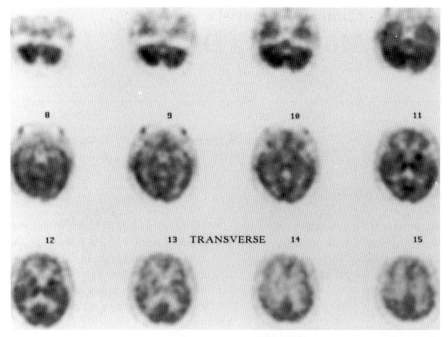

CASE FIG. 5.34D

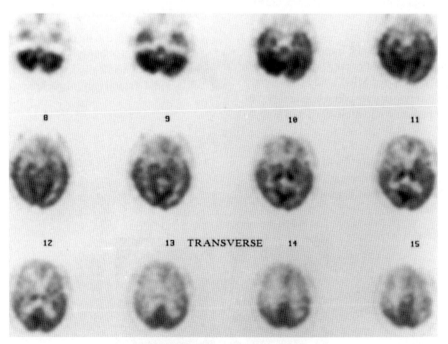

CASE FIG. 5.34E

Clinical Diagnosis:

Bilateral Moyamoya Disease and a Left Frontal Infarction

CONTRIBUTORS:

Rashid Fawwaz, M.D.,
Jeffrey Naiman, M.D.
Institution: New York Presbyterian Medical
Center

IMAGING DATA:

PET Scanner: Picker PRISM 3000
Tracer: ^{99m}Tc ECD $\times$ 2

Collimator: LEUHR fan-beam
Dose: 22 mCi, 23 mCi

This 58-year-old woman has moyamoya disease and a left frontal infarction who presented with profound cognitive and speech problems. She underwent encphalo-duro-arterio-synangiosis (EDAS) surgery, followed by improved mental status.

A postsurgical CT (Case Fig. 5.35A) revealed evidence of an old infarction of the territory of the left anterior cerebral artery and the region of surgical intervention.

Initial transverse-plane brain ECD SPECT images (Case Fig. 5.35B) were obtained prior to EDAS surgery. This image reveals a large region of near absent radioracer activity in the right frontal lobe with some associated decrease of tracer activity to the right frontal region. These findings are consistent with a diagnosis of moyamoya disease. A postoperative brain ECD SPECT scan shown in the transverse plane (Case Fig. 5.35C) reveals an overall improvement in radiotracer activity to the frontal regions bilaterally as compared with the initial ECD brain SPECT findings.

Teaching Point:

Subarachnoid hemorrhage associated with intraventricular hemorrhage will be associated with moderate to severe global hypoperfusion.

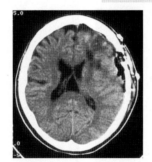

CASE FIG. 5.35A

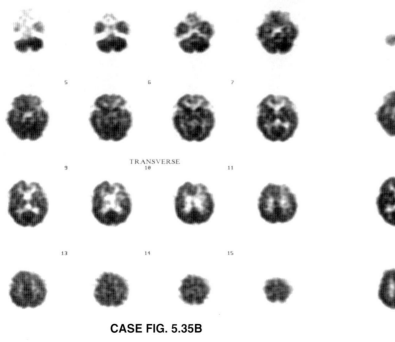

CASE FIG. 5.35B

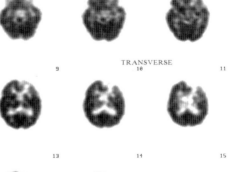

CASE FIG. 5.35C

Clinical Diagnosis:

Moyamoya Disease with Bilateral Cerebrovascular Dilatory Insufficiency

CONTRIBUTOR:	IMAGING DATA:	
David H. Lewis, M.D.	**PET Scanner:** Picker PRISM 3000	**Collimator:** High-resolution fan-beam
Institution: Harborview Medical Center	**Tracer:** 99mTc ECD	**Dose:** 25 mCi × 2

This 35-year-old woman was asymptomatic but had a family history (siblings) of moyamoya disease.

Angiography revealed severe bilateral ICA and MCA stenoses. Reconstitution of distal vessels occurred via extensive scalp and leptomeningeal collaterals. Superficial temporal arteries were small but patent. CT was normal.

99mTc ECD brain SPECT studies (Case Fig. 5.36A, B) were performed before (rows 2 and 4) and after 1 g acetazolamide (rows 1 and 2) intravenous infusion. Sagittal images (images go from right to left) reveal bilateral relative hypoperfusion of the frontal and temporal lobes, more on the left.

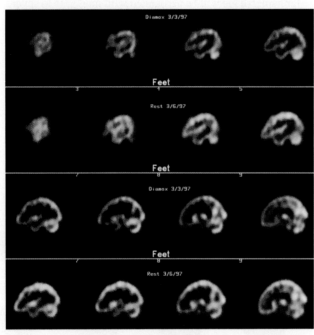

CASE FIG. 5.36A

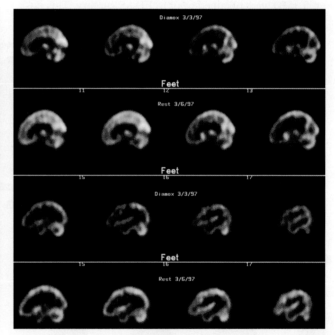

CASE FIG. 5.36B

CASE 5-37   **Clinical Diagnosis:**

Moyamoya Disease with Cerebrovascular Dilatory Insufficiency

CONTRIBUTOR:	IMAGING DATA:	
David H. Lewis, M.D.	**PET Scanner:** Picker PRISM 3000	**Collimator:** High-resolution fan-beam
Institution: Harborview Medical Center	**Tracer:** 99mTc ECD	**Dose:** 25 mCi × 2

This 39-year-old woman has progressive aphasia and episodes of hemiparesis.

Angiography revealed a stenosis of the left middle cerebral artery in a pattern consistent with moyamoya disease. CT revealed a left frontal hypodensity in a watershed territory and mild left cerebral hemispheric volume loss.

99mTc ECD brain SPECT studies were performed before and after intravenous infusion of 1 g acetazolimide. Coronal ECD brain SPECT images (Case Fig. 5.37A) reveal perfusion defects in the left temporal and superior frontal lobes in the MCA, ACA, and the watershed region of the MCA/ACA territory with Diamox that resolve at rest. These findings are consistent with left hemispheric vascular insufficiency. There is a fixed defect on the most superior aspect of the left frontal lobe that correlates with the area of known infarct. Diamox ECD SPECT in the transverse plane (Case Fig. 5.37B), rows 2 and 4, shows improvement the left hemisphere's vascular reserve after

the superior temporal artery (STA-MCA) bypass as compared to the presurgical Diamox study (rows 1 and 3). There is a fixed defect at the most superior aspect of the transverse images that correlates with the area of hypodensity on the CT scan.

Teaching Points:

1. Brain SPECT may be useful for evaluating cerebrovascular dilatory reserve in patients with occlusive and stenotic cerebrovascular diseases such as moyamoya.

2. Functional imaging may indicate areas of brain that may be at risk from ischemic episodes that are hemodynamic rather than embolic in origin.

3. The effects of bypass procedures on cerebrovascular reserve can also be assessed with brain SPECT by comparing pre- and postsurgical Diamox studies.

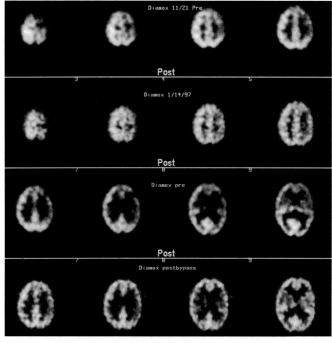

CASE FIG. 5.37A

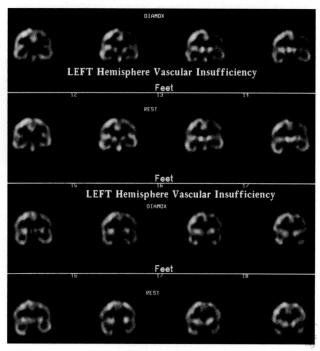

CASE FIG. 5.37B

117

Clinical Diagnosis:

Vasospasm After Clipping of a Left Posterior Communicating Artery Aneurysm

CONTRIBUTOR:	IMAGING DATA:	
David H. Lewis, M.D.	**Camera:** GE 400 AT	**Collimator:** LEAP
Institution: Harborview Medical Center	**Tracer:** ^{99m}Tc HMPAO	**Dose:** 30.0 mCi

This 46-year-old woman became progressively more lethargic 4 days following the surgical clipping of an aneurysm of the left posterior communicating artery. A CT scan at that time revealed residual subarachnoid hemorrhage.

On the day of the first SPECT study, the patient was observed to be severely obtunded. The initial HMPAO SPECT study (Case Fig. 5.38A) revealed a diffuse decrease in radiotracer activity that was more marked on the left.

A transcranial Doppler (TCD) study revealed a marked decrease in the velocity of flow bilaterally consistent with severe vasospasm in both the internal carotid and middle cerebral arteries bilaterally.

A bilateral cerebral arteriogram (Case Fig. 5.38B) confirmed the presence of severe vasospasm involving multiple segments in the right and left internal carotid (*arrows*) and middle cerebral arteries (*arrows*). Repeat bilateral cerebral arteriograms (Case Fig. 5.38C), following balloon angioplasty revealed a significant decrease in the degree of vasospasm.

Following the balloon angioplasty, the patient's clinical status rapidly improved. At the time of the follow-up SPECT study, she was alert and without evidence of focal neurologic deficits.

The follow-up HMPAO SPECT (Case Fig. 5.38D) study revealed markedly improved radiotracer uptake bilaterally.

Published with permission from Lewis DH, Eskridge JM, Newell DW et al. Brain SPECT and the effect of cerebral angioplasty in delayed ischemia due to vasospasm. *J Nucl Med* 1992;33:1789–1796.

Teaching Point:

Cerebral SPECT imaging can be extremely useful in the pre- and postoperative evaluation of subarachnoid hemorrhage. In particular, SPECT is complementary to TCD in the noninvasive assessment of patients with vasospasm.

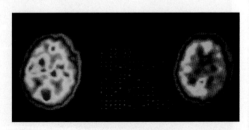

CASE FIG. 5.38A

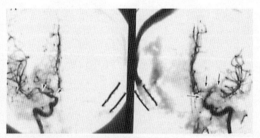

CASE FIG. 5.38B

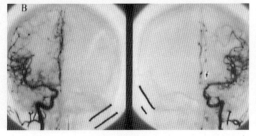

CASE FIG. 5.38C

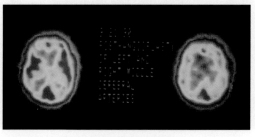

CASE FIG. 5.38D

Clinical Diagnosis:

Aneurysm of the Left (Petrosal Cavernous) Carotid Artery

CONTRIBUTOR:	IMAGING DATA:	
Ronald L. Van Heertum, M.D.	**Camera:** GE Neurocam	**Collimator:** Ultra-high-resolution
Institution: Columbia-Presbyterian Medical Center	**Tracer:** ^{99m}Tc HMPAO	**Dose:** 21.0 mCi

This 31-year-old woman, a schoolteacher, was referred for further evaluation of a left internal carotid (cavernous) artery aneurysm. The patient had previously sustained left facial bone fracture in a motor vehicle accident several years prior to her current presentation.

An MRA study revealed an aneurysm of the left internal carotid (cavernous) artery.

The patient was injected with ^{99m}Tc HMPAO at the time of a temporary balloon occlusion of the left internal carotid artery. The HMPAO SPECT study (Case Fig. 5.39) in the transaxial plane revealed an overall decrease in radiotracer uptake in the left cerebral hemisphere. In addition, a focal area of decreased radiotracer activity was noted in the right frontal cortex.

Teaching Point:

Performing cerebral SPECT at the time of temporary balloon occlusion of the internal carotid artery can be useful for determining whether patients will be able to tolerate permanent carotid artery occlusion. In this particular case, the study demonstrated decreased radiotracer activity in the left cerebral hemisphere after balloon occlusion, indicative of an inadequate collateral circulation supply from the right side. As a result, a decision was made to change the clinical management from carotid occlusion to obliteration of the aneurysm with GDC coils. This decision was based on the SPECT results coupled with the observation of a very small ophthalmic collateral on a subsequent cerebral arteriogram.

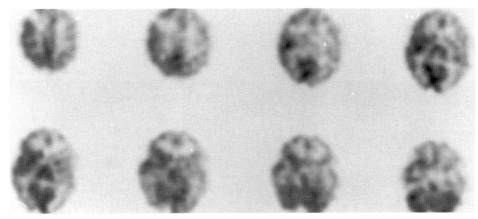

CASE FIG. 5.39

Clinical Diagnosis:

Aneurysm of the Right Cavernous Carotid Artery

CONTRIBUTOR:	IMAGING DATA:	
Frederick J. Bonte, M.D.	**Camera:** Toshiba GCA 9300	**Collimator:** High-resolution, fan-beam
Institution: University of Texas-Southwestern Medical Center	**Tracer:** ^{99m}Tc HMPAO	**Dose:** 21.0 mCi

This 59-year-old woman was referred for evaluation of double vision associated with right third-and fourth-nerve palsies.

CT and MRI were both reported to be negative. However, a cerebral arteriogram showed a small aneurysm of the right cavernous carotid artery. After angiography, the patient was observed to be lethargic, aphasic, and hemiparietic on the right side, but she recovered uneventfully.

An HMPAO SPECT study (**A** in (Case Fig. 5.40, *upper row*) revealed slight reduction of radiotracer uptake in the distribution of the right internal carotid artery.

A follow-up HMPAO SPECT study (**B** in Case Fig. 5.40, *lower row*) performed at the time of a test balloon occlusion of the right internal carotid revealed a marked decrease in radiotracer activity throughout the territory of the right internal carotid artery with a concomitant decrease in radiotracer activity in the left cerebellar hemisphere, consistent

with crossed cerebellar diaschisis, which was thought to have occurred immediately following the cessation of input from the corticopontine cerebellar tracts.

At the time of the test balloon occlusion, the patient lost consciousness for approximately 15 sec, while the balloon was inflated.

Teaching Points:

1. Crossed cerebellar diaschisis can be observed immediately following the loss of an afferent stimulus (deafferentiation).

2. Cerebral SPECT in conjunction with temporary balloon occlusion of the carotid artery is a very useful technique for accurately assessing the integrity of the collateral cerebral circulation.

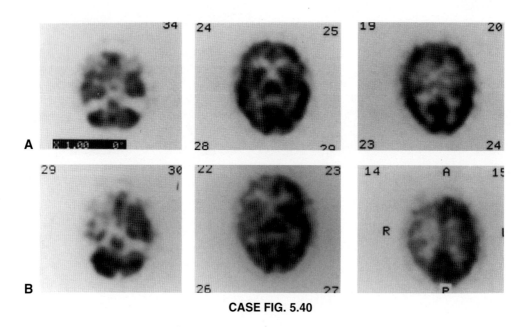

CASE FIG. 5.40

CASE 5-41　　　**Clinical Diagnosis:**

Infarction of the Left Cerebellar Hemisphere

CONTRIBUTOR:	IMAGING DATA:	
William L. Ashburn, M.D.	**Camera:** Elscint APEX 409AG-ECT; APEX	**Collimator:** LEAP
Institution: UCSD Medical Center	009 Precursor	**Dose:** 3.0 mCi
	Tracer: ^{123}I IMP	

This 57-year-old man was referred for evaluation of dizziness of 6 months' duration.

A CT scan was negative.

A cerebral SPECT study (Case Fig. 5.41) in the transaxial plane showed a marked decrease in tracer deposition in the left cerebellar hemisphere (*arrows*) that was compatible with ischemia or infarction in that region.

A follow-up cerebral arteriogram revealed absent flow to the left cerebellar hemisphere due to complete occlusion of the left vertebral artery and 60% stenosis of both ICAs.

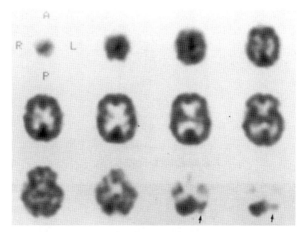

CASE FIG. 5.41

CASE 5-42　　　　**Clinical Diagnosis:**
Infarction of the Left Basal Ganglia

CONTRIBUTOR:	IMAGING DATA:	
Thomas C. Hill, M.D.	**Camera:** Strichman SME-810	**Collimator:** High-resolution
Institution: New England Deaconess Hospital	**Tracer:** [123]I IMP	**Dose:** 3.0 mCi

This patient was referred for evaluation of an acute left cerebrovascular accident.

A CT scan (Case Fig. 5.42A), performed without intravenous contrast, showed an oval low-density area involving the left basal ganglia and internal capsule.

A cerebral SPECT study (Case Fig. 5.42B) in the transaxial plane showed that tracer deposition was absent in the left caudate nucleus (*arrow*). In addition, there was a slight decrease of tracer activity in the adjacent cortical gray matter (*arrowhead*). The overall findings were consistent with a left lacunar infarction and a concomitant decrease in the adjacent cerebral cortex was felt to be secondary to cortical diaschisis.

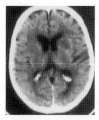

CASE FIG. 5.42A

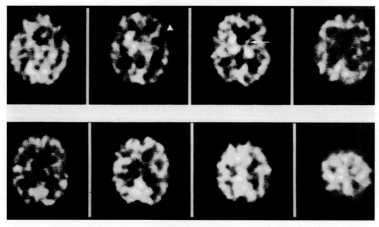

CASE FIG. 5.42B

CASE 5-43

Clinical Diagnosis:

Acute Left Hemispheric Stroke Before and After Tissue Plasminogen Activator

CONTRIBUTORS:	IMAGING DATA:	
Paul Hoffer, M.D.	**Camera:** Picker PRISM 3000	**Collimator:** High-resolution, fan-beam
David Moon, M.D.	**Tracer:** ^{99m}Tc HMPAO	**Dose:** 20 mCi
Institution: Yale University of Medicine		

This 35-year-old man presented for evaluation immediately following the acute onset of right-sided weakness. An initial CT scan at the time of presentation was negative for acute hemorrhage or infarction.

The initial HMPAO SPECT study, performed on the same day as the CT scan (Case Fig. 5.43A) in the transaxial plane, revealed a significant decrease in radiotracer activity throughout much of the left hemisphere, corresponding to the territory of the left middle cerebral artery. In addition, crossed cerebellar diaschisis, with diminished radiotracer activity in the right cerebellar hemisphere, was noted. Immediately following this study, tissue plasminogen activator was administered to the patient.

A follow-up HMPAO SPECT study performed 2 days later (Case Fig. 5.43B) revealed an overall improvement in the radiotracer uptake throughout the left hemisphere. Focal increased activity, felt to be secondary to luxury perfusion, was observed in the left frontal temporal region. In addition, a focal deficit was observed in the left lenticular nucleus and adjacent left insular cortex, corresponding to a residual area of infarction noted on a follow-up MRI exam.

Teaching Point:

This case illustrates the potential value of cerebral SPECT in the assessment of a variety of therapeutic interventions in patients with acute stroke.

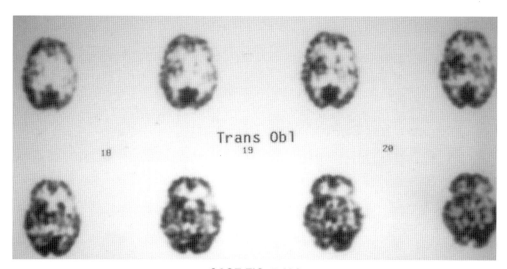

CASE FIG. 5.43A

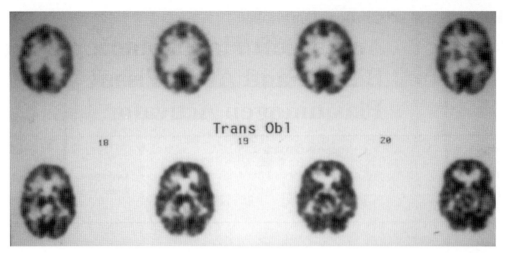

CASE FIG. 5.43B

CASE 5-44

CONTRIBUTORS:

Jacques Dacourt, M.D., Ph.D.

Ismael Mena, M.D.

Institution: University of Nice (France) and

Harbor-UCLA Medical Center

Clinical Diagnosis:
Luxury Perfusion Following a Migraine Attack

IMAGING DATA:

Camera: GE 400T   **Collimator:** LEAP

Tracer: ^{99m}Tc HMPAO   **Dose:** 20.0 mCi

This 24-year-old woman was referred for evaluation of a migraine headache with an associated left hemiplegia. At the time of evaluation, the patient's migraine headache had resolved but the patient remained hemiplegic.

MRI examination (Case Fig. 5.44, *right*), was normal.

An HMPAO SPECT study (Case Fig. 5.44, *left*) revealed an intense increase in radiotracer uptake throughout the right hemisphere, which was most marked in the frontal lobe. Overall, the SPECT pattern was felt to be most compatible with luxury perfusion following a migraine crisis.

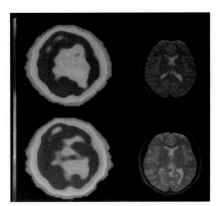

CASE FIG. 5.44

125

Clinical Diagnosis:
Progressive Aphasia

CONTRIBUTORS:

James M. Mountz, M.D., Ph.D.,
Elmer C. San Pedro, M.D.
Institution: The University of Alabama at
                Birmingham Medical Center

IMAGING DATA:

Camera: PRISM 3000 XP
Tracer: ^{99m}Tc HMPAO

Collimator: LEUHR parallel-hole
Dose: 30 mCi

Three elderly patients where diagnosed with primary progressive aphasia by standard cognitive and linguistic examinations.

Case Figure 5.45 demonstrates anterior temporal perfusion deficits as opposed to posterior deficits, seen in

Alzheimer's disease. Deficits can involve the right hemisphere (*left figure*), both hemispheres (*middle figure*), or left hemisphere (*right figure*).

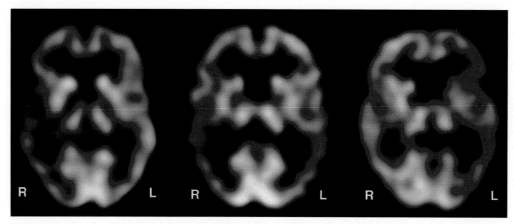

CASE FIG. 5.45

Functional Cerebral SPECT and PET Imaging, Third Edition,
edited by R.L.Van Heertum and R.S. Tikofsky,
Lippincott Williams & Wilkins, New York © 2000.

CHAPTER 6

Dementia

Ronald L. Van Heertum, Ronald S. Tikofsky, and Alan B. Rubens

There has been a rapid increase in the utility of single-photon-emission computed tomography (SPECT) and positron-emission tomography (PET) scanning in the diagnosis and understanding of dementia and its underlying disordered brain function (1–4). PET imaging has demonstrated characteristic alterations in cerebral perfusion and metabolism in Alzheimer's disease.

SPECT imaging, which is still more readily available than PET, demonstrates the same patterns of perfusion and metabolic alteration as those seen with PET (5,6). It distinguishes Alzheimer's disease from other types of dementia, such as multi-infarct dementia, hydrocephalus, progressive supranuclear palsy, and various frontal lobe dementias (7–13). It also helps differentiate Alzheimer's disease from the cognitive impairments associated with depression.

In PET and SPECT images, the pattern of abnormality generally associated with the presence of dementia is that of reduced tracer uptake. However, in certain types of dementia—i.e., multi-infarct dementia—regions of absent tracer uptake are observed. The distribution of decreased uptake provides information relative to the severity of disease and most prevelant type of cognitive impairment seen on clinical and neuropsychological examination (14–19). A characteristic pattern of alterations in regional cerebral perfusion and glucose metabolism is observed in dementia of the Alzheimer's type. This pattern is not seen in other forms of dementia with the exception of diffuse Lewy body disease, Lewy body variant disease, and Parkinson's disease. The salient features of this pattern include relatively preserved blood flow and metabolism to the subcortical gray matter, sensorimotor and

occipital cortices, and cerebellum. There is significant reduction of cerebral perfusion and metabolism to the temporal and posterior parietal lobes and in more advanced cases, the frontal lobes. Wide variations in the perfusion/metabolic patterns of PET and SPECT imaging studies of Alzheimer's disease patients are seen; these patterns often correlate significantly with the patient's neurobehavioral symptoms.

In younger patients and also early in the course of the disease, patients may manifest unilateral or more asymmetric radiotracer distribution patterns on both PET and SPECT. In such cases, there tends to be a good correlation between the asymmetry seen on PET and SPECT and the cognitive deficits noted on neuropsychological testing.

The second most common type of dementia is the ischemic vascular type, which may be due to multiple infarcts, diffuse small vessel disease, or infarcts in strategic locations such as the medial thalamic nucleus (20). MID is characterized by a random, multifocal distribution of infarcts and abnormalities associated with specific vascular territories. MID may also be characterized by unilateral hemispheric reductions of tracer uptake.

The third major form of dementia, which is being recognized with increasing frequency, is the entity of mixed dementia. Although there is a wide spread spectrum of possible causes for mixed dementia, the most common is combined Alzheimer's and vascular disease.

There are other types of dementia: specifically, a broad spectrum of neurodegenerative disorders some of which are associated with movement disorders such as Parkinson's disease. Other causes include alcohol or other forms of substance abuse, frontal temporal lobe dementia, hydrocephalus, and infectious causes such as AIDS-related dementia. Both PET and SPECT (21,22) imaging are helpful in the differentiation of the pathophysiologic patterns seen in the various forms of dementia. They are useful in establishing physiologic subgroups that correlate with the different clinical presentations seen in patients with Alzheimer's and other diseases.

R. L. Van Heertum: Department of Radiology, Columbia University College of Physicians and Surgeons, New York, New York 10032.

R. S. Tikofsky: Department of Radiology, Columbia University College of Physicians and Surgeons, Harlem Hospital Center, New York, New York 10032.

A. B. Rubens: Department of Neurology, University of Arizona College of Medicine, Tucson, Arizona 85725.

PET imaging, with its superior resolving power and radiopharmaceuticals as compared to SPECT, still has some advantages for the early detection of dementia. However, the general availability, relative simplicity, and affordability of SPECT make it a valuable technique in the assessment of patients with dementia. SPECT will continue to play a significant role in the early diagnosis and longitudinal study of patients with dementia.

At present, reports in the literature indicate that PET and SPECT (23) are reliable tools for differentiating persons with moderate to severe dementia from normals. In addition, the scans reflect the type and severity of the cognitive deterioration associated with the disease. Even with the newer SPECT instruments, it is still unclear whether the minimal changes in regional cerebral blood flow (rCBF), which may be associated with early onset of dementing disease, can be detected. PET however, has been shown to be reliable in this setting. The development of methods for assessing tracer-receptor activity, cognitive activation, and quantitative SPECT should help in this differentiation. In spite of any current concerns, SPECT is still a valuable diagnostic tool for the initial evaluation of persons with suspected dementia. At present, it also appears that quantitative SPECT has the potential to assess the effects of pharmacologic treatments on dementia patients. Recent developments using tracer imaging techniques are proving useful in clarifying clinical distinctions among a number of neurodegenerative disorders. Patients with movement disorders such as Parkinson's and Huntington's disease often have a clinical presentation that includes a component of cognitive dysfunction. In some cases, these patients manifest some evidence of dementia. Tracer imaging can contribute to the early detection of these disorders in this patient population. These new imaging applications are also useful in the study of dementia. For example, in using ^{123}I iomazenil SPECT (24), there was a significant change in estimated bensodiazepine receptors volume distribution (BZR Vd) in all but the occipital cortex in a small sample of probable Alzheimer's disease patients as compared to normals. In another study, SPECT ^{123}I iomazenil imaging 3 hr postinjection appeared to demonstrate decreased perfusion more clearly than imaging with ^{99m}Tc HMPAO (25). Similarly, there is a good correlation between ^{123}I iomazenil imaging and performance on the Mini-Mental State Examination (26). Developing clinical research supports the concept that receptor imaging with BZR is an excellent diagnostic imaging tool for the detection of brain changes associated with Alzheimer's disease. This approach may, in fact, be more sensitive than traditional SPECT imaging techniques for demonstrating the pathophysiologic aspects of the disease that are most closely associated with the severity of cognitive decline.

REFERENCES

1. Tikofsky RS, Hellman RS, Parks RW. Single photon emission computed tomography and applications to dementia. In: Parks RW, Zec RF, Wilson RS eds. *Neuropsychology of Alzheimer's disease and other dementias*. New York: Oxford University Press, 1993:489–510.

2. Mielke R, Pietrzyk U, Jacobs A, et al. HMPAO SPET and FDG PET in Alzheimer's disease and vascular dementia: comparison of perfusion and metabolic pattern. *Eur J Nucl Med* 1994;21:1052–1060.

3. Jagust WJ, Eberling JL, Reed BR, et al. Clinical studies of cerebral blood flow in Alzheimer's disease. *Ann NY Acad Sci* 1997;826:254–262.

4. Jobst KA, Barnetson LP, Shepstone BJ. Accurate prediction of histologically confirmed Alzheimer's disease and the differential diagnosis of dementia: the use of NINCDS-ADRA and DSM-III-R criteria, SPECT, x-ray CT, and Apo E4 in medial temporal lobe dementias. Oxford Project to Investigate Memory and Aging. *Int Psychogeriatr* 1998;10:271–302.

5. Johnson KA, Holman BL, Rosen J, et al. Iofetamine I-123 single photon emission computed tomography is accurate in the diagnosis of Alzheimer's disease. *Arch Intern Med* 1990;150:752–756.

6. Holman BL, Johnson KA, Gerada B, et al. The scintigraphic appearance of of Alzheimer's disease: a prospective study using technetium-99m-HMPAO SPECT. *J Nucl Med* 1992;33:181–185.

7. Neary D, Snowden JS, Shields RA, et al. Single photon emission tomography using ^{99m}Tc-HM-PAO in the investigation of dementia. *J Neurol Neurosurg Psychiatry* 1987;50:1101–1109.

8. Jagust WJ, Budinger TF, Reed BR. The diagnosis of dementia with single photon emission computed tomography. *Arch Neurol* 1987;44:258–262.

9. Antuono PG, Tikofsky RS, Hellman RS, Saxena VK. Single photon emission computed tomography (SPECT) in the evaluation of the dementias. *Mind* 1990;4:6–8.

10. Bartolini A, Gasparetto B, Loeb C. Assessment of SPECT features in the differential diagnosis between degenerative and multiinfarct dementia. In: Battistin L, Gerstenbrand F, eds. *Aging and dementia: new trends in diagnosis and therapy*. New York: Wiley-Liss, 1990;441–438.

11. Cohen, MB, Graham LS, Lake R, et al. Diagnosis of Alzheimer's disease and multiple infarct dementia by tomographic imaging of iodine-123 IMP. *J Nucl Med* 1986;27:769–774.

12. Masdeu JC, Yudd A, Van Heertum RL, et al. Single-photon emission computed tomography in human immunodeficiency virus encephalopathy: a preliminary report. *J Nucl Med* 1991;32:1471–1475.

13. Read SL, Miller DL, Mena I, et al. SPECT in dementia: clinical and pathological correlation. *J Am Geriatr Soc* 1995;43:1243–1247.

14. Goldenberg G, Podreka I, Suess E, Deecke L. The cerebral localization of neuropsychological impairment in Alzheimer's disease: a SPECT study. *J Neurol* 1989;236:131–138.

15. Hellman RS, Antuono PG, Tikofsky RS, et al. Correlation between regional reductions in cerebral blood flow (SPECT/IMP) and neuropsychological test scores in dementia patients (abstr). *J Nucl Med* 1990;31:731.

16. Johnson KA, Mueller ST, Walshe TM, et al. Single photon emission computed tomography in Alzheimer's disease: abnormal iofetamine I 123 uptake reflects dementia severity. *Arch Neurol* 1988;45:392–396.

17. Montaldi D, Brooks DN, McColl JH, et al. Measurements of regional cerebral blood flow and cognitive performance in Alzheimer's disease. *J Neurol Neurosurg Psychiatry* 1990;53:33–38.

18. Tikofsky RS, Hellman RS, Antuono PA, et al. Boston naming test (BNT) and enhanced quantitative SPECT HMPAO in Alzheimer's disease (abstr). *Radiology*. (Supp) 1991;181P:174.

19. Elfgren LI, Ryding E, Passant U. Performance on neuropsychological tests related to single photon emission computerized tomography findings in frontotemporal dementia. *Br J Psychiatry* 1996;169:416–422.

20. Sabri O, Schneider R, Buell U. Comparison of PET, SPET, neuropsychological and morphological findings in vascular dementia. *Eur J Nucl Med* 1997;24:348–349.

21. Mayberg H. Clinical correlates of PET- and SPECT-identified defects in dementia. *J Clin Psychiatry* 1994;55(Suppl):12–21.

22. Davis PC, Mirra SS, Alazraki N. The brain in older persons with and without dementia: findings on MR, PET, and SPECT images. *AJR* 1994;162:1267–1278.

23. Hellman RS, Tikofsky RS, Van Heertum R, et al. A multi-institutional study of interobserver agreement in the evaluation of dementia with rCBF/SPECT technetium-99m exametazime (HMPAO). *Eur J Nucl Med* 1994;21:306–313.

24. Soricelli A, Postiglione A, Grivet-Fojaja MRI, et al. Reduced cortical distribution volume of iodine-123 iomazenil in Alzheimer's disease as a measure of loss of synapses. *Eur J Nucl Med* 1996;23:1323–1328.
25. Fukuchi K, Hashikawa K, Seike Y, et al. Comparison of iodine-123-iomazenil SPECT and technetium-99m-HMPAO-SPECT in Alzheimer's disease. *J Nucl Med* 1997;38:467–470.
26. Kitamura S, Koshi Y, Komiyama T, et al. Benzodiazepine receptor and cerebral blood flow in early Alzheimer's disease—SPECT study using ^{123}I-iomazenil and ^{123}I-IMP. *Kaku Igaku (Jpn J Nucl Med)* 1996; 33:49–56.

SUGGESTED READINGS

Dewan MJ, Gupta S. Toward a definite diagnosis of Alzheimer's disease. *Comp Psychiatry* 1992;33:282–290.
Eberling JL, Reed BR, Baker MG, Jagust WJ. Cognitive correlates of regional cerebral blood flow in Alzheimer's disease. *Arch Neurol* 1993;50:761–766.
Ishii K, Sasaki M, Kitagaki H, et al. Reduction of cerebellar glucose metabolism in advanced Alzheimer's disease. *J Nucl Med* 1997;38:935–928.
Holman BL, Nagel JS, Johnson KA, Hill TC. Imaging dementia with SPECT. *Ann NY Acad Sci* 1991;629:165–174.
Launes J, Sulkava R, Erkinjuntti T, et al. 99Tcm-HMPAO SPECT in suspected dementia. *Nucl Med Commun* 1991;12:757–765.
Ohnishi T, Hoshi H, Nagamachi S, et al. Regional cerebral blood flow study with 123I-IMP in patients with dementia. *Am J Neuroradiol* 1991; 12:513–520.

Pearlson GD, Harris GJ, Powers RE, et al. Quantitative changes in mesial temporal volume, regional cerebral blood flow, and cognition in Alzheimer's disease. *Arch Gen Psychiatry* 1992;49:402–408.
Rosci MA, Pigorini F, Bernabei A, et al. Methods for detecting early signs of AIDS dementia complex in asymptomatic HIV-1-infected subjects. *AIDS* 1992;6:1309–1316.
Sabri O, Hellwig D, Schreckenberger M, et al. Correlation of neuropsychological, morphological, and functional (regional cerebral blood flow and glucose utilization) findings in cerebral microangiopathy. *J Nucl Med* 1998;39:147–154.
Tikofsky RS, Ichise M, Seibyl JP, Verhoeff NPLG. Functional brain SPECT imaging: 1999 and beyond. In: Freeman LM, ed. *Nucl Med Ann* New York: Lippincott Williams & Wilkins. 1999;193–264.
Tozzi V, Narciso P, Galgani S, et al. Effects of zidovudine in 30 patients with mild to end-stage AIDS dementia complex. *AIDS* 1993;7: 683–692.
Tranquart F, Ades P.E, Groussin P, et al. Postoperative assessment of cerebral blood flow in subarachoid haemorrhage by means of 99mTc-HMPAO tomography. *Eur J Nucl Med* 1993;20:53–58.
Wyper D, Teasdale E, Patterson J, et al. Abnormalities in rCBF and computed tomography in patients with Alzheimer's disease and in controls. *Brit J Radiol* 1993;66:23–27.
Yoshida T, Kuwabara Y, Ichiya Y, et al. Cerebral muscarinic acetylcholinergic receptor measurement in Alzheimer's disease patients on 11C-N-methyl-4-piperidyl benzilate—comparison with cerebral blood flow and cerebral glucose metabolism. *Ann Nucl Med* 1998; 12:35–42.

CASE 6-1

Clinical Diagnosis:
Dementia, Possible Alzheimer's Disease

CONTRIBUTORS:	IMAGING DATA:	
Robert S. Hellman, M.D.,	**Camera:** GE Neurocam	**Collimator:** High-resolution
Ronald S. Tikofsky, M.D.	**Tracer:** ^{99m}Tc HMPAO	**Dose:** 30.0 mCi
Institution: Medical College of Wisconsin		

This 79-year-old woman was referred by the Memory Disorders Clinic for evaluation of signs and symptoms of dementia. At the time of evaluation, her Mini-Mental State Examination score was 17/30. The patient's symptoms, which had started 2 years previously, began with mood changes and hallucinations, inability to handle finances, and the progressive inability to operate her TV remote control.

No CT or MRI studies had been performed

A hexamethylpropyleneamine-okime (HMPAO) SPECT study (Case Fig. 6.1) in the transaxial **(A)**, coronal **(B)**, and sagittal **(C)** planes revealed decreased radiotracer in the right frontal, temporoparietal, and left posterior parietal regions. These findings are consistent with Alzheimer's disease.

Teaching Point:

HMPAO SPECT can be useful in the evaluation of suspected Alzheimer's disease. The pattern of reduced tracer uptake is similar to that of ^{123}I IMP SPECT and F-18 fluorodeoxyglucose (^{18}FDA) PET studies.

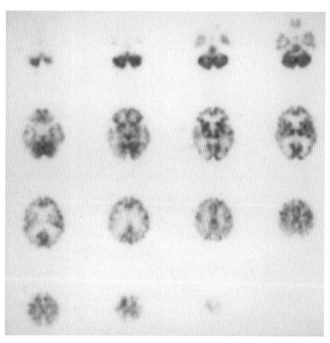

CASE FIG. 6.1A

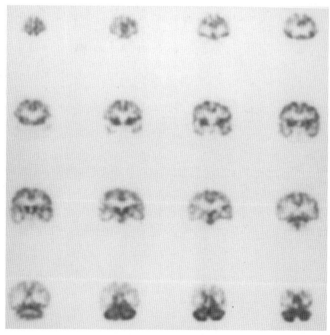

CASE FIG. 6.1B

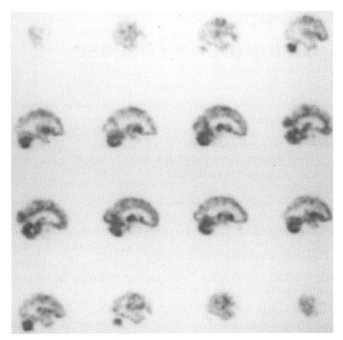

CASE FIG. 6.1C

Clinical Diagnosis:
Alzheimer's Disease

CONTRIBUTORS:

James M. Mountz, M.D., Ph.D.,
Michael V. Yester, Ph.D.
Institution: The University of Alabama at
Birmingham Medical Center

IMAGING DATA:

Coincidence Imaging
Camera: Picker PRISM 3000 XP
Tracer: ^{99m}Tc HMPAO

Collimator: Parallel-hole
Dose: 30 mCi

This 61-year-old woman had a clinical history of Alzheimer's disease.

Two ^{99m}Tc HMPAO SPECT scans are shown, one of a normal 60-year-old woman (Case Fig. 6.2). Her scan shows uniform tracer distribution throughout the cortex, with slight "hyperperfusion" in the basal ganglia—clear delineation of low perfusion to white matter. The image labeled "Alzheimer's) on this figure is that of a 61 year old woman with a clinical diagnosis of Alzheimer's disease. Her ^{99m}Tc HMPAO SPECT scan is characterized by globally decreased perfusion throughout the cortex relative to the cerebellum. The most prominent areas of decreased perfusion are in the posterior temporoparietal regions (*arrows*) with relative sparing of the basal ganglia, somatosensory cortex, and cerebellum. These findings are characteristic of the cerebral perfusion deficit patterns reported for Alzheimer's disease.

Teaching Points:

1. Alzheimer's disease, especially in patients with very characteristic perfusion patterns, can be diagnosed accurately.

2. This observation is important, since acetylcholinesterase inhibitors are currently available for therapy and have been shown to decrease or reverse the cognitive decline.

3. Reports have shown that there is decrease or reversal of the regional perfusion deficits in patients who respond to treatment.

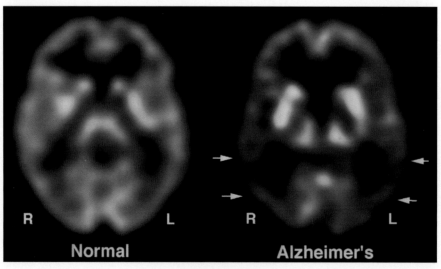

CASE FIG. 6.2

Clinical Diagnosis:
Possible Alzheimer's Disease

CONTRIBUTOR:	IMAGING DATA:	
Matthew Bloom, M.D.	**Camera:** Picker PRISM 3000	**Collimator:** Ultra-high-resolution fan-beam
Institution: Columbia-Presbyterian Medical Center	**Tracer:** ^{99m}Tc HMPAO	**Dose:** 30 mCi

This 68-year-old woman with an 8-year history of anomia, fluctuating antisocial behavior, and violent outbursts was referred for evaluation of progressive short-term memory loss.

MRI (T2-weighted) revealed mild generalized atrophy and a small lacunar infarct in the right cerebral peduncle.

At the time of the SPECT study, the patient was quite agitated and uncooperative. As a result, a shortened SPECT acquisition was performed. HMPAO SPECT (Case Fig. 6.3) in the coronal (**A**) and sagittal (**B**) planes revealed an overall decrease in radiotracer uptake that was most marked in the posterior-parietal-temporal and frontal lobes bilaterally. There is relative sparing of the sensorimotor area and the subcortical structures, including basal ganglia and thalami.

Teaching Point:

Cerebral SPECT can be very useful in the evaluation of dementia, particularly in patients who are difficult to evaluate with clinical neuropsychological testing, such as this patient with anomia. This study further demonstrates the value of shortening the total SPECT acquisition time in agitated or uncooperative patients.

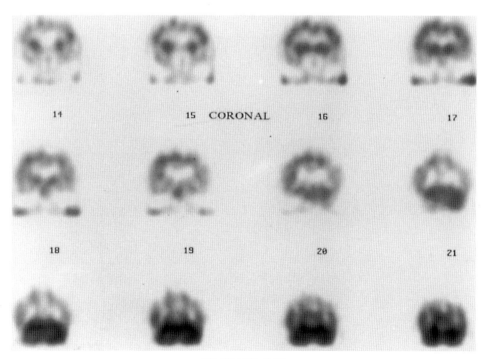

CASE FIG. 6.3A

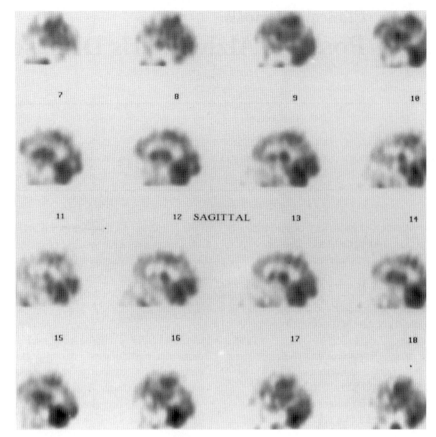

CASE FIG. 6.3B

Clinical Diagnosis:

Amnestic Syndrome, Possible Alzheimer's Disease

CONTRIBUTORS:	IMAGING DATA:	
Robert S. Hellman, M.D.,	**Camera:** GE 400 AC/T;Star	**Collimator:** High-resolution
Ronald S. Tikofsky, M.D.	**Tracer:** ^{99m}Tc HMPAO	**Dose:** 30 mCi
Institution: Medical College of Wisconsin		

This 74-year-old woman with a known history of three motor vehicle accidents and alcohol/phenobarbital abuse was referred for evaluation of progressive memory changes. Her memory changes were first noted in 1983, following the third motor vehicle accident. Although her Mini-Mental State Examination at the present time was within the normal range (29/30), she did show a mild impairment on the Blessed Dementia rating scale (8.5/16). The brief psychiatric rating scale and Hachinski cerebral ischemia score were within normal range. The criteria used for amnestic syndrome were those of the National Institute of Neurological and Communicative Disorders and Stroke (NINCDS/ADRDA).

An MRI scan showed diffuse cerebral atrophy with mild senescent white matter changes.

An HMPAO SPECT study (Fig. 6.4) in the transaxial plane revealed decreased case tracer activity in the mesial anterior temporal and posterior frontal lobes. In addition, mild decreased tracer activity was noted bilaterally, right greater than left, in the posterior parietal lobes.

Teaching Points:

1. This is an atypical presentation for Alzheimer's disease. However, repeat scans will typically show the progression of the disease over time.

2. Approximately 80% of patients with amnestic syndrome progress to Alzheimer's disease within 5 years of onset.

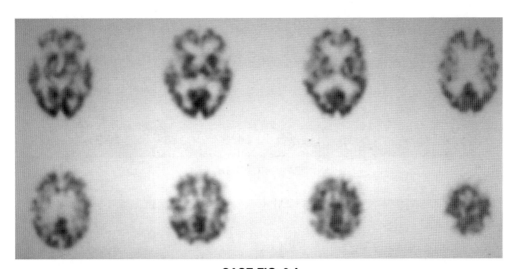

CASE FIG. 6.4

Clinical Diagnosis:
Dementia of Unknown Etiology

CONTRIBUTORS:

Masanori Ichise, M.D.,
Morris Freedman, M.D.
Institution: Mount Sinai Hospital, Baycrest
Center for Geriatric Care,
Toronto, Canada

IMAGING DATA:

Camera: Picker PRISM 3000
Tracer: ^{99m}Tc ECD

Collimator: Ultra-high-resolution fan-beam
Dose: 20 mCi

This 59-year-old woman was referred for the evaluation of memory problems. Her mental status examination showed that she was disoriented to dates and place, did not know current events, and was unable to copy figures. Her remote memory was also poor.

MRI revealed mild cortical atrophy.

The ^{99m}Tc ECD SPECT study (transverse and sagittal images, (Case Figs. 6.5A, B) shows bilateral posterior temporoparietal perfusion deficits with relative sparing of the sensorimotor region.

Teaching Point:

Characteristic perfusion deficits seen in Alzheimer's disease will typically include sparing of primary cortices.

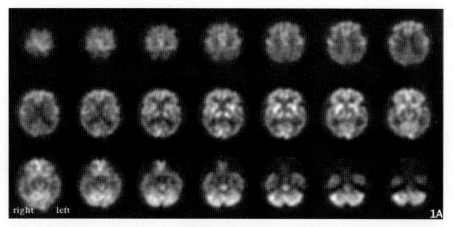

CASE FIG. 6.5A

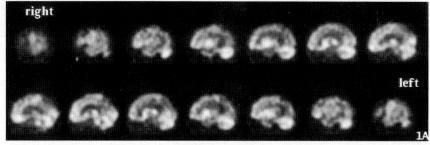

CASE FIG. 6.5B

Clinical Diagnosis:
Dementia of Unknown Etiology

CONTRIBUTOR:	IMAGING DATA:	
Masanori Ichise, M.D.	**Camera:** Picker PRISM 3000	**Collimator:** Ultra-high-resolution fan-beam
Institution: Mount Sinai Hospital, Toronto, Canada	**Tracer:** ⁹⁹ᵐTc ECD	**Dose:** 20 mCi

This 53-year-old man was referred for the evaluation of disorientation and forgetfulness.

A CT scan point to a subdural hematoma (Fig. 6.6, *top*).

The transverse images from this ⁹⁹ᵐTc ECD SPECT study (Fig. 6.6, *bottom*) showed an extraaxial distortion of the left frontal lobe, but underlying cortical perfusion was intact.

Teaching Points:

1. Subdural hematoma may cause "dementia."

2. Correlation with anatomic images such as CT is important in the evaluation of brain perfusion SPECT studies.

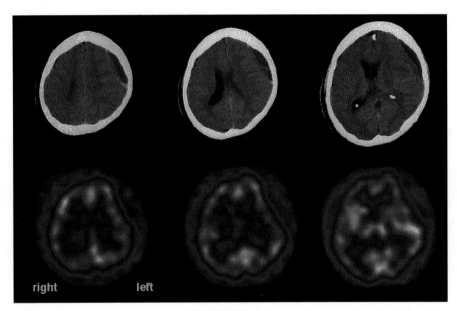

CASE FIG. 6.6

Clinical Diagnosis:
Alzheimer's Disease

CONTRIBUTORS:	IMAGING DATA:	
Masonori Ichise, M.D.,	**Camera:** Picker PRISM 3000	**Collimator:** Ultra-high-resolution fan-beam
Morris Freedman, M.D.	**Tracer:** ^{99m}Tc ECD	**Dose:** 20 mCi
Institution: Mount Sinai Hospital, Baycrest Center for Geriatric Care, Toronto, Canada		**Attenuation Correction:** Chang

This 65-year-old woman had a 2-year history of gradual cognitive deterioration; she was referred for evaluation of suspected Alzheimer's disease. Her cognitive assessment showed attentional difficulties, memory problems, difficulties in reading and writing, and poor performance on visuospatial tests (visual agnosia). Her cognitive function declined progressively over the 3 years since her initial referral.

CT revealed mild ventriculomegally.

The ECD SPECT study in the transverse plane from 1996 (Case Fig. 6.7A) showed perfusion deficits in the left posterior temporoparietal lobes. The second ECD SPECT study in 1997 showed some progression of perfusion deficits, now involving both sides but worse on the left (Case Fig. 6.7B). The third ECD SPECT in 1998 showed almost symmetric bilateral posterior temporoparietal perfusion deficits (Case Fig. 6.7C).

Teaching Point:

Alzheimer's disease may show asymmetric perfusion deficits that progress to involve bilateral posterior temporoparietal lobes.

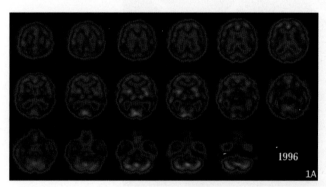

CASE FIG. 6.7A

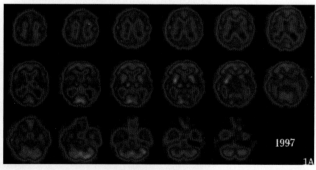

CASE FIG. 6.7B

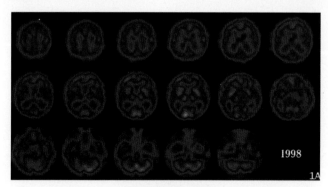

CASE FIG. 6.7C

Clinical Diagnosis:
Dementia

CONTRIBUTORS:	IMAGING DATA:	
Alan Waxman, M.D.,	**Camera:** Picker Prism 3000	**Collimator:** LEUHR
Hart Cohen, M.D.	**Tracer:** ⁹⁹ᵐTc Bicisate	**Dose:** 20.0 mCi
Institution: Cedars-Sinai Medical Center		**Attenuation Correction Method:** Chang 11

This 78-year-old man initially presented with loss of memory and speech fluency and a gradually developing inability to articulate his thoughts. He had been profoundly depressed for approximately 1 year following his retirement. For the past 2 1/2 years, he has noted a progressive increase in memory loss and further erosion of speech. Mild, bilateral upper extremity tremor was noted on physical examination. The patient appeared depressed and his speech showed word-finding difficulty.

MRI showed mild, diffuse atrophy.

Initial SPECT studies (Case Fig. 6.8A) showed minimally decreased tracer activity bilaterally in the posterior parietal regions; this was greater on the right. Repeat SPECT performed 27 months later demonstrates progressive reduction of tracer activity in these regions consistent with progression of the disease process (Case Fig. 6.8B).

Teaching Points:

1. The ⁹⁹ᵐTc Bicisate study was able to detect an Alzheimer's pattern relatively early in the patient's clinical course and changes in tracer activity parallel disease progression.

2. SPECT scans will often reveal major abnormalities early in the clinical course of Alzheimer's disease and demonstrate disease progression on serial studies.

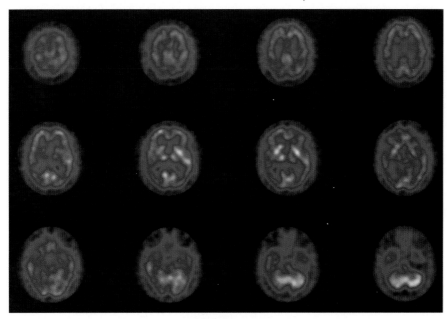

CASE FIG. 6.8A

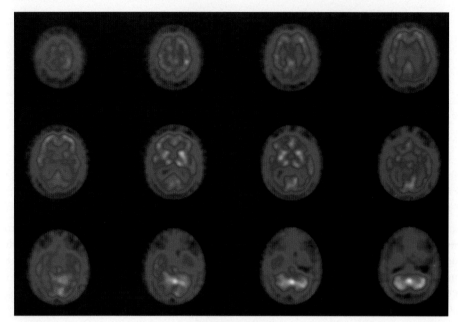

CASE FIG. 6.8B

Clinical Diagnosis:
Dementia and Depression

CONTRIBUTORS:	IMAGING DATA:	
Ronald S. Tikofsky, Ph.D.,	**Camera:** PRISM 3000	**Collimator:** High-resolution fan-beam
Chaitali Bagchi, M.D.,	**Tracer:** ^{99m}Tc ECD	**Dose:** 24.9 mCi
Deepika Singh, M.D.		
Institution: Columbia University, Harlem Hospital Center		

This 82-year-old woman presented with hypertension, degenerative joint disease, cataracts, and a recent onset of dementia and depression.

CT scan of the brain done the same day as the SPECT study revealed mild atrophy, with periventricular white matter lucencies and a small right occipital cortical infarction (Case Fig. 6.9A).

The transverse plane of the SPECT ECD study reveals significantly decreased perfusion bilaterally in the temporoparietal regions, left greater than right (Case Fig. 6.9B). This finding is consistent with the presence of de-

menting disease. In addition, there is a region of absent radiotracer uptake in the right occipital lobe consistent with the CT findings. Radiotracer uptake throughout the brain is somewhat decreased. The width of the interhemispheric and sylvian fissures is suggestive of atrophy.

Teaching Points:

SPECT perfusion patterns in elderly patients who present with clinical findings of decreased cognitive function suggestive of dementia and depression will often show overall decreased cortical perfusion and, more significantly, decreased tracer uptake in the temporoparietal regions.

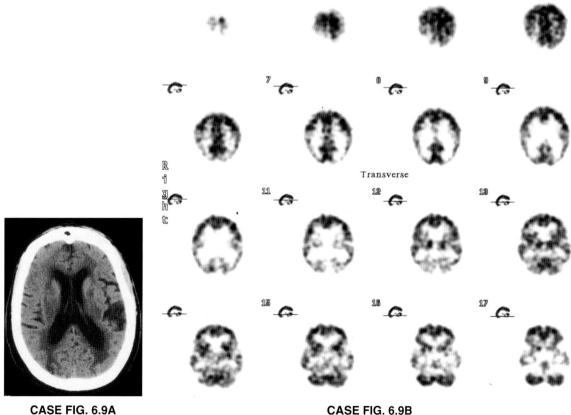

CASE FIG. 6.9A

CASE FIG. 6.9B

Clinical Diagnosis:
Progressive Dementia

CONTRIBUTOR:	IMAGING DATA:	
Betty Triantafillou, M.D.	**PET Scanner:** Siemens XACT 47	**Attenuation Correction**
Institution: New York Presbyterian Medical Center	**Tracer:** [18]FDG	**Method:** Autoattenuation
		Dose: 9.52 mCi

This 52-year-old woman presented with a history of progressive memory disorder of 1 year's duration.

MRI (Case Fig. 6.10A) reveals diffuse cortical atrophy which is most pronounced in the frontal and temporal lobes.

PET images in the transverse, coronal, and sagittal planes reveal diffuse reduction of radiotracer activity in the frontal and temporal lobes (Case Fig. 6.10 A–D), which is disproportionate to the degree of atrophy seen on MRI.

Teaching Point:

This study demonstrates the characteristic pattern of hypometabolism visualized in patients with frontotemporal dementia.

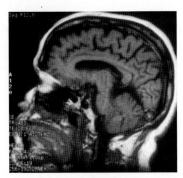

CASE FIG. 6.10A

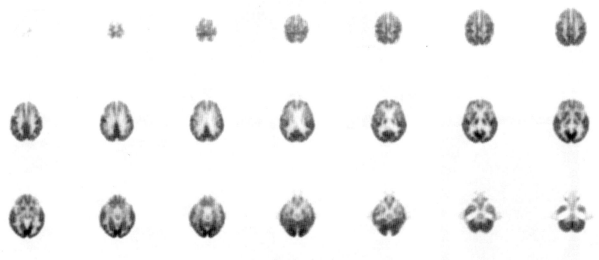

CASE FIG. 6.10B

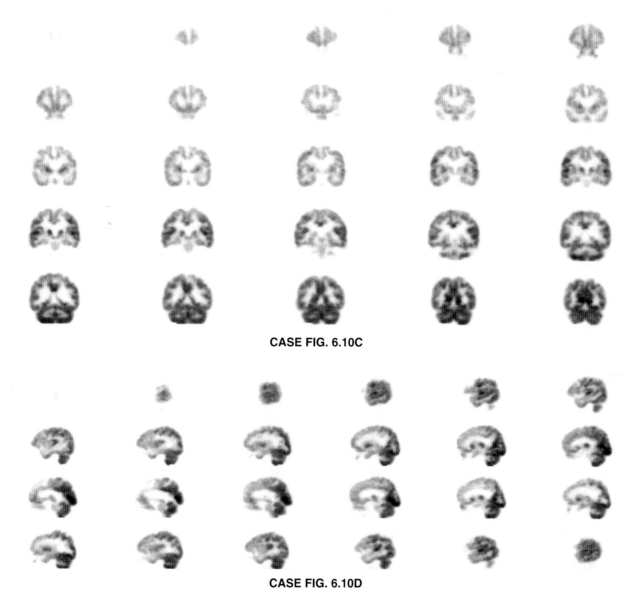

CASE FIG. 6.10C

CASE FIG. 6.10D

Clinical Diagnosis:
Progressive Language Dysfunction

CONTRIBUTORS:	IMAGING DATA:	
Ronald L. Van Heertum, M.D.,	**PET Scanner:** Siemens XACT 47	**Attenuation Correction**
Betty Triantafillou, M.D.	**Tracer:** [18]FDG	**Method:** Autoattenuation protocol
Institution: The Kreitchman PET Center,		**Dose:** 9.76 mCi
New York Presbyterian Medical		
Center		

This 58-year-old man had a 3 1/2-year history of progressive language dysfunction and memory impairment.

A brain MRI on 5/7/97 (Case Fig. 6.11A) demonstrated mild ventricular prominence.

PET images in the transverse, coronal, and sagittal planes reveal moderately decreased metabolism in the bilateral temporal and parietal lobes with relative sparing of the sensorimotor cortex (Case Figs. 6.11 B–D). These findings are most consistent with Alzheimer's disease.

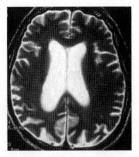

CASE FIG. 6.11A

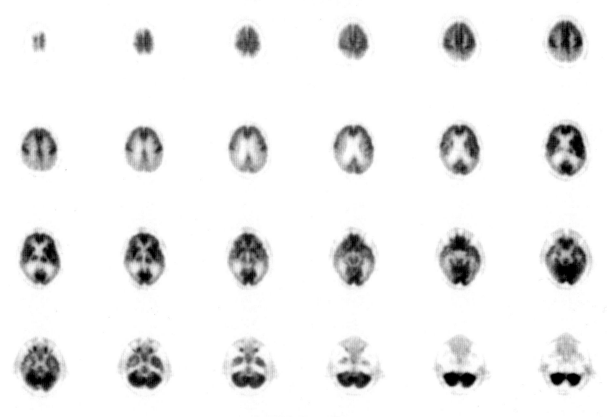

CASE FIG. 6.11B

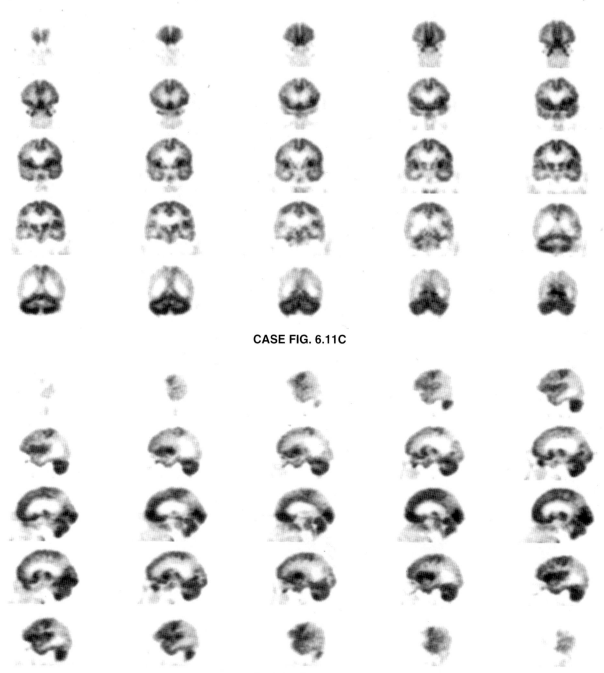

CASE FIG. 6.11C

CASE FIG. 6.11D

CASE 6-12

Clinical Diagnosis:
Progressive Memory Disorder

Ronald S. Van Heertum, M.D.,

CONTRIBUTOR:	IMAGING DATA:	
Jeffrey Plutchok, M.D.	**PET Scanner:** Siemens XACT 47	**Attenuation Correction**
Institution: New York Presbyterian Medical Center	**Tracer:** ^{18}FDG	**Method:** Autoattenuation
		Dose: 9.83 mCi

This 70-year-old man had a history of progressive memory dysfunction and incontinence. He appeared to be lethargic and experiencing generalized weakness. A brain SPECT (Case Fig. 6.12A, *axial view*) suggested frontotemporal hypoperfusion.

MRI shows signs of cortical atrophy and large ventricles for age (Case Fig. 6.12B).

Transverse, coronal, and sagittal reconstructed images of the brain (Case Fig. 6.12 C–E) reveal a severe, left greater than right, temporal, frontal, and parietal hypometabolism with relative sparing of the sensorimotor strip. These findings demonstrate a pattern consistent with Alzheimer's disease.

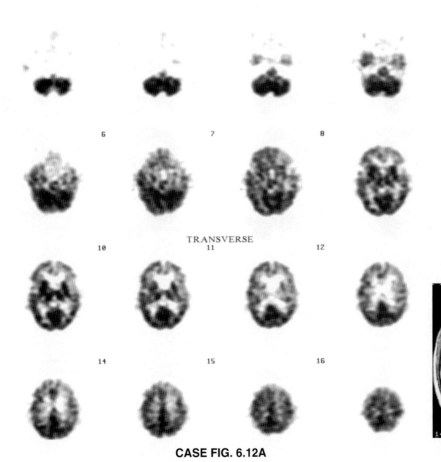

CASE FIG. 6.12A

CASE FIG. 6.12B

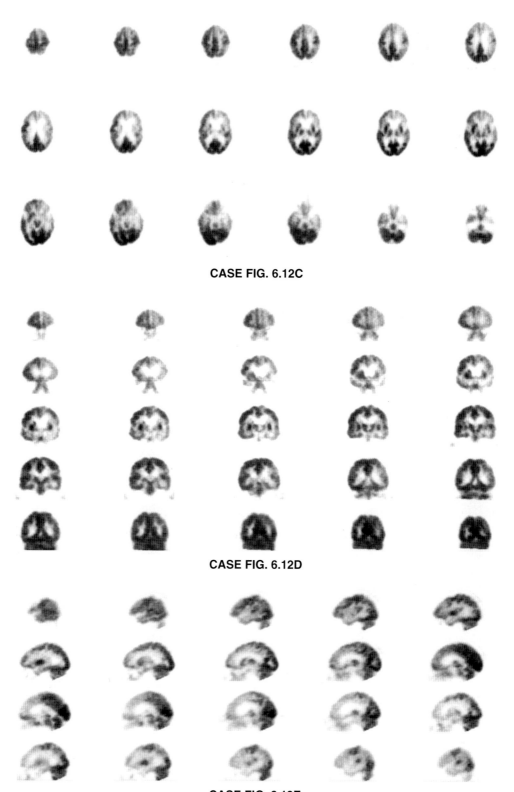

CASE FIG. 6.12C

CASE FIG. 6.12D

CASE FIG. 6.12E

CASE 6-13

Clinical Diagnosis:
Progressive Memory Loss

CONTRIBUTOR:	IMAGING DATA:	
Angela Lignelli, M.D.	**PET Scanner:** Siemens XACT 47	**Attenuation Correction**
Institution: New York Presbyterian Medical Center	**Tracer:** [18]FDG	**Method:** Autoattenuation
		Dose: 9.91 mCi

This 60-year-old woman presented with progressive short-term memory loss of 5 years' duration. The patient's symptoms are exaggerated in stressful situations, during which she becomes confused and depressed and often has difficulty understanding directions.

MRI (Case Fig. 6.13A) reveals mild atrophy.

PET images in the transverse, coronal, and sagittal planes reveal reduced radiotracer uptake throughout the posterior parietal, temporal, and frontal cortices with relatively preserved radiotracer activity in the subcortical, sensorimotor, and occipital areas (Case Figs. 6.13 B–D).

Teaching Point:

This pattern of radiotracer uptake is quite characteristic of dementia and similar for blood flow and metabolic brain imaging studies.

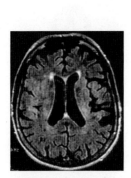

CASE FIG. 6.13A

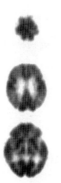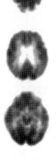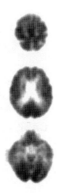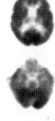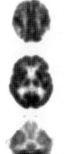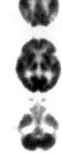

CASE FIG. 6.13B

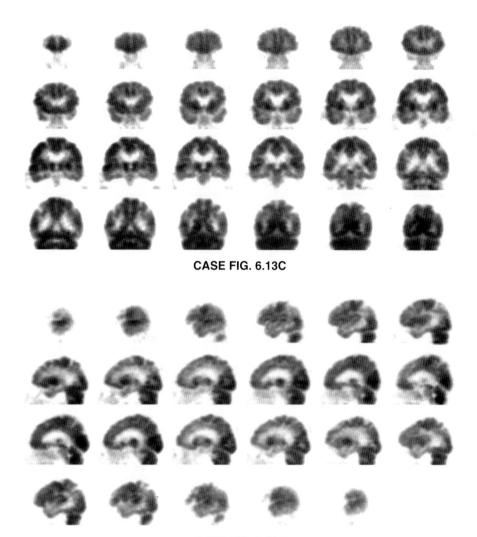

CASE FIG. 6.13C

CASE FIG. 6.13D

Clinical Diagnosis:
Corticobasal Degeneration

CONTRIBUTOR:	IMAGING DATA:	
Murray Becker, M.D., Ph.D.	**PET Scanner:** Siemens XACT 47	**Attenuation Correction**
Institution: New York Presbyterian Medical	**Tracer:** [18]FDG	**Method:** Autoattenuation
Center		**Dose:** 10.26 mCi

This 84-year-old woman presented with right arm weakness, difficulty walking, dizziness, and memory loss of approximately a year's duration. She was initially thought to have Parkinson's disease, but was unresponsive to Sinemet (carbidopa-levodopa) and Artane (trihexyphenidyl).

MRI showed diffuse atrophy.

PET images in the transverse, coronal, and sagittal planes reveal focal decreased tracer uptake in the left mesial frontal lobe and the right posterior temporal lobe (Case Figs. 6.14A–C).

Teaching Point:

PET imaging can be very helpful in distinguishing corticobasal degeneration from Parkinson's disease.

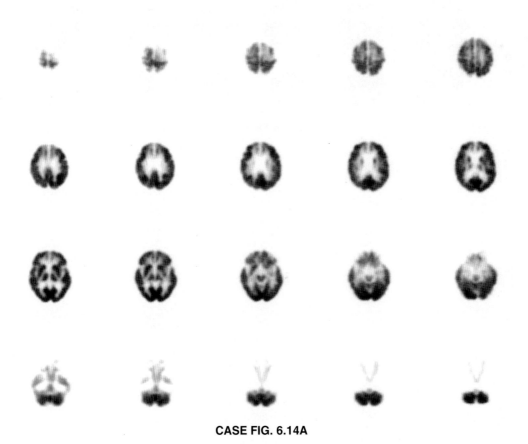

CASE FIG. 6.14A

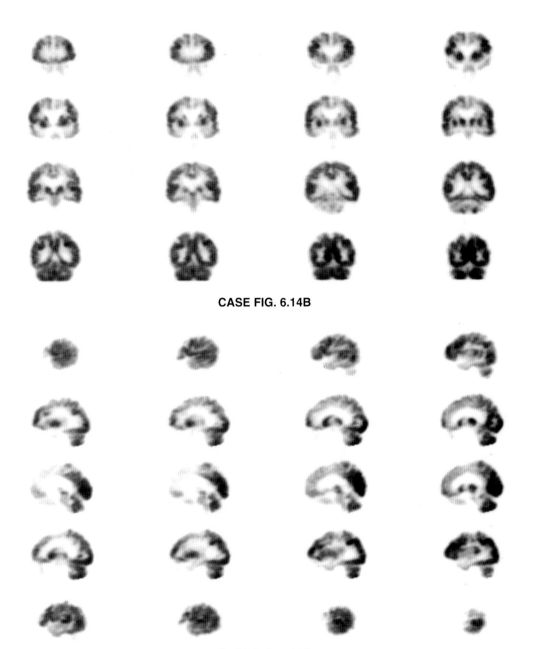

CASE FIG. 6.14B

CASE FIG. 6.14C

CASE 6-15

Clinical Diagnosis:

Olivopontine Cerebellar Degeneration

CONTRIBUTOR:	IMAGING DATA:	
Ronald L. Van Heertum, M.D.	**PET Scanner:** Siemens XACT 47	**Attenuation Correction**
Institution: New York Presbyterian Medical Center	**Tracer:** [18]FDG	**Method:** Autoattenuation
		Dose: 10.19 mCi

This 62-year-old man with a past history of lymphoma presented with gait impairment, slurred speech, and progressive cognitive deficits of approximately 10 months duration. MRI (Case Fig. 6.15A), electroencephalography (EEG), and cerebrospinal fluid (CSF) studies were unremarkable.

PET images in the transverse, coronal, and sagittal planes reveal marked decrease of radiotracer activity in the cerebellum and pons (Case Fig. 6-15B–D).

Teaching Point:

The PET pattern of reduced radiotracer activity in olivopontine cerebellar degeneration is quite characteristic of dementia.

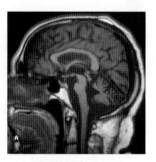

CASE FIG. 6.15A

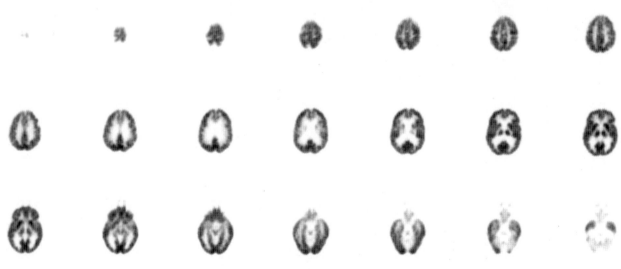

CASE FIG. 6.15B

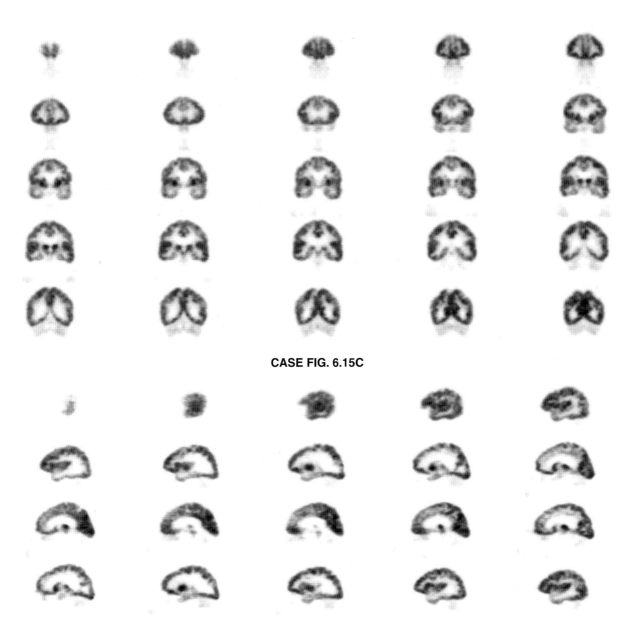

CASE FIG. 6.15C

CASE FIG. 6.15D

Clinical Diagnosis:
Multi-Infarct Dementia

CONTRIBUTOR:

Ronald L. Van Heertum, M.D.
Institution: St. Vincent's Hospital and
Medical Center

IMAGING DATA:

Camera: GE 400 AC/T;Star II
Tracer: [123]I IMP

Collimator: High-resolution
Dose: 3.0 mCi

This 64-year-old woman with known multi-infarct dementia (MID) was referred for evaluation of the recent onset of hemiplegia.

The CT scan (Case Fig. 6.16A) demonstrated a large area of infarction involving the left occipital lobe. In addition, cortical atrophy and bilateral white matter hypodensity were noted, suggesting microvascular disease.

A cerebral SPECT study (Case Fig. 6.16B), in the transaxial (**A**), coronal (**B**), and sagittal (**C**) planes, showed that

tracer deposition was absent in the left occipital lobe (*arrows*), left frontal lobe (*arrowheads*), and left basal ganglia.

> **Teaching Point:**
>
> In cases of MID, the cerebral SPECT study will frequently be more useful than a CT scan and, in some cases, MRI for defining the full extent of disease.

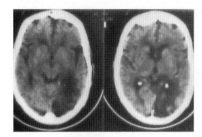

CASE FIG. 6.16A

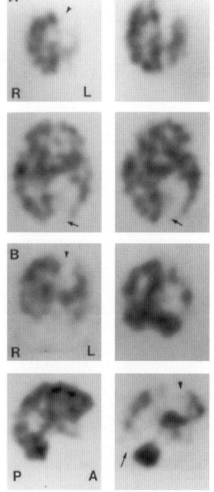

CASE FIG. 6.16B

Clinical Diagnosis:
Bilateral Posterior Parietotemporal Infarctions

CONTRIBUTOR:	IMAGING DATA:	
Ronald L. Van Heertum, M.D.	**Camera:** Picker PRISM 3000	**Collimator:** Ultra-high-resolution fan-beam
Institution: Columbia-Presbyterian Medical Center	**Tracer:** ^{99m}Tc HMPAO	**Dose:** 20.0 mCi

This 78-year-old man was referred for further evaluation of progressive memory loss. The patient had a known prior history of cerebrovascular disease.

A CT scan (Case Fig. 6.17A) revealed bilateral temporoparietal hypodensities consistent with infarctions.

An HMPAO SPECT study (Case Fig. 6.17B–D) in the transaxial (**B**), coronal (**C**), and sagittal (**D**) planes revealed absent radiotracer activity bilaterally in the areas of infarction seen on the prior CT scan.

Teaching Point:

This case emphasizes the importance of correlating the SPECT scan results with an anatomic study (CT or MRI), as not all bilateral temporoparietal defects are due to Alzheimer's disease.

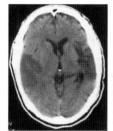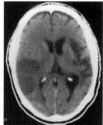

CASE FIG. 6.17A

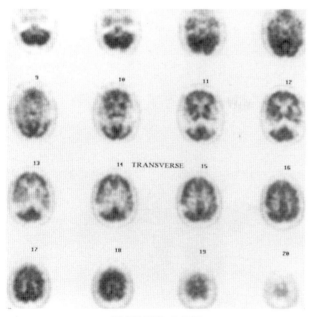

CASE FIG. 6.17B

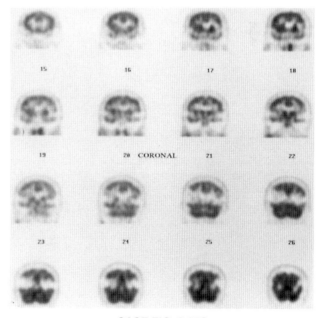

CASE FIG. 6.17C

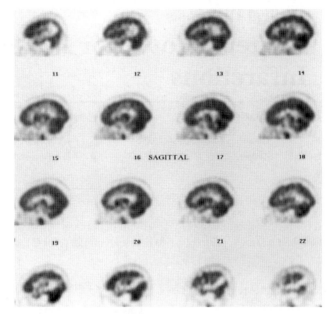

CASE FIG. 6.17D

Clinical Diagnosis:

Dementia and Prior History of Stroke and Alcohol Abuse

CONTRIBUTORS:	IMAGING DATA:	
Ronald S. Tikofsky, Ph.D.	**Camera:** PRISM 3000	**Collimator:** High-resolution fan-beam
Candido Quinones, M.D.	**Tracer:** ^{99m}Tc ECD	**Dose:** 31.8 mCi
Institution: Columbia University, Harlem Hospital Center		

This 49-year-old woman presented with a new-onset of dementia. The patient had a stroke a year prior to onset of the present change in mental status. The referring physician states that the prior stroke does not account for the severity of the patient's current mental status.

A CT scan of the brain revealed a left and right temporoparietal infarction.

The transverse, coronal, and sagittal SPECT ECD images (Case Figs. 6-18A–C) reveal a large deficit of absent radiotracer activity in right frontal lobe and decreased radiotracer activity in the right parietal lobe. In addition, there was absent radiotracer activity in the distribution of the left middle cerebral artery extending into the basal ganglia and thalamus. These radiotracer deficits are larger than the defects seen on CT. The presence of changes in the temporoparietal regions maybe new findings that are contributing to the increased severity of the patients altered mental status.

Teaching Points:

SPECT perfusion patterns in patients with multiple infarction and alterations in mental status may be indicative of changes in brain cerebral blood flow that are representative of vascular or MID.

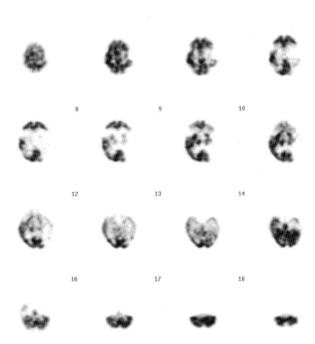

CASE FIG. 6.18A

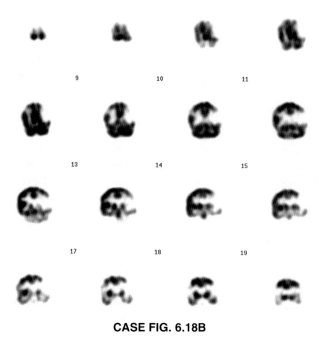

CASE FIG. 6.18B

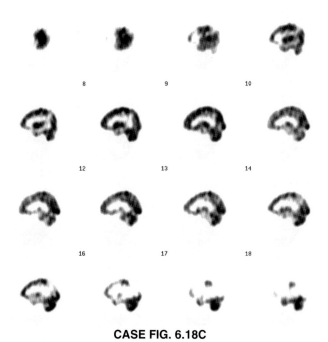

CASE FIG. 6.18C

Clinical Diagnosis:

Vascular Dementia

CONTRIBUTORS:	IMAGING DATA:	
Robert S. Hellman, M.D.,	**Camera:** GE Neurocam	**Collimator:** High-resolution
Ronald S. Tikofsky, M.D.	**Tracer:** 99mTc HMPAO	**Dose:** 30 mCi
Institution: Medical College of Wisconsin		

This 68-year-old woman was referred by a geriatric psychiatrist for a cerebral SPECT scan as part of an Alzheimer's disease workup. No other history was available at the time of the SPECT study. At the time of the SPECT study, no anatomic imaging exams had been performed.

The HMPAO/SPECT study (Case Figs. 6.19 A,B), in the transaxial (**A**) and coronal (**B**) planes, revealed a sharply defined defect in the left occipital and posterior temporal region that was felt to be consistent with an area of infarction involving the posterior circulation. No crossed cerebellar diaschisis was seen. These findings were not consistent with the provisional diagnosis of possible Alzheimer's disease. Correlation with CT or MRI was recommended.

A follow-up CT scan (Case Fig. 6.19C) showed diffuse brain atrophy consistent with the patient's age. In addition,

an old left posterior parietooccipital infarction was observed. No intracranial mass, acute hemorrhage, or acute infarction was reported.

Teaching Points:

1. When used as an initial screen in patients suspected of Alzheimer's disease, the cerebral SPECT scan may reveal focal deficits compatible with areas of infarction or other abnormalities that do not conform with the original diagnosis.

2. When regions of absent perfusion are observed, CT or MR imaging studies should be requested to clarify the diagnosis further.

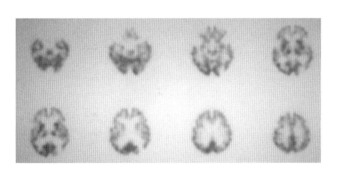

CASE FIG. 6.19A

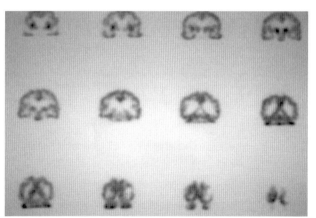

CASE FIG. 6.19B

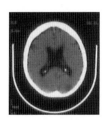

CASE FIG. 6.19C

CASE 6-20

Clinical Diagnosis:
Pick's Disease

CONTRIBUTORS:

Robert S. Hellman, M.D.,
Ronald S. Tikofsky, M.D.
Institution: Medical College of Wisconsin

IMAGING DATA:

Camera: GE Neurocam
Tracer: ^{99m}Tc HMPAO

Collimator: High-resolution
Dose: 30 mCi

This 65-year-old man began to manifest progressively more bizarre behavior approximately 6 to 7 years prior to referral for evaluation. His long-term memory was reported to be intact, but recent memory was impaired. The patient had no significant past medical or psychiatric history. Neuropsychological testing, performed 2 years prior to his current evaluation, showed a normal cognitive performance except for the Wisconsin Card Sorting Test, which was suggestive of frontal lobe dysfunction. An EEG study was normal, and clinical examination was suggestive of frontal lobe syndrome with a high likelihood of Pick's disease. Repeat neuropsychological examination showed a minimal decline from the previous testing with significant impairment noted on the Wisconsin Card Sorting Test with preservation. The overall findings were considered highly suggestive of a frontal lobe syndrome such as Pick's disease.

An MRI study revealed atrophy in the temporal and possibly frontal lobes.

An HMPAO SPECT (Case Fig. 6.20), in the transaxial plane, showed decreased radiotracer uptake in the frontal lobes bilaterally.

Teaching Point:

Bilateral decreased radiotracer uptake in the frontal lobes is a typical SPECT finding scan in frontal lobe dementias. This finding correlates well with neuropsychological performance deficits indicative of frontal lobe dysfunction. This combination of findings is often indicative of Pick's disease.

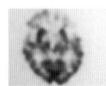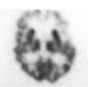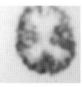

CASE FIG. 6-20

Clinical Diagnosis:
Pick's Disease

CONTRIBUTORS:

Masanori Ichise, M.D.,

Morris Freedman, M.D.

Institution: Mount Sinai Hospital, Baycrest
Center for Geriatric Care,
Toronto, Canada

IMAGING DATA:

Camera: Picker PRISM 3000
Tracer: ^{99m}Tc ECD

Collimator: Ultra-high-resolution fan-beam
Dose: 20 mCi
Attenuation Method: Chang

This elderly patient was referred for the evaluation of his progressive neurobehavioral problems. The patient was almost mute, being able to say only "S" and "F." He did not seem to recognize family members.

Frontal lobe atrophy CT reveals.

This man's ECD SPECT study (transverse and sagittal images, (Case Figs. 6.21A,B) showed marked frontal lobe perfusion deficits bilaterally, sparing sensory motor cortices.

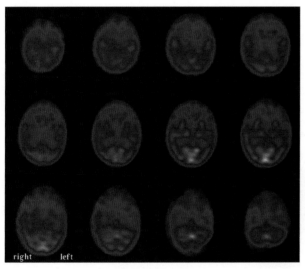

CASE FIG. 6.21A

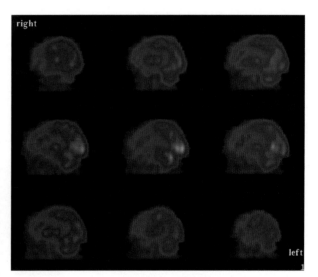

CASE FIG. 6.21B

CASE 6-22

Clinical Diagnosis:
Frontal Temporal Dementia

CONTRIBUTORS:

Marco Pagani, M.D.,
Lennart Thurfjell, Ph.D.,
Prof. Hans Jacobsson
Institution: Karolinska Hospital and Centre
for Image Analysis, Uppsala
University

IMAGING DATA:

Camera: Trionix Triad XLT 20
Tracer: ^{99m}Tc HMPAO

Collimator: LEUHR
Dose: 37 mCi

This 76-year-old man presented with progressive dementia of 10 years' duration and recent episodes of syncope and vomiting. The patient also had a long-standing history of hypertension of over 20 years' duration.

CT revealed diffuse cortical and cerebellar atrophy (Case Fig. 6.22A,B).

Transverse and sagittal-plane SPECT images as compared to a normal brain atlas data-base reference image reveal a pronounced decrease in tracer activity in the frontal cortex (Case Figs. 6.22C,D).

Teaching Points:

The decreased radiotracer uptake in frontal lobes is highlighted by the subtraction image (Ref-Pat). The reference image represents data from 12 age-matched controls. The SPECT studies have been coregistered to the computerized brain atlas (CBA).

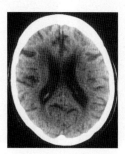

CASE FIG. 6.22A

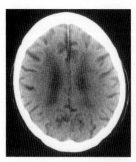 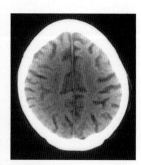

CASE FIG. 6.22B

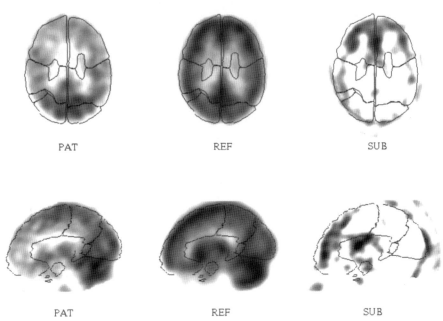

PAT REF SUB

PAT REF SUB

CASE FIG. 6.22C

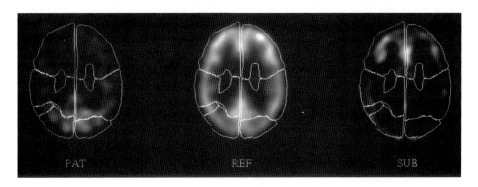

PAT REF SUB

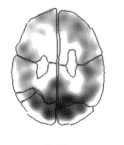 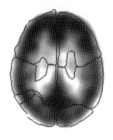 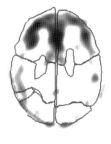

PAT REF SUB

CASE FIG. 6.22D

Clinical Diagnosis:

Primary Degenerative Dementia: Pick's Disease vs. Frontal Lobe Dementia; Parkinsonism Secondary to Primary Degenerative Dementia

CONTRIBUTORS:	IMAGING DATA:	
Robert S. Hellman, M.D.,	**Camera:** GE Neurocam	**Collimator:** High-resolution
Ronald S. Tikofsky, M.D.	**Tracer:** ^{99m}Tc HMPAO	**Dose:** 30 mCi
Institution: Medical College of Wisconsin		

This 76-year-old woman with a 2-year history of mental deterioration was admitted to the behavioral psychiatry unit for further evaluation. Neuropsychological evaluation was suggestive of senile dementia of the Alzheimer's type (SDAT). At the time of evaluation, her speech showed perserveration and echolalia. Rehospitalizations in 1992 and 1993 indicated that Parkinson's disease had developed secondary to the primary dementia and that she was showing further decline in cognitive and motor functions suggestive of frontal lobe dysfunction.

An MRI showed marked atrophy with enlarged ventricles.

An HMPAO SPECT study (Case Fig. 6.23) in the transaxial (**A**) and saggital (**B**) planes showed a significant decrease in radiotracer uptake in the frontal lobes bilaterally, which was felt to be consistent with frontal lobe dementia, possibly Pick's disease.

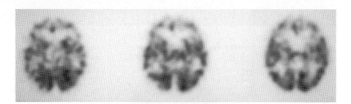

CASE FIG. 6.23A

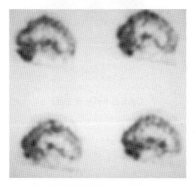

CASE FIG. 6.23B

Clinical Diagnosis:
Huntington's Disease

CONTRIBUTOR:	IMAGING DATA:	
Ronald L. Van Heertum, M.D.	**PET Scanner:** Siemens XACT 47	**Attenuation Correction**
Institution: New York Presbyterian Medical Center	**Tracer:** [18]FDG	**Method:** Autoattenuation
		Dose: 9.45 mCi

This 50-year-old man presented with choreiform movements. A PET scan was requested to help distinguish between Huntington's disease and corticobasal ganglionic degeneration.

MRI (Case Fig. 6.24A) revealed generalized atrophy and focal atrophy of the caudate nuclei.

Transverse, coronal, and sagittal plane PET images reveal marked symmetrically decreased radiotracer uptake in the caudate nuclei (Case Fig. 6-24 B–D).

> **Teaching Point:**
>
> This pattern of decreased significant hypometabolism involving the caudate nuclei is characteristic of Huntington's disease.

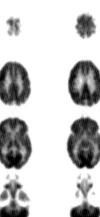
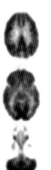
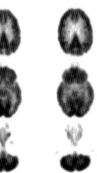
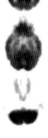
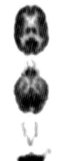
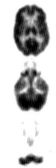

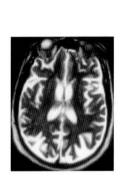

CASE FIG. 6.24A   **CASE FIG. 6.24B**

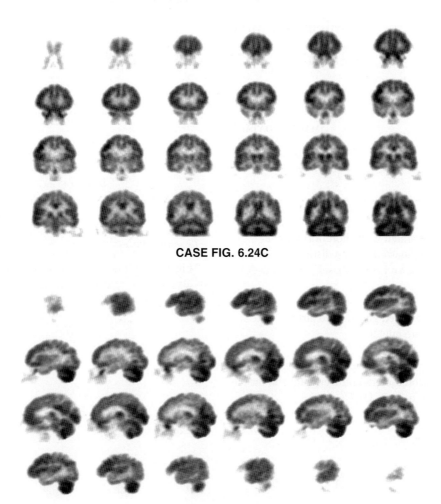

CASE FIG. 6.24C

CASE FIG. 6.24D

Clinical Diagnosis:
Huntington's Disease

CONTRIBUTOR:

Ronald L. Van Heertum, M.D.
Institution: St. Vincent's Hospital and
Medical Center

IMAGING DATA:

Camera: GE 400 AC/T;Star II
Tracer: ^{123}I IMP

Collimator: High-resolution
Dose: 3.0 mCi

This 55-year-old man was referred for an ongoing evaluation of his known Huntington's disease with mild dementia of 9 years' duration.

A CT scan (Case Fig. 6.25A) showed diffuse atrophy of the cerebral cortex.

The cerebral SPECT study (Case Fig. 6.25B) in the transaxial (**A**), coronal (**B**), and sagittal (**C**) planes revealed decreased tracer deposition throughout the cerebral cortex and periventricular white matter, corresponding to the cortical atrophy noted on the CT scan. In addition, tracer deposition was absent bilaterally in the caudate nuclei *(arrows).*

Teaching Point:

Absent or markedly diminished tracer activity in the caudate nuclei is a frequent and characteristic pattern observed in patients with Huntington's disease.

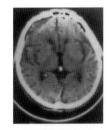

CASE FIG. 6.25A

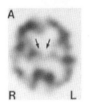 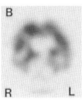 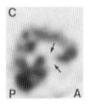

CASE FIG. 6.25B

Clinical Diagnosis:
Huntington's Disease

CONTRIBUTORS:

Robert S. Hellman, M.D.,
Ronald S. Tikofsky, M.D.
Institution: Medical College of Wisconsin

IMAGING DATA:

Camera: GE Neurocam
Tracer: ^{99m}Tc HMPAO

Collimator: High-resolution
Dose: 30 mCi

This 40-year-old woman was referred for further evaluation of a long history of Huntington's disease with progressive dementia.

A CT scan (Fig. 6.26 A,B) showed diffuse cerebral atrophy with mild dilation of the lateral and third ventricles. In addition, the caudate nuclei were indistinctly visualized.

An HMPAO study (Fig. 6.26C) in the transaxial plane revealed markedly decreased tracer uptake in the caudate nuclei. The decrease in tracer activity was greater on the left. There is also decreased tracer uptake in the right inferior frontal lobe.

Teaching Points:

1. The caudate nuclei will not be well visualized in Huntington's disease.

2. SPECT images will reflect either absent tracer uptake or various degrees of reduced tracer uptake. These findings may be asymmetric.

3. The presence of decreased tracer uptake in the cortex typically occurs with changes in cognitive function.

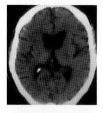 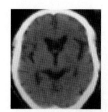

CASE FIG. 6.26A   **CASE FIG. 6.26B**

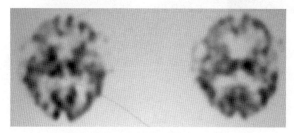

CASE FIG. 6.26C

Clinical Diagnosis:
Huntington's Disease

CONTRIBUTORS:

Robert S. Hellman, M.D.,
Ronald S. Tikofsky, M.D.
Institution: Medical College of Wisconsin

IMAGING DATA:

Camera: GE Neurocam
Tracer: ^{99m}Tc HMPAO

Collimator: High-resolution
Dose: 30 mCi

This 33-year-old woman with a known history of Huntington's disease was referred for evaluation of an exacerbation of symptoms. At the time of presentation, the patient's symptoms had progressed, with a recent increase in uncontrollable movements and episodes of choking during eating.

An MRI (Case Fig. 6.27A,B) demonstrated atrophic caudate nuclei bilaterally consistent with the patient's diagnosis of Huntington's disease. There was also a subtle increase in signal intensity in the putamen bilaterally.

An HMPAO SPECT study (Case Fig. 6.27C) in the transaxial plane showed decreased tracer uptake in both caudate nuclei, right greater than left. Decrease in tracer uptake was also observed in the right temporal region. These findings are compatible with the diagnosis of Huntington's disease.

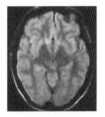 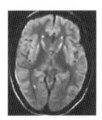

CASE FIG. 6.27A   **CASE FIG. 6.27B**

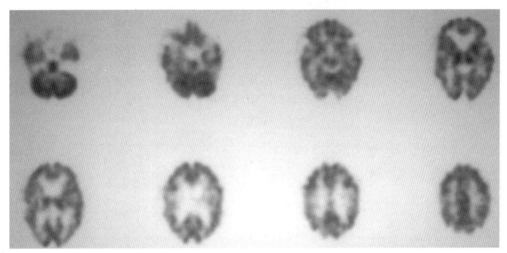

CASE FIG. 6.27C

Clinical Diagnosis:

HIV Encephalopathy: Pre- and Postazodithymidine Therapy

CONTRIBUTOR:	IMAGING DATA:	
Ronald L. Van Heertum, M.D.	**Camera:** GE 3000 XCT	**Collimator:** Ultra-high-resolution
Institution: Columbia-Presbyterian Medical Center	**Tracer:** ⁹⁹ᵐTc HMPAO	**Dose:** (1) 21.0 mCi; (2) 20.5 mCi

This 30-year-old known HIV-seropositive man presented for evaluation of progressive memory loss.

CT scan was negative.

The initial HMPAO SPECT (Case Fig. 6.28A) in the coronal (**A**) and sagittal (**B**) planes, revealed a mild overall reduction in radiotracer uptake with a heterogeneous distribution throughout the cortex.

Subsequent to the initial SPECT scan, the patient was placed on azodithymidine, with significant clinical improvement.

A follow-up HMPAO SPECT study (Case Fig. 6.28B) in the coronal (**A**) and sagittal (**B**) planes revealed an overall improvement in radiotracer distribution.

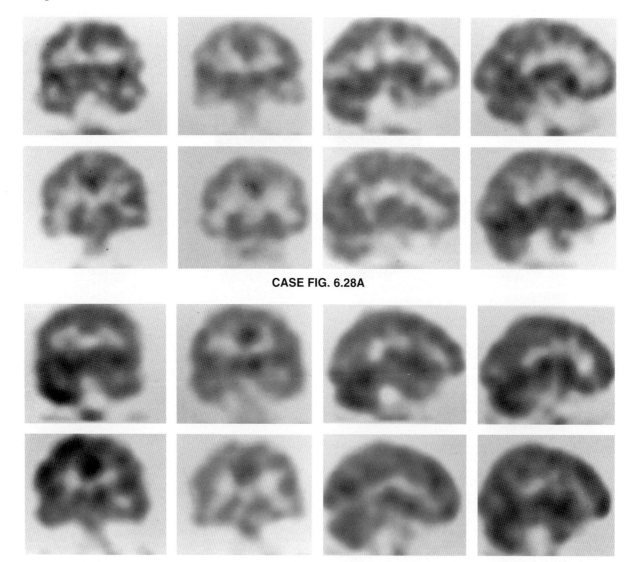

CASE FIG. 6.28A

CASE FIG. 6.28B

CASE 6-29

Clinical Diagnosis:
AIDS-Related Dementia

CONTRIBUTOR:	**IMAGING DATA:**	
Ronald L. Van Heertum, M.D.	**Camera:** GE 400 AC/T;Star II	**Collimator:** High-resolution
Institution: St. Vincent's Hospital and Medical Center	**Tracer:** ^{123}I IMP	**Dose:** 3.0 mCi

This 37-year-old bisexual man was referred for evaluation of the acute onset of dementia; he also complained of blurred vision and generalized headaches. His neurologic examination revealed a right hemiparesis and an expressive aphasia. Laboratory tests showed him to be seropositive for the HIV antigen.

A CT scan (Case Fig. 6.29A) was negative.

A SPECT study (Case Fig. 6.29B) in the transaxial (**A**), coronal (**B**), and sagittal (**C**) planes showed a decreased tracer deposition in the left frontal and parietooccipital lobes (*arrowheads*), with a slight decrease in tracer activity in the right parietal-occipital lobe (*open arrow*). Radiotracer deposition was also decreased in then thalamus, particularly on the left side (*arrow*).

Teaching Point:

As shown in this case, the cerebral SPECT study may be positive despite a negative CT or MRI scan. The typical pattern in AIDS-related dementia shows random cortical defects combined with subcortical defects.

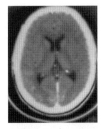

CASE FIG. 6.29A

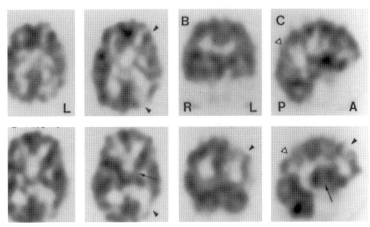

CASE FIG. 6.29B

CASE 6-30

Clinical Diagnosis:
HIV Encephalopathy

CONTRIBUTOR:	IMAGING DATA:	
Scott Miller, M.D.	**Camera:** GE Neurocam	**Collimator:** Ultra-high-resolution
Institution: Columbia-Presbyterian Medical Center	**Tracer:** 99mTc HMPAO	**Dose:** 21.7 mCi

This 42-year-old woman with known AIDS was referred for evaluation of a progressive alteration in her mental status characterized by increasing apathy, confusion, and progressive memory loss.

An MRI examination revealed mild cortical atrophy.

HMPAO SPECT (Case Fig. 6.30), in the transaxial (**A**), coronal (**B**), and sagittal (**C**) planes revealed an overall decrease in radiotracer uptake with a superimposed markedly heterogeneous distribution pattern throughout the cerebral cortex.

Published with permission from Van Heertum RL, Miller SH, Moesson R. SPECT brain imaging in neurologic disease. *Radiol Clin North Am* 1993;31:881–907.

Teaching Point:

Cerebral SPECT is a highly sensitive technique for the detection of HIV encephalopathy.

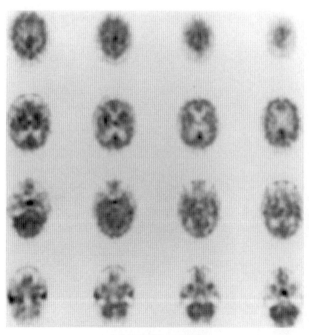

CASE FIG. 6.30A

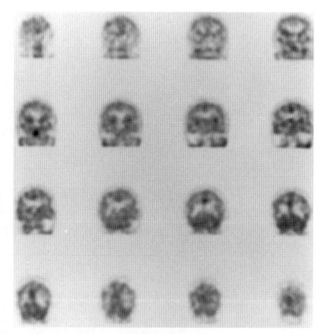

CASE FIG. 6.30B

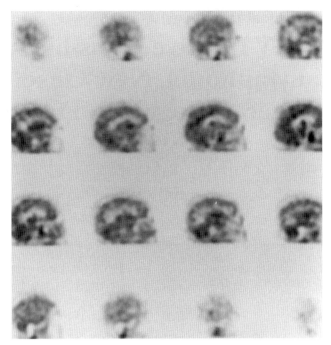

CASE FIG. 6.30C

Clinical Diagnosis:

HIV-Positive, Possible Atypical Lymphoma, New-Onset Seizures, and Altered Cognitive Function

CONTRIBUTORS:	IMAGING DATA:	
Ronald S. Tikofsky, Ph.D.,	**Camera:** Prism 3000	**Collimator:** High-resolution fan-beam
Roberta C. Locko, M.D.	**Tracer:** ^{99m}Tc ECD	**Dose:** 3.23 mCi ^{201}Tl 29.6 mCi (ECD)
Institution: Columbia University, Harlem Hospital Center		

This 33-year-old man had a history or hypertension and end-stage renal disease; he is HIV/AIDS (CDC-4) positive. The patient presented with a new onset of seizures and altered cognitive function.

An MRI revealed abnormalities in periventricular white matter signal as well as a focal abnormality in the left parietal lobe, which could represent toxoplasmosis or lymphoma. An anterior cerebral artery infarction (ACA) infarct was also part of the differential (Case Fig. 6-31A,B). A contrast CT scan of the brain showed edema of the left frontal periventricular white matter extending to involve the cortex medially, with mass effect on the frontal horn. Findings suggested lymphoma vs. infarct, less likely toxoplasmosis. A ^{201}Tl SPECT scan performed to evaluate the possibility of lymphoma was negative.

The SPECT ECD study shows a heterogenous pattern of decreased tracer up take throughout the brain. The most prominent regions of decreased perfusion are seen in the posterior temporoparietal regions, right greater than left (Case Fig. 6.31C). This perfusion pattern is often seen in patients with HIV/AIDS dementia.

Teaching Point:

The combination of ^{201}Tl and ^{99m}Tc SPECT imaging may be helpful in establishing the presence of lymphoma and AIDS-related dementia.

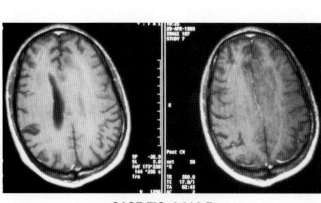

CASE FIG. 6.31A,B

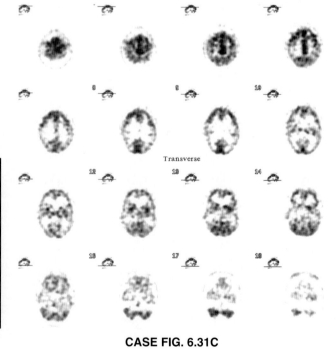

Transverse

CASE FIG. 6.31C

Clinical Diagnosis:
HIV Dementia

CONTRIBUTORS:	IMAGING DATA:	
Ronald S. Tikofsky, Ph.D.,	**Camera:** PRISM 3000	**Collimator:** High-resolution fan-beam
Candido Quinones, M.D.,	**Tracer:** ^{99m}Tc ECD	**Dose:** 21.7, 28.2, 30.5 mCi
Vladimir Berthaud, M.D.		
Institution: Columbia University, Harlem		
Hospital Center		

This 37-year-old man was admitted with markedly altered mental status. He was unresponsive, and there was a question as to whether he had toxoplasmosis or central nervous system (CNS) lymphoma. After being placed on antitoxoplasmosis medication, he demonstrated steady improvement in mental status and was discharged to a long-term care facility. At time of discharge, the patient was coherent and ambulatory.

An initial CT scan of the brain showed multiple lucencies. Follow-up CT scan of the brain revealed a significant reduction in the lucencies (Case Fig. 6-32A,B). A ^{201}TI scan was negative for lymphoma.

This patient had three SPECT ECD scans and one ^{201}Tl scan. The initial SPECT scan showed marked heterogeneity of radiotracer uptake, which is markedly decreased for age. In addition, there is some evidence of areas of absence or near-absence radiotracer activity in the right frontal and parietal regions. There is also gross distortion of the right frontal lobe, consistent with the CT findings. Mild crossed cerebellar diaschisis (decreased activity in the left cerebellar hemisphere) is present. There is near-normal radiotracer

uptake to the basal ganglia, thalamus, and occipital cortex. A follow-up ECD SPECT 2 weeks after the initial scan shows marked improvement of radiotracer uptake. The crossed cerebellar diaschisis is resolved and there is near-normal but still heterogenous radiotracer uptake to both hemispheres except for the temporoparietal regions, left greater than right. The distortion of the frontal lobes is almost completely resolved. The patient's mental state was significantly improved at this time. A final follow-up ECD SPECT scan showed continue improvement with only minor decreases in radiotracer uptake. This is consistent with the improved findings on CT and the patient's clinical status. The course of these changes is shown in the transverse (Case Fig. 6.32C) and sagittal images (Case Fig. 6.32D).

Teaching Point:

SPECT imaging in patients with AIDS dementia and presumed toxoplasmosis or lymphoma can be useful in ruling out lymphoma and monitoring the effectiveness of antitoxoplasmosis therapy.

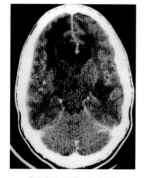 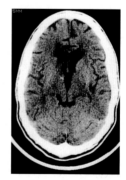

CASE FIG. 6.32A   **CASE FIG. 6.32B**

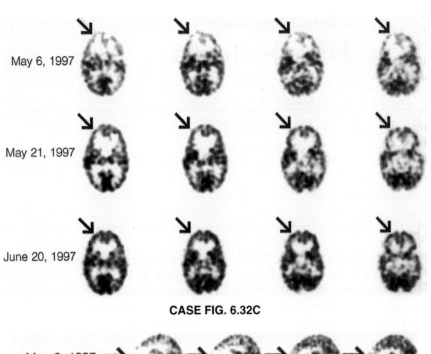

May 6, 1997

May 21, 1997

June 20, 1997

CASE FIG. 6.32C

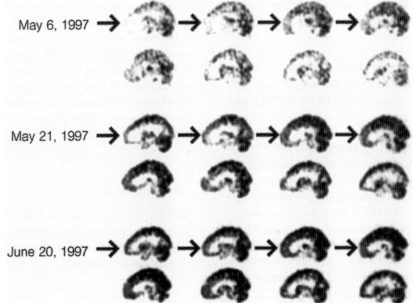

May 6, 1997

May 21, 1997

June 20, 1997

CASE FIG. 6.32D

CASE 6-33

Clinical Diagnosis:
Brain Lymphoma

CONTRIBUTOR:	IMAGING DATA:	
Dominique Delbeke, M.D., Ph.D.	**PET Scanner:** Siemens ECAT 933 and	**Collimator:** High-energy fan-beam method:
Institution: Vanderbilt University Medical	Elscint Varicam	**Dose:** 10 mCi
Center	**Tracer:** ^{18}FDG	

This 33-year-old man with AIDS presented with increasing confusion.

A gadolinium-enhanced T1-weighted MRI image demonstrates a large enhancing mass in the left frontal lobe (Case Fig. 6.33A).

A corresponding PET image demonstrates marked ^{18}FDG uptake in the lesion (Case Fig. 6.33B) indicative of lymphoma rather than toxoplasmosis. Fluorodeoxy glucose

SPECT images (Case Fig. 6.33C) also demonstrate marked ^{18}FDG uptake; however, the image quality suffers from the limited sensitivity of the technique.

Teaching Point:

Fluorodeoxyglucose imaging can differentiate lymphoma from toxoplasmosis in AIDS patients.

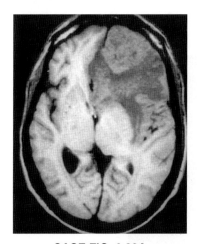

CASE FIG. 6.33A

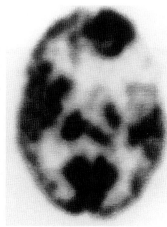

CASE FIG. 6.33B

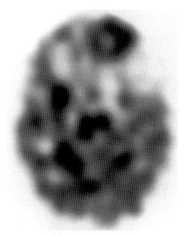

CASE FIG. 6.33C

Clinical Diagnosis:
Parkinson's Disease and Memory Problems

CONTRIBUTORS:

James M. Mountz, M.D., Ph.D.,
Michael V. Yester, Ph.D.
Institution: The University of Alabama at
Birmingham Medical Center

IMAGING DATA:

Camera: Picker PRISM 3000 XP
Tracer: [99m]Tc HMPAO

Collimator: LEUHR parallel-hole
Dose: 30 mCi

This 59-year-old man with a long-standing history of Parkinson's disease is now showing signs of memory problems. Parkinson's disease's a movement disorder associated with degeneration of the substantia nigra and dysfunction of the nigrostriatal pathways with resulting decrease in dopamine presence at the synapse of the globus pallidus. An associated characteristic of this disease is parkinsonian dementia.

A transverse-plane HMPAO SPECT scan (Case Fig. 6.34) reveals that parkinsonian dementia has a perfusion pattern on SPECT scans that is similar to that of Alzheimer's disease except that there is relative sparing of the frontal lobes and greater accentuation of the decreased perfusion to the temporal parietal regions (*arrows*).

Teaching Points:

Parkinson's dementia can be diagnosed on ^{99m}Tc HMPAO brain SPECT scans. It remains to be seen if Parkinson's dementia responds to the acetylcholinesterase inhibitors, which are currently approved for therapeutic use in Alzheimer's disease.

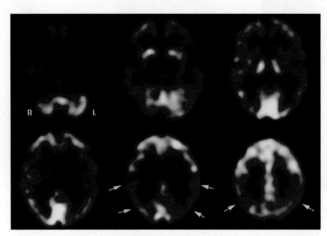

CASE FIG. 6.34

Clinical Diagnosis:
Parkinson Syndrome

CONTRIBUTOR:	IMAGING DATA:	
John P. Seibyl, M.D.	128 × 128 matrix, two-dimensional	**Attenuation Correction**
Institution: Yale University School of Medicine	Butterworth filter then ramp filter for back projection	**Method:** Chang 0 algorithm
	Camera: Picker PRISM 3000 XP	**Collimator:** Fan-beam
	Tracer: [123]I beta-CIT	**Dose:** 6.0 mCi

Eleven years earlier, this 39-year-old woman had a left thalamic and anterior midbrain arteriovenous malformation (AVM) treated with proton-beam radiation and subsequent gamma-knife irradiation to the left midbrain for recurrent hemorrhage. The patient now presents with a 1-year history of hemiparkinsonian symptoms, including right upper and lower extremity bradykinesia and gait disturbance.

Arteriovenous malformation in left midbrain with decreased flow to left substantia nigra.

Images show marked unilateral reduction of dopamine transporters in the left basal ganglia (Case Fig. 6.35).

Teaching Points:

This patient with unilateral loss of dopamine nigra cells, presumably in the context of AVM and its treatment, now presents with mild parkinsonian symptoms. SPECT demonstrated a marked unilateral reduction in dopamine transporter binding consistent with the patient's clinical findings.

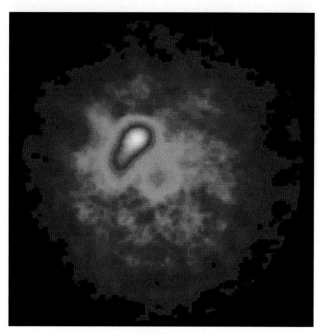

CASE FIG. 6.35

Clinical Diagnosis:
Idiopathic Parkinson's Disease

CONTRIBUTOR:	IMAGING DATA:
Ferruccio Fazio, M.D.	**PET Scanner:**
Institution: Universitá Di Milano—Polo H.S.	**Tracer:** I 123 beta-CIT
Raffaele, Instituto D'Scienze	
Radiologiche, Cattedra Di	
Medicina Nucleare (Milan)	

This is a patient with a clinical history of idiopathic Parkinson's disease.

Transaxial SPECT images of the distribution of dopamine reuptake site in the basal ganglia. Case Fig. 6.36 shows re-duced tracer uptake in the basal ganglia, which is particularly pronounced in the putamen rather than the caudate nucleus.

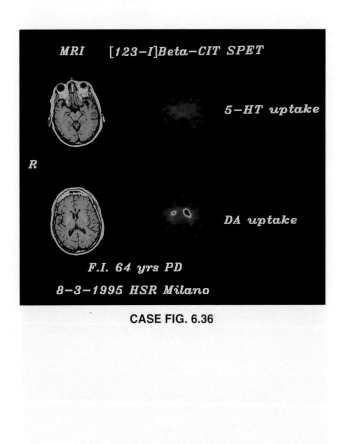

CASE FIG. 6.36

Clinical Diagnosis:

Hoehn-Yahr Stage 1 Parkinson's Disease, Hoehn-Yahr Stage 4 Parkinson's Disease, and a Healthy Control

CONTRIBUTOR:

John P. Seibyl, M.D.

Institution: Yale University School of Medicine

IMAGING DATA:

64 × 64 matrix, two-dimensional Butterworth filter then ramp filter for back projection

Camera: Ceraspect SPECT tomograph, Digital Scintigraphics, Inc.

Tracer: [123]I beta-CIT

Correction Method: Chang 0 algorithm

Collimator: Parallel-hole

Dose: 6.0 mCi

Images show normal and symmetric appearance of the basal ganglia in a healthy control subject. The stage 1 Parkinson's disease (PD) subject demonstrates hemiparkinsonian symptoms on the left side, contralateral to the side of greatest reduction in DA transporters on the SPECT scan. This scan also shows changes on the side ipsilateral to the motor symptoms, indicating that SPECT is sensitive to changes prior to the development of clinical symptoms. There is greater involvement of the putamen relative to the caudate, consistent with postmortem findings. The stage 4 patient shows marked bilateral reduction of tracer uptake consistent with the degree of functional motor impairment. These features are seen in Case Fig. 6.37.

Teaching Points:

Dopamine transporter imaging with ^{123}I beta-CIT SPECT shows reductions in striatal binding, which correlate with the degree of motor impairment. SPECT imaging demonstrates preclinical alterations in brain in patients with early PD.

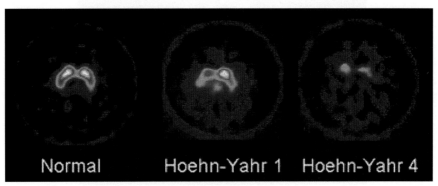

CASE FIG. 6.37

CASE 6-38

Clinical Diagnosis:
Multiple System Atrophy (MSA)

CONTRIBUTOR:	**IMAGING DATA:**	
John P. Seibyl, M.D.	128 × 128 matrix, two-dimensional	**Attenuation Correction**
Institution: Yale University School of Medicine	Butterworth filter then ramp filter for back projection	**Method:** Chang 0 algorithm
	Camera: Picker PRISM 3000XP	**Collimator:** Fan-beam
	Tracer: ¹²³I beta-CIT	**Dose:** 6.0 mCi

This 64-year-old man presented with motor and gait disturbance and autonomic dysregulation.

Images show marked bilateral reduction of radiotracer uptake in the striatum (Case Fig. 6.38).

Teaching Points:

Multiple system atrophy, a parkinsonionan syndrome is characterized by reduction of radiotracer uptake in the striatum. While this entity is difficult to distinguish on the basis of the SPECT study from idiopathic Parkinson's disease (PD), the uptake tends to be more symmetrically reduced. There is also less of a putamen-to-caudate gradient in MSA as compared with PD.

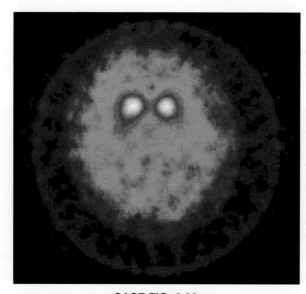

CASE FIG. 6.38

Clinical Diagnosis:
Parkinson's Disease Dementia

CONTRIBUTOR:	IMAGING DATA:	
Angela Lignelli, M.D.	**PET Scanner:** Siemens XACT 47	**Attenuation Correction**
Institution: New York Presbyterian Medical Center	**Tracer:** ^{18}FDG	**Method:** Autoattenuation
		Dose: 9.35 mCi

This 60-year-old woman presented with progressive cognitive impairment of 4 years' duration. Her symptoms had become more pronounced over the preceding several months. The patient had also recently been treated for a movement disorder, with some improvement.

T1- and T2-weighted MRI (Case Fig. 6.39A) reveals mild diffuse atrophy.

PET images in the transverse, coronal, and sagittal planes reveal reduced radiotracer activity in the posterior parietal, temporal (right greater than left), and right occipital cortex with relative preservation of radiotracer activity in the subcortical and sensorimotor structures (Case Fig. 6.39B–D).

Teaching Points:

In the Lewy body disease variant of Alzheimer's disease, disorders such as Parkinson's disease frequently reveal evidence of occipital cortex involvement.

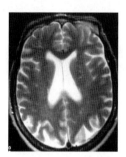

CASE FIG. 6.39A

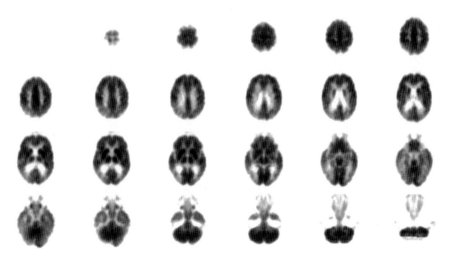

CASE FIG. 6.39B

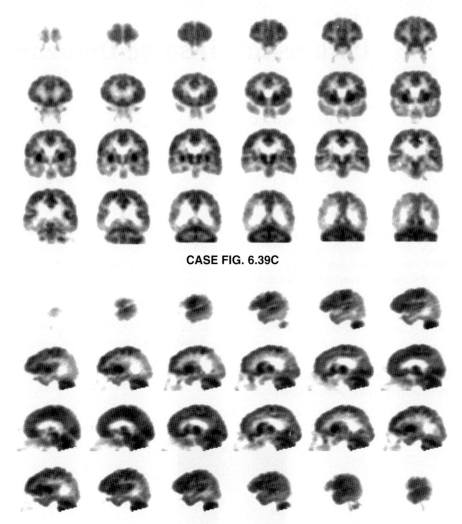

CASE FIG. 6.39C

CASE FIG. 6.39D

Clinical Diagnosis:

Meningioma; Possible Alzheimer's Disease

CONTRIBUTOR:	IMAGING DATA:	
Ramy Nour, M.D.	**Camera:** GE Neurocam	**Collimator:** High-resolution
Institution: Columbia-Presbyterian Medical Center	**Tracer:** ^{99m}Tc HMPAO	**Dose:** 21.6 mCi

This 71-year-old woman with a known hypertension and diabetes mellitus, presented with a 1-year history of progressive cognitive decline. In particular, she was noted to have profound short- and long-term memory loss, language dysfunction, and impaired abstract reasoning.

An MRI scan (Case Fig. 6.42A,B) in the axial (**A**) and coronal (**B**) planes demonstrated a mass lesion consistent with a meningioma adjacent to the left temporal lobe.

The finding of a meningioma was felt to be incidental and unrelated to the patient's cognitive decline. As a result, the patient had been given a provisional clinical diagnosis of Alzheimer's disease.

An HMPAO SPECT study (Case Fig. 6.42C) in the transaxial plane revealed a focal area of increased radiotracer activity corresponding to the meningioma seen on the MRI study.

Teaching Point:

This case demonstrates the importance of correlating the SPECT and MRI studies. Other causes of focal increase in radiotracer activity include other tumors, seizure disorders, and luxury perfusion.

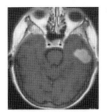

CASE FIG. 6.42A

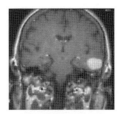

CASE FIG. 6.42B

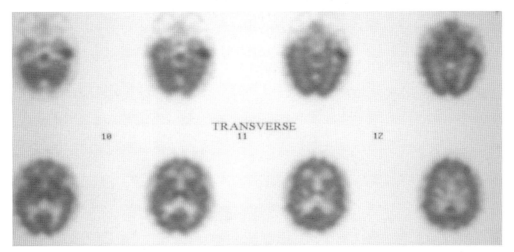

TRANSVERSE

10   11   12

CASE FIG. 6.42C

Functional Cerebral SPECT and PET Imaging, Third Edition,
edited by R.L.Van Heertum and R.S. Tikofsky,
Lippincott Williams & Wilkins, New York © 2000.

CHAPTER 7

Seizure Disorders

Ronald S. Tikofsky and Ronald L. Van Heertum

Devous reports that approximately 50,000 persons in the United States have medically refractory seizures (1). At least 500 patients per year undergo surgical treatment to eliminate or reduce the frequency and/or severity of their seizures. Many patients electing this therapeutic option as a technique for localizing the seizure focus improve.

Essential to the success of these surgical interventions is the accurate localization of the seizures. The clinical application of single-photon-emission computed tomography (SPECT) and position-emission tomography (PET) imaging to the study of patients with complicated epilepsy, both children and adults, is becoming increasingly common in centers where surgical intervention for the treatment of complex partial seizures is performed (2–4). When seizure patients are referred for SPECT/PET imaging, it is essential that the type of seizure pattern and its clinical localization should have been determined. This knowledge will help in the evaluation of the images, since many epileptic patients present with more than one type of seizure pattern. It is essential, therefore, that nuclear medicine physicians performing functional imaging studies on these patients appreciate the variation in the presentation of seizure disorders. In 1989, the International League Against Epilepsy (ILAE) proposed a universal classification system for the epilepsies. This classification system is still commonly used by epileptologists.

The epilepsies are gererally divided into two major groups. The first distinguishes epilepsies characterized by generalized seizures from those involving focal or partial seizures. Focal and partial seizures are "localization-related partial or focal epilepsies." The second major group distinguishes be-

tween epilepsies with a known etiology (called symptomatic or "secondary") and the idiopathic (primary) and cryptogenic epilepsies (whose etilogy is unclear or occult).

"Temporal lobe syndromes" represent the most common seizure pattern referred to the nuclear medicine laboratory for imaging. Typically, the components of the syndrome are simple partial complex seizures, complex partial seizures, and possibly also generalized seizures. Some patients exhibit a combination of these features. It is important to distinguish between simple partial seizures, whose features are autonomic, possibly including psychic symptoms and/or sensory experiences, and complex partial seizures, which often begin with motor arrest followed by automatisms. These seizures usually last less than 1 min and are followed by postictal confusion, amnesia, and gradual recovery.

Patients with two other types of temporal lobe seizures are frequently referred for functional imaging. One is the amygdalohippocampal type, sometimes called a mesiobasal limbic or rhinencephalic seizure. These disorders are similar to the other types of temporal lobe seizures described above, but patients with this type of seizure pattern rarely show auditory symptoms. Rather, they are characterized by epigastric distress, marked autonomic signs, fear, panic, and olfactory-gustatory hallucinations. The other group comprises what have been termed *lateral temporal seizures* (LTS). Patients with simple LST seizures tend to have audiotory hallucinations or illusions and dream-like states as well as linguistic and visual misperceptions. The particular pattern depends on the hemisphere involved. If there is seizure propagation to the mesial temporal or extratemporal structures, the simple seizure can evolve into a complex partial seizure.

Frontal lobe epilepsies constitute another major group of seizure patterns. These seizures can present as simple, complex partial, secondarily generalized, or any combination of these patterns. Frontal lobe seizures tend to occur frequently in the course of the day and may even occur during sleep. Status epilepticus is a frequent complication. The seizures in

R. S. Tikofsky: Department of Radiology, Columbia University College of Physicians and Surgeons, Harlem Hospital Center, New York, New York 10037.

R. L. Van Heertum: Department of Radiology, Columbia University College of Physicians and Surgeons, New York, New York 10032.

this group tend to be short; if they are of the partial complex type, postictal confusion is rarely observed. Tonic or postural motor manifestations with complex gestural automatisms are frequently seen at seizure onset, and when there are bilateral discharges, falling is common. The specific pattern presented by a given patient is related to the particular region of seizure activity in the various frontal lobe territories (supplementary motor, cingulate, motor cortex, etc.). Seizures arising from the parietal and/or occipital lobes are less frequently seen.

Research reports demonstrate that SPECT and PET imaging can play a major role in the identification of epileptogenic foci in patients with medically intractible complex partial seizures who are candidates for temporal lobe resection (5–9). These studies focus on SPECT/PET imaging in the interictal (baseline) state. Two other approaches to presurgical seizure localization with SPECT/PET are in current use. One is to perform "ictal" studies. This involves injection of the tracer at or during ictus (10,11). The other is to inject the tracer in the immediate postictal state (12,13). The choice of options and imaging approaches, SPECT or PET, is somewhat dependent upon institutional logistics in performing the studies and the stability and half-life of the tracers. Tracers that do not have good stability over time or have very short half-lives are difficult to prepare and deliver to a seizure unit and still capture a seizure in progress (ictus), since seizure duration is typically very brief. The availability of stable (up to 6 hr) tracers makes it more likely that one can inject at or during ictus. The most efficient situation for injecting during ictus is to have the tracer available in the seizure unit with a member of the epilepsy team trained to inject the tracer as soon as seizure activity is detected. This represents the ideal conditions for ictal studies, which capture the brain's perfusion and metabolic activity at a key point in time. Postictal injections (within 5 min postictus) are the more frequent occurrence. These studies can yield clinically useful information for seizure localization. Injection of tracers at ictus or in the postictal state provides a "snapshot" of the brain's activity at the time of injection. In the case of SPECT imaging, current radiopharmaceuticals remain fixed in the brain; thus, patients can be imaged as soon as they stabilize after a seizure or several hours postinjection without significant changes in tracer perfusion. This allows sufficient time for patients to be brought to the imaging area and increases the probability of identifying the physiologic changes associated with an active seizure focus. Seizure patterns on SPECT and PET have been shown to be similar (7,14).

During the interictal period, the seizure focus is identified by an area of reduced perfusion/metabolism in approximately 50% of patients. Baseline (interictal) scans will often have a normal appearance. During an active seizure (ictus), there will be an area of increased perfusion/metabolism that marks the site of the active seizure focus in approximately 80–90% of patients. Scans obtained with an immediate postical injection show a significant reduction of perfusion/metabolic activity, often in the medial temporal lobe. This may be accompanied by a spread of decreased perfusion/metabolic activity to the remaining temporal lobe. In some instances, changes in

perfusion/metabolism are seen in the opposite cerebral hemisphere or in the entire ipsilateral hemisphere. In addition to temporal lobe changes, there have been reports in both the SPECT and PET literature of hypoperfusion in subcortical regions in documented cases of unilateral mesial temporal lobe seizures (15,16). Findings of thalamic hypoperfusion during interictal SPECT studies of patients with temporal lobe epilepsy have now been reported (17). This phenomenon can be expected to occur in about 25% of cases. In addition, crossed cerebellar diaschisis has been observed during ictal imaging (18) in SPECT studies. It is possible that such occurrences will aid in seizure lateralization. The mechanisms underlying the observed changes in perfusion are not well understood. However, such findings can be expected in interictal or ictal SPECT or PET images.

SPECT imaging, because it has been more widely available at clinical sites, is becoming increasingly accepted as an important method for identifying single and multiple seizure foci. Similarly, as PET imaging capabilities expand into clinical settings, PET too will become accepted as a means for presurgical localization of epileptic foci. The combination of SPECT/PET with computed tomography (CT), magnetic resonance imaging (MRI), and electroencephalographic studies increases the accuracy of noninvasive lesion localization and improves the rate of surgical success (9,19,20). A recent metanalysis of SPECT brain imaging in epilepsy concludes that SPECT imaging has an important role to play in the management of refractory epilepsy by uniquely offering "the possibility of visualizing regional cerebral blood flow at all stages of a seizure" (21). The authors of the study assert that for temporal lobe epilepsy, this leads to an accuracy of approximately 90% in localizing the focus of the seizure. They do point out that the current literature is not in total support of their claim because of insufficient ictal SPECT studies.

SPECT imaging has also been used in conjunction with mapping the distribution of amobarbital sodium in intracarotid WADA testing to identify eloquent cortex. A critical issue in the performance of WADA testing is to be certain that the amobarbital sodium reaches the intended site. By injecting a radiotracer such as as Technetium 91-hexamethylopropyleneamine-oxime (^{99m}Tc-HMPAO) or ^{99m}Tc-Ethylcysteinate dimer (ECD) and performing SPECT imaging, the distribution of amobarbital can be more accurately traced. Jeffery et al. (22) reported on 25 patients studied using this approach. Their findings and those Biersack et al. (23) demonstrate that it is possible to determine the distribution of amobarbital when it is used in tandem with the WADA test procedure. Similar findings have been reported by Hietala et al. (24). The integration of SPECT imaging into protocols for routine WADA testing has not been widely adapted; however, it is still considered a useful application for determining the adequacy of the WADA injection. Duncan et al. (4) used PET mapping in lieu of WADA testing or intraoperative cortical stimulation to identify eloquent brain areas in children with seizures. Their results indicate that nonivasive PET brain mapping performed prior to surgery has the potential to reduce surgical risk and thus lead to an improved clinical outcome.

REFERENCES

1. Devous MD Sr. Comparison of SPECT applications in neurology and psychiatry. *J Clin Psychiatry* 1992;53(suppl):13–19.
2. Devous MD Sr. Leroy RF, Homan RW. Single photon emission computed tomography in epilepsy. *Sem Nucl Med* 1990;20:325–342.
3. Duncan R, Patterson, Hadley DM, et al. CT, MRI, and SPECT imaging in temporal lobe epilepsy. *J Neurol Neurosurg Psychiatry* 1990;53:11–15.
4. Duncan JD, Moss SD, Bandy DJ, et al. Use of positron emission tomography for presurgical localization of eloquent brain areas in children with seizures. *Pediatr Neurosurg* 1997;26:144–156.
5. Rowe CC, Bercovic SF, Sia STB, et al. Localization of epileptic foci with postictal single photon emission computed topography. *Ann Neurol* 1989;26:660–668.
6. Harvey AS, Hopkins IJ, Bowe JM, et al. Frontal lobe epilepsy: clinical seizure characteristics and localization with ictal 99m Tc-HMPAO SPECT. *Neurology* 1993;43:1966–1980.
7. Markand ON, Salanova V, Worth R, et al. Comparative study of interictal PET and ictal SPECT in comples partial seizures. *Acta Neurol Scand* 1997;95:129–136.
8. Gaillard WD, White S, Malow B, et al. FDG-PET in children and adolescents with partial seizures: role in epilepsy surgery evaluation. *Epilepsy Res* 1995;20:77–84.
9. Theodore WH, Sato S, Kufta CV, et al. FDG-positron emission tomography and invasive EEG: seizure focus detection and surgical outcome. *Epilepsia* 1997;38:81–86.
10. Newton MR, Austin MC, Chan JG, et al. Ictal SPECT using technetium-99m-HMPAO: methods for rapid preparation and optimal deployment of tracer during spontaneous seizures. *J Nucl Med* 1993;34:666–670.
11. Theodore WH, Balish M, Leiderman D, et al. Effect of seizures on cerebral blood flow measured with ^{15}O-H$_2$O and positron emission tomography. *Epilepsia* 1996;37:796–802.
12. Newton MR, Berkovic SF, Austin MC, et al. Postctal switch in blood flow distribution and temporal lobe seizures. *J Neurol Neurosurg Psychiatry* 1992;55:891–894.
13. Rowe CC, Berkovic SF, Austin MC, et al. Patterns of postictal cerebral blood flow in temporal lobe epilepsy: quantitative and qualitative findings. *Neurology* 1991;41:1096–1103.
14. Ryvlin P, Phiippon B, Cinotti L, et al. Functional neuroimaging strategy in temporal lobe epilepsy: a comparative study of 18 FDG-PET and 99mTc-HMPAO-SPECT. *Ann Neurol* 1990;27:162–166.
15. Sperling MR, Gur RC, Alavi A, et al. Subcortical metabolic alterations in partial epilepsy. *Epilepsia* 1990;31:145–155.
16. Rausch R, Henry TR, Ary CM, et al. Asymmetric interictal glucose hypometabolism and cognitive performance in epileptic patients. *Arch Neurol* 1994;51:139–144.
17. Yune MJ, Lee JD, Ryu YH, et al. Ipsilateral thalamic hypoperfusion on interictal SPECT in temporal lobe epilepsy. *J Nucl Med* 1998;39:281–185.
18. Duncan R, Patterson J, Bone I, et al. Tc99m HMPAO single photon emission tomography in in temporal lobe epilepsy. *Acta Neuol Scand* 1990;81:287–293.
19. Tikofsky RS, Morris GL, Hellman RS, et al. rCBF/.SPECT seizure evaluation in surgical candidates. Reader agreement and relation to surgical site (abstr). *Epilepsia* 1992;34(suppl);134.
20. Delbeke D, Lawrence SK, Abou-Khalil BW, et al. Postsurgical outcome of patients with uncontrolled complex partial seizures and temporal lobe hypometabolism on 18FDG-positron emission tomography. *Invest Radiol* 1996;31:261–266.
21. Devous MD Sr, Thisted RA, Morgan GF, et al. SPECT brain imaging in epilepsy: a meta-analysis. *J Nucl Med* 1998;39:285–293.
22. Jeffery PJ, Monsieu LH, Szabo Z, et al. Mapping the distribution of amobarbital sodium in the intracarotid Wada test for use of Tc-99m HMPAO with SPECT. *Radiology* 1991;178:847–850.
23. Biersack HJ, Linke D, Brassel F, et al. Technetium-99m-HMPAO brain SPECT in epileptic patients before and during unilateral hemispheric anesthesia (Wada test): Report of three cases. *J Nucl Med* 1987;28:1763–1767.
24. Hietala S-O, Sivenius H, Aasley J, et al. Brain perfusion with intracarotid injection of 99m-Tc-HMPAO in partial complex epilepsy during amobarbital testing. *Eur J Nucl Med* 1990;16:683–687.

SUGGESTED READINGS

Chugani HT. The use of positron emission tomography in the clinical assessment of epilepsy. *Semin Nucl Med* 1992;22:247–253.

Devous MD Sr, Leroy RF, Homan RW. Single photon emission computed tomography in epilepsy. *Sem Nucl Med* 1990;20:325–341.

Hotta SS. 18F-labeled 2-deoxy-2-fluoro-D-glucose positron-emission tomography scans for the localization of the epileptogenic foci. *Health Technol Assess Rep* 1998;12:1–17.

Juni JE, Waxman AD, Devous MD Sr, et al. Procedure guidelines for brain perfusion SPECT using technetium-99m radiopharmaceuticals. Society of Nuclear Medicine. *J Nucl Med* 1998;39:923–926.

Kuzniecky RI. Neuroimaging in pediatric epilepsy. *Epilepsia* 1996; 37(suppl 1):S10–S21.

Lamusuo S, Ruottienen HM, Knuuti J, et al. Comparison of [^{18}F] FDG-PET, [^{99m}Tc]-HMPAO-SPECT, and [^{123}I]-iomazenil-SPECT in localising the epileptogenic cortex. *J Neurol Neurosurg Psychiatry* 1997;63:743–748.

Sadzot B. Neuroimaging in epilepsy: is there a future for positron emission tomography? *Epilepsia* 1996;37:511–514.

Sperling MR. Neuroimaging in epilepsy. *Neurol Clin* 1993;11:883–903.

Clinical Diagnosis:
Medically Intractable Seizure Disorder

CONTRIBUTOR:	IMAGING DATA:	
James Mountz, M.D., Ph.D.	**Camera:** ADAC dual-headed Genesys	**Collimator:** High-resolution
Institution: University of Alabama Hospital	**Tracer:** ^{99m}Tc HMPAO	**Dose:** 15 mCi

This 10-year-old boy with known seizures since age 2 1/2 years was referred for evaluation of progressively increasing seizure activity uncontrolled by medication. At the time of referral, the patient averaged 30–40 seizures per day. The seizures were characterized by tonic extension of the left arm and nonpurposeful movement of the arm with preservation of consciousness. Repeat electroencephalographys (EEGs) showed mild background slowing with occasional sharp discharges and slow-wave activity in the right frontocentroparietal region interictally.

Multiple CT and MRI examinations were performed, and all were negative (Fig. 7.1A).

An HMPAO SPECT study (Fig. 7.1B) in the transaxial plane obtained during ictus revealed a focus of increased tracer activity in the right premotor cortex. This finding was felt to represent the site of the seizure focus. This region was surgically excised; pathologic tissue examination revealed cortical dysplasia.

Teaching Point:

As with ^{123}I IMP SPECT, ^{99m}Tc HMPAO SPECT studies will frequently demonstrate foci of increased radiotracer deposition at the site of the seizure focus at the time of ictus.

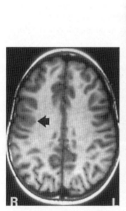

CASE FIG. 7.1A

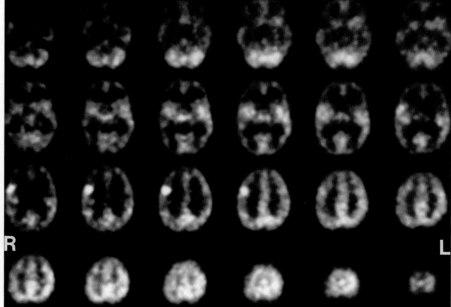

CASE FIG. 7.1B

Clinical Diagnosis:
Partial Complex Intractable Seizures

CONTRIBUTORS:	IMAGING DATA:	
Ronald L. Van Heertum, M.D.,	**PET Scanner:** Siemens XACT 47	**Attenuation Correction Method:**
Angela Lignelli, M.D.	**Tracer:** [18]FDG labeled	Autoattenuation protocol
Institution: New York Presbyterian Medical		**Dose:** 1.17 mCi
Center		

This 1-year-old girl with right hemimyencephaly and a history of infantile spasms since age 1 month had a recent change in seizure type to partial complex. She was poorly controlled with gabapentin, phenobarbital, and phenytoin and continued to have five to six seizures per day.

A video EEG study was reported to show a right temporal seizure focus. An MRI study (Fig. 7.2A) revealed right hemimyencephaly with indistinct right frontoparietal gyri (dysplasia) and right cerebral white matter changes, hypoplastic splenium, as well as slight left cerebral atrophy.

At the time of the intravenous injection of 1.7 mCi of [18]FDG labeled, the patient was seizing, with flexion of all extremities and face contortion for approximately 3 min. Approximately 15 min later, she was again observed to be seizing. The patient experienced a similar episode 20 minutes postinjection; at this time, she was sedated with 200 mg po of chloral hydrate. This study revealed (Fig. 7.2B–D) revealed a focal area of significantly increased tracer uptake in the right middle temporal lobe. Some increase in tracer uptake was also noted in the adjacent region of the posterior frontal lobe. In addition, regions of increased tracer uptake were observed in the posterior left temporal lobe extending to the left occipital lobe and in a small region of the left anterior frontal lobe.

Teaching Point:

Ictal PET scans may uncover more than a single hypermetabolic focus. The larger regions of hypermetabolic activity are the ones most often consistent with ictal seizure foci.

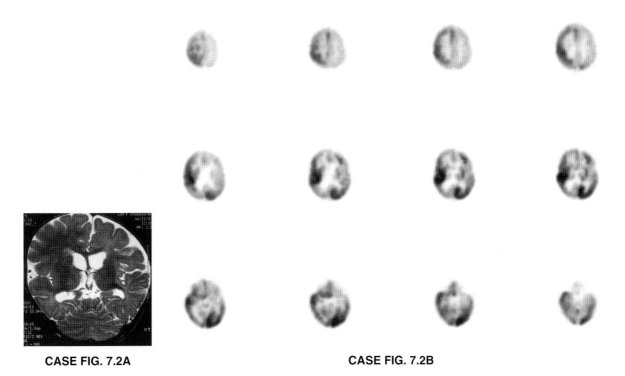

CASE FIG. 7.2A

CASE FIG. 7.2B

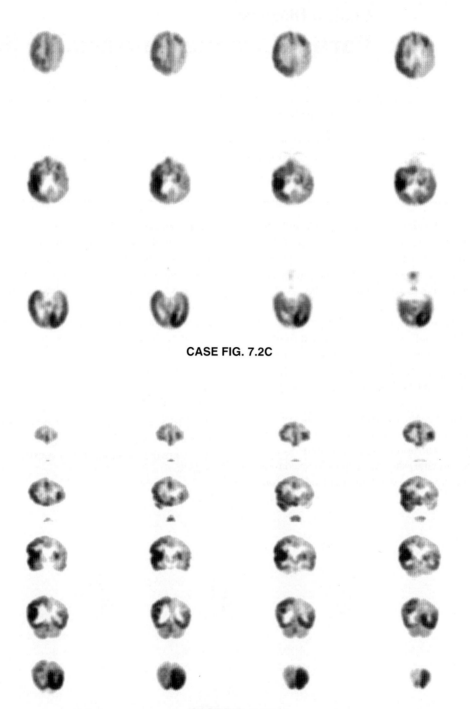

CASE FIG. 7.2C

CASE FIG. 7.2D

Clinical Diagnosis:
Intractable Epilepsy

CONTRIBUTORS:	IMAGING DATA:	
James M. Mountz, M.D., Ph.D.,	**Camera:** Picker PRISM 3000XP	**Collimator:** low-energy, high-resolution,
Elmer C. San Pedro, M.D.	**Tracer:** ^{99m}Tc HMPAO	parallel hole
Institution: The University of Alabama at		**Dose:** 18 mCi
Birmingham Medical Center		

This 14-year-old boy had a history of intractable epilepsy.

The transverse sections of ^{99m}Tc HMPAO ictal and interictal SPECT scans (Fig. 7.3A) are shown. The ictal scan was performed first and reveals an area of intense hyperemia in the right frontal lobe (*arrow*). The second scan, interictal, was performed to confirm the site of epileptic focus. This scan was coregistered with the ictal scan; a normal perfusion pattern is seen in the same region of the right frontal lobe.

Teachinig Points:

Comparing ictal ^{99m}Tc HMPAO or ^{99m}Tc ECD brain SPECT to the interictal SPECT significantly increases confidence in identifying an epileptogenic focus.

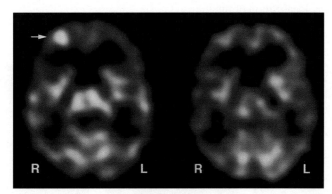

CASE FIG. 7.3

Clinical Diagnosis:
Intractable Epilepsy

CONTRIBUTORS:	IMAGING DATA:	
James M. Mountz, M.D., Ph.D.,	**Camera:** Picker PRISM 3000XP	**Collimator:** low-energy, high-resolution,
Elmer C. San Pedro, M.D.	**Tracer:** 99mTc HMPAO	parallel hole
Institution: The University of Alabama at		**Dose:** 18 mCi
Birmingham Medical Center		

This 9-year-old boy had a history of intractable epilepsy of 6 years' duration at the time of the study.

The patient's MRI study was normal for age (Fig. 7.4A).

Figure 7.4B (*arrow*) shows the transverse section of a 99mTc HMPAO scan performed 2 hr after bedside injection and 3 sec after seizure onset (the seizure lasted 25 sec). This ictal scan shows a focal area of intense tracer uptake in the right frontal lobe. Figure 7.4C (*arrow*) shows a "fusion image" of coregistered SPECT and MRI scans to yield more precise anatomic-physiologic localization of the

seizure focus in the frontal lobe. Based on the fusion image, the anatomic location was determined, the epileptogenic focus was surgically excised, and the patient is now seizure-free.

Teaching Point:

Ictal 99mTc HMPAO or 99mTc ECD brain SPECT for the identification of extra–temporal lobe seizures has extremely high accuracy (i.e., sensitivity and specificity).

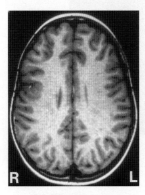

CASE FIG. 7.4A

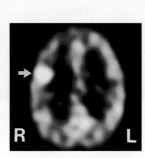

CASE FIG. 7.4B

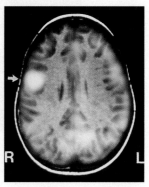

CASE FIG. 7.4C

Clinical Diagnosis:

Hypothalamic Hamartoma and Intractable Epilepsy

CONTRIBUTORS:

James M. Mountz, M.D., Ph.D.,

Elmer C. San Pedro, M.D.

Institution: The University of Alabama at
              Birmingham Medical Center

IMAGING DATA:

Camera: Picker PRISM 3000XP

Tracer: ^{99m}Tc HMPAO

Collimator: low-energy, high resolution,
            parallel hole

Dose: 18.5 mCi

This 16-year-old girl with a hypothalamic harmatoma presented with intractable seizures.

MRI reveals a hypothalamic hamartoma (Case Fig. 7.5, *arrow*).

An interictal transverse and sagittal ^{99m}Tc HMPAO SPECT image has a normal appearance (Case Fig. 7.5A, B). The ictal transverse and sagittal plane ^{99m}Tc HMPAO images reveal increased radiotracer uptake in the region of the hamartoma to best advantage (Case Fig. 7.5 C, D; *arrow*).

Teaching Points:

A comparison of the ^{99m}Tc HMPAO brain SPECT to the interictal SPECT can assist in determining whether the harmatoma was the likely origin of the seizures.

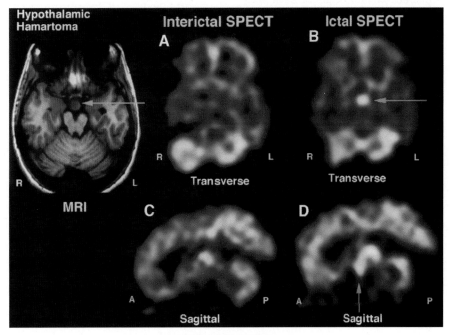

CASE FIG. 7.5A-D

Clinical Diagnosis:
Partial Epilepsy Due to Hypothalamic Hamartoma

CONTRIBUTOR:	IMAGING DATA:	
David H. Lewis, M.D.	**Camera:** Picker PRISM 3000	**Collimator:** Ultra-high-resolution fan-beam
Institution: Harborview Medical Center	**Tracer:** ^{99m}Tc ECD	**Dose:** 25 mCi × 2

This 12-year-old girl has had epilepsy since early childhood. It has recently become more serious, with the development of atonic episodes. She has gelastic seizures and precocious puberty due to a hypothalamic hamartoma.

MRI shows a hypothalamic hamartoma (Case Fig. 7.6A–C).

SPECT ECD studies were performed during an interictal period (Case Fig. 7.6D) and with ictus (Case Fig. 7.6E). Overlay display of MRI and SPECT (Case Fig. 7.6F) shows that there is ECD tracer uptake in the region of the hypothalamic hamartoma during ictus that is not present interictally. This implies that the seizures originate from the

hypothalamic hamartoma. Options for treatment might include surgery or radiation therapy for this benign neoplasm.

Teaching Points:

1. High-resolution brain SPECT can resolve very small lesions if there is uptake in them with ictus that is not present in the interictal period in epilepsy.

2. Image fusion and advanced computer techniques (as shown here on a Hermes work station from Nuclear Diagnostics) enable a direct comparison of functional and anatomic images and also comparison of different states in the same individual (e.g., ictal vs. interictal injections).

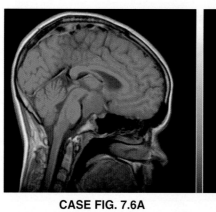
CASE FIG. 7.6A

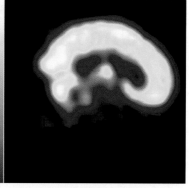
CASE FIG. 7.6D

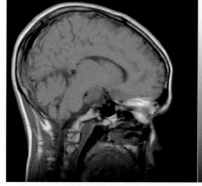
CASE FIG. 7.6B

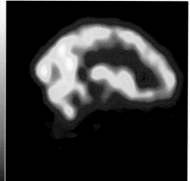
CASE FIG. 7.6E

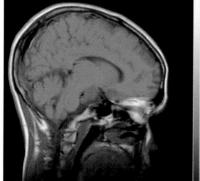
CASE FIG. 7.6C

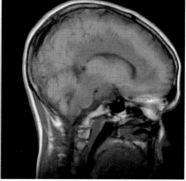
CASE FIG. 7.6F

Clinical Diagnosis:
Uncontrolled Seizures

CONTRIBUTORS:

Ronald L. Van Heertum, M.D.,

Jeffrey Naiman, M.D.

Institution: New York Presbyterian Medical
Center

IMAGING DATA:

PET Scanner: Siemens XACT 47

Tracer: [18]FDG labeled

Attenuation Correction Method:
Autoattenuation protocol

Dose: 2.25 mCi

This 6-year-old boy had poorly controlled seizure activity.

Transverse- and coronal-plane PET images (Case Fig. 7.7A–C) reveal decreased tracer uptake in the left temporal cortex, extending from the anterior to the posterior cortex. The seizure focus encompasses more of the temporal lobe than is typically seen.

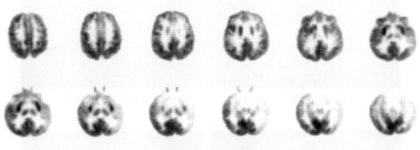

CASE FIG. 7.7A

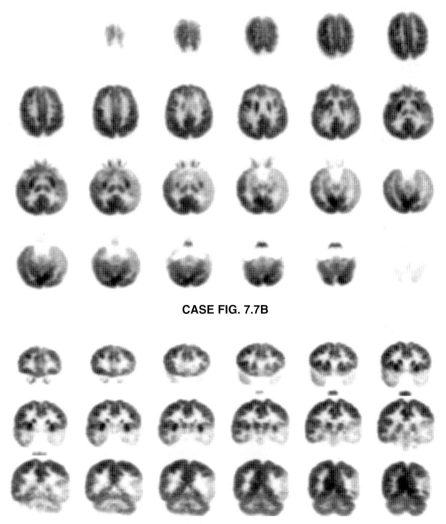

CASE FIG. 7.7B

CASE FIG. 7.7C

Clinical Diagnosis:
Complex Partial Seizures

CONTRIBUTORS:

Ronald L. Van Heertum, M.D.,
Jongwon Lee, M.D.
Institution: New York Presbyterian Medical
Center

IMAGING DATA:

PET Scanner: Siemens XACT 47
Tracer: [18]FDG

Attenuation Correction Method:
Autoattenuation protocol
Dose: 5.88 mCi

This 11-year-old right-handed boy had a history of seizures starting in June 1997. He appeared to have a complex partial seizure disorder with secondary generalization and atypical absence spells.

The EEG was suspicious for a left frontotemporal focus. An MRI was reported as normal (Case Fig. 7.8A).

Transverse-,coronal-, and sagittal-plane [18]FDG PET images (Case Figs. 7.8 B–D) reveal a marked decrease in tracer uptake in the inferior left frontal lobe, left anterior, and predominantly mesial midtemporal region compatible with a seizure focus.

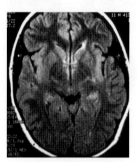

CASE FIG. 7.8A

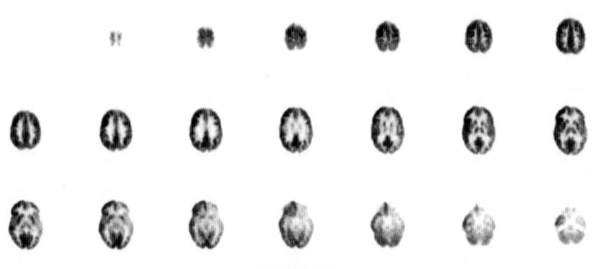

CASE FIG. 7.8B

202

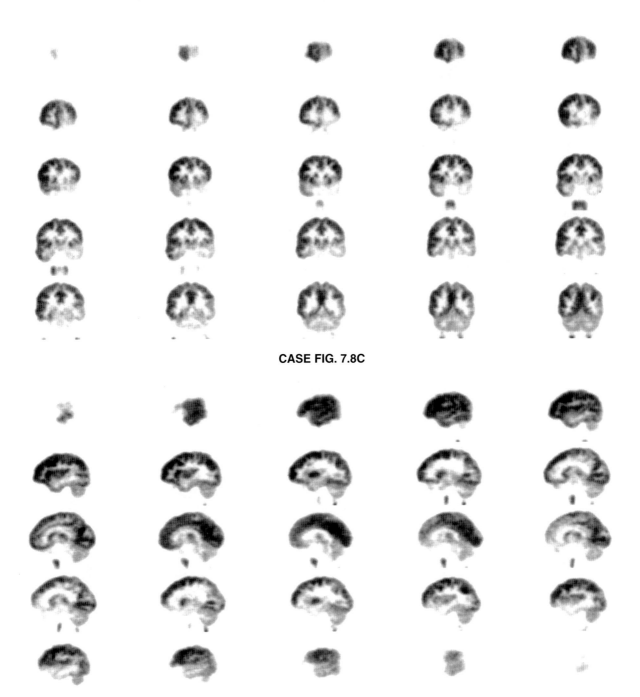

CASE FIG. 7.8C

CASE FIG. 7.8D

CASE 7-9

Clinical Diagnosis:
Seizures

CONTRIBUTORS:	IMAGING DATA:	
Ronald L. Van Heertum, M.D., Jongwon Lee, M.D.	**PET Scanner:** Siemens XACT 47	**Attenuation Correction Method:**
Institution: New York Presbyterian Medical Center	**Tracer:** ^{18}FDG	Autoattenuation protocol
		Dose: 2.81 mCi

This 4 1/2 year old girl had a history of seizures since 3 years of age. The workup of seizures showed right hemimegalencephaly. She has seizure episodes one or two times a month despite medications.

The EEG revealed a potential seizure focus in the right frontal region.

The patient was sedated with 1200 mg pochloral of hydrate prior to scanning. The transverse- and coronal-plane ^{18}FDG

PET images (Case Fig. 7.9 A,B), shown here reveal an enlarged right cerebral hemisphere consistent with a history of right hemimegalencephaly. There is moderately diffuse decreased radiotracer uptake throughout the right cerebral hemisphere, including the gray and white matter as well as right thalamus and basal ganglia. No discrete focus is seen. The left cerebellum has decreased tracer uptake consistent with crossed cerebellar diaschisis.

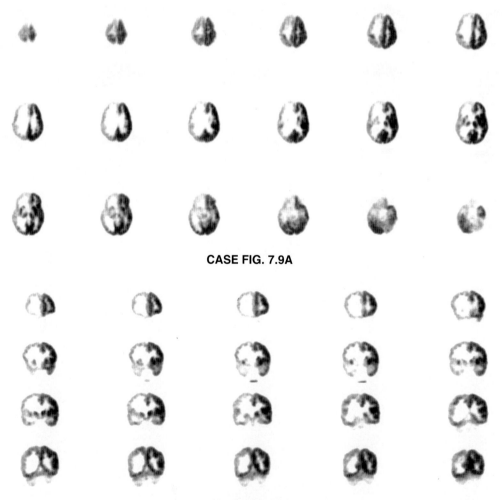

CASE FIG. 7.9A

CASE FIG. 7.9B

Clinical Diagnosis:
Medically Intractable Seizures

CONTRIBUTORS:	IMAGING DATA:	
Ronald L. Van Heertum, M.D.,	**PET Scanner:** Siemens XACT 47	**Attenuation Correction Method:**
Jongwon Lee, M.D.	**Tracer:** ¹⁸FDG-labeled	Autoattenuation protocol
Institution: New York Presbyterian Medical Center		**Dose:** 1.8 mCi

CONTRIBUTORS:

Ronald L. Van Heertum, M.D.,

Jongwon Lee, M.D.

Institution: New York Presbyterian Medical
Center

This 22-month-old boy had medically intractable seizures since 14 months of age. The mother states that he has three to six seizures per day, characterized by eye twitching and jerking of the left arm and leg with occasional loss of consciousness.

An EEG study was suspicious for a left temporal/parietal seizure focus. An MRI (Case Fig. 7.10A) study was interpreted as negative.

The study reveals diffuse moderate decreased tracer accumulation involving the entire left temporal lobe and posterior parietal lobe (Case Fig. 7.10B–D). No other region of decreased tracer accumulation is seen.

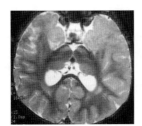
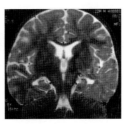

CASE FIG. 7.10A

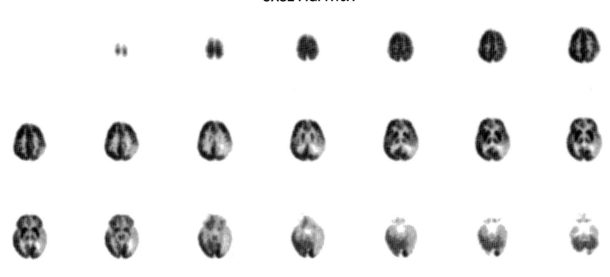

CASE FIG. 7.10B

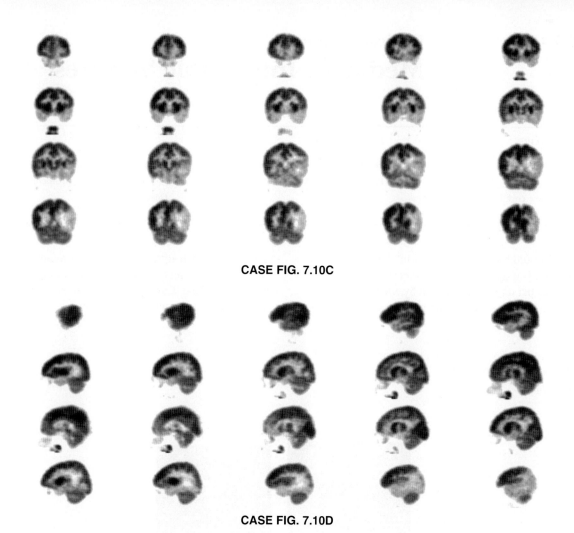

CASE FIG. 7.10C

CASE FIG. 7.10D

Clinical Diagnosis:
Refractory Seizures

CONTRIBUTORS:

Ronald L. Van Heertum, M.D.,
Murray Becker, M.D.
Institution: New York Presbyterian Medical
      Center

IMAGING DATA:

PET Scanner: Siemens XACT 47
Tracer: [18]FDG

Attenuation Correction Method:
    Autoattenuation protocol
Dose: 1.85 mCi

This 22-month-old girl had medically refractory seizures.

The MRI revealed multiple subcortical tubers.

Transverse-, coronal-, and sagittal-plane [18]FDG PET images reveal multiple hypometabolic foci in both cerebral hemispheres (Case Figs. 7.11A–C). The largest is identified within the left occipital lobe and appear to extend into the posterior left temporal lobe. These areas correspond to the MRI findings.

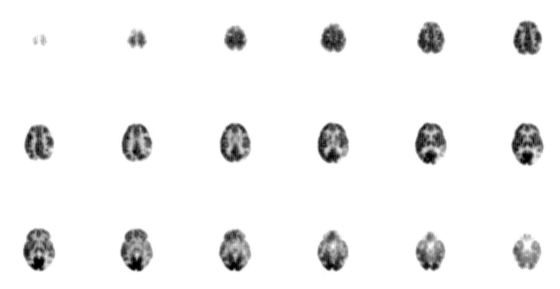

CASE FIG. 7.11A

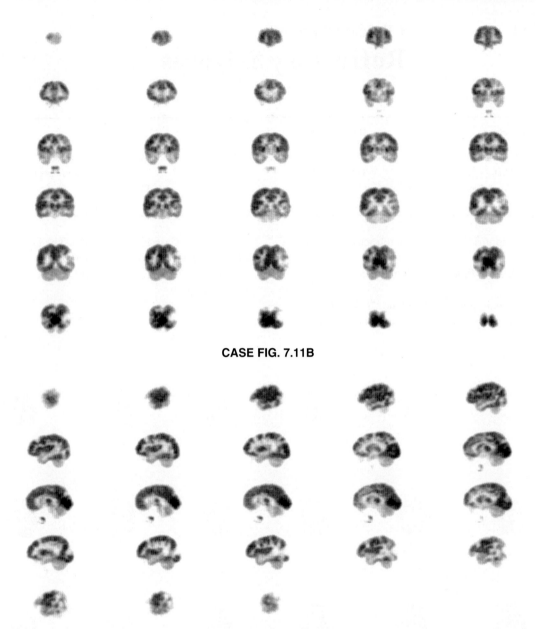

CASE FIG. 7.11B

CASE FIG. 7.11C

Clinical Diagnosis:
Status Epilepticus

CONTRIBUTOR:	IMAGING DATA:	
Thomas C. Hill, M.D.	**Camera:** Strichman SME-810	**Collimator:** High-resolution
Institution: New England Deaconess Hospital	**Tracer:** ^{123}I IMP	**Dose:** 3.0 mCi

This 94-year-old woman was referred for evaluation of status epilepticus. Her seizure activity began 8 hr before her hospital admission. There was no history of a prior seizure disorder.

An EEG showed continuous bursts of left frontotemporal seizure activity. At the time of admission, the patient was started on intravenous phenytoin, which was continued over the next 2 days; she slowly became more responsive but was still disoriented.

An emergency CT scan (Fig. 7.12A) was unremarkable except for a benign calcification in the left temporal lobe.

Four days after admission, a cerebral SPECT study (Fig. 7.12b) in the transaxial plane showed an intense focus of increased tracer deposition in the left frontal lobe (*arrowhead*). As a result, the patient's medication was adjusted and she became more oriented and alert.

Teaching Point:

In this case, the cerebral SPECT study was very helpful in determining the presence of persistent seizure activity despite what were thought to be adequate dosage levels of anticonvulsant medication.

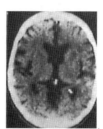

CASE FIG. 7.12A

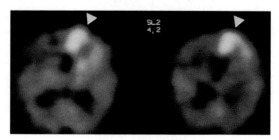

CASE FIG. 7.12B

Clinical Diagnosis:

Intractable Seizures

CONTRIBUTORS:	IMAGING DATA:	
Ronald L. Van Heertum, M.D.,	**PET Scanner:** Siemens XACT 47	**Attenuation Correction Method:**
Angela Lignelli, M.D.	**Tracer:** ^{18}FDG	Autoattenuation protocol
Institution: New York Presbyterian Medical		**Dose:** 10.43 mCi
Center		

This 45-year-old man had intractable partial seizures which were primarily nocturnal.

Video EEG reveals a questionable right frontal localization with rapid spread of seizure activity. MRI reveals right mesial temporal lobe sclerosis (Case Fig. 7.13A).

Transverse- and coronal-plane ^{18}FDG PET images (Case Figs. 7.13B–C) reveal a focal area of decreased radiotracer uptake in the right anterior and mesial temporal lobe.

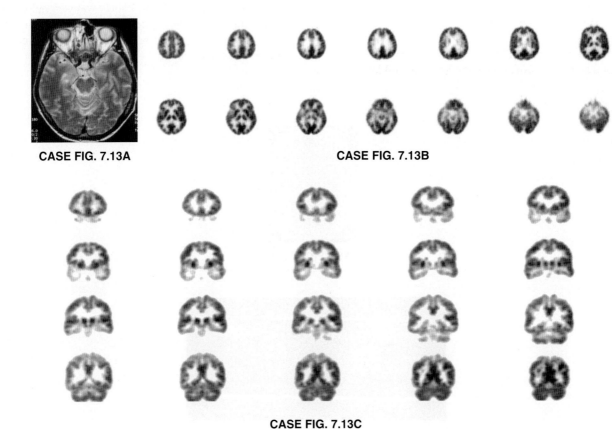

CASE FIG. 7.13A   CASE FIG. 7.13B

CASE FIG. 7.13C

Clinical Diagnosis:

Seizures

CONTRIBUTORS:	IMAGING DATA:	
Ronald L. Van Heertum, M.D.,	**PET Scanner:** Siemens XACT 47	**Attenuation Correction Method:**
Betty Triantafillou, M.D.	**Tracer:** ^{18}FDG	Autoattenuation protocol
Institution: New York Presbyterian Medical		**Dose:** 9.99 mCi
Center		

This 22-year-old man had a history of seizures that first started when he was 17 years of age. Seizures were characterized by left arm movement and tight posturing.

Video EEG revealed slowing in the right hemisphere with several simple partial seizures from the right anterior region. MRI revealed right cerebral hemiatrophy with central dysplasia involving the opercular portion of the frontal, parietal, and temporal lobes (Case Fig. 7.14A).

Transverse and coronal plane ^{18}FDG PET images (Case Figs. 7.14,B,C) shown here reveal markedly decreased radiotracer activity throughout the right anterior and midtemporal lobe, extending posteriorly, which is compatible with a seizure focus. The decreased size and deformity of the right hemisphere seen in the PET images is consistent with the MRI findings.

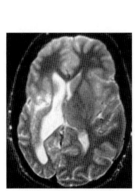

CASE FIG. 7.14A

CASE FIG. 7.14B

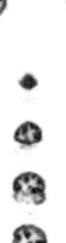
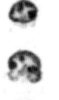

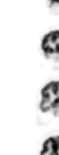

CASE FIG. 7.14C

Clinical Diagnosis:
Intractable Seizures

CONTRIBUTORS:

Rashid A. Fawwaz, M.D.,
Betty Triantafillou, M.D.
Institution: New York Presbyterian Medical
Center

IMAGING DATA:

PET Scanner: Siemens XACT 47
Tracer: [18]FDG labeled

Attenuation Correction Method:
Autoattenuation protocol
Dose: 9.55 mCi

This 45-year-old woman had a history of seizures since she was 2 years of age. They were not adequately controlled by medication.

MRI was normal (Case Fig. 7.15A), but an EEG demonstrated an epileptiform focus in the left anterior temporal lobe.

Transverse- and coronal-plane 18FDG PET images (Case Figs. 7.15B,C) reveal an area of diffuse decreased radiotracer uptake in the left anterior and midtemporal lobe region consistent with the EEG findings of an interictal seizure focus.

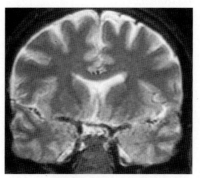

CASE FIG. 7.15A

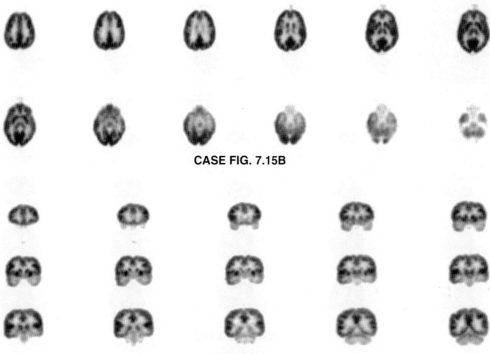

CASE FIG. 7.15B

CASE FIG. 7.15C

Clinical Diagnosis:
Intractable Seizures

CONTRIBUTORS:	IMAGING DATA:	
Philip Alderson, M.D.,	**PET Scanner:** Siemens XACT 47	**Attenuation Correction Method:**
Jeffrey Plutchok, M.D.	**Tracer:** [18]FDG	Autoattenuation protocol
Institution: New York Presbyterian Medical Center		**Dose:** 11.67 mCi

This 42-year-old woman had a seizure disorder since 1974. A PET scan was requested to confirm the localization of a seizure focus prior to surgery.

A video EEG showed seizure activity arising from the right temporal lobe. An outside MRI was normal.

[18]FDG PET images transverse, coronal and oblique axial temporal planes (Case Figs. 7.16A–C), reveal significant hypometabolism in the right anteromedial temporal lobe. These findings are consistent with an interictal seizure focus in the right temporal lobe.

Teaching Point:

Presurgical PET imaging can assist in determining the seizure focus in patients being considered for surgical treatment of intractable seizures.

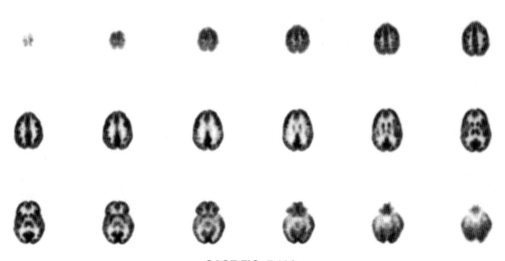

CASE FIG. 7.16A

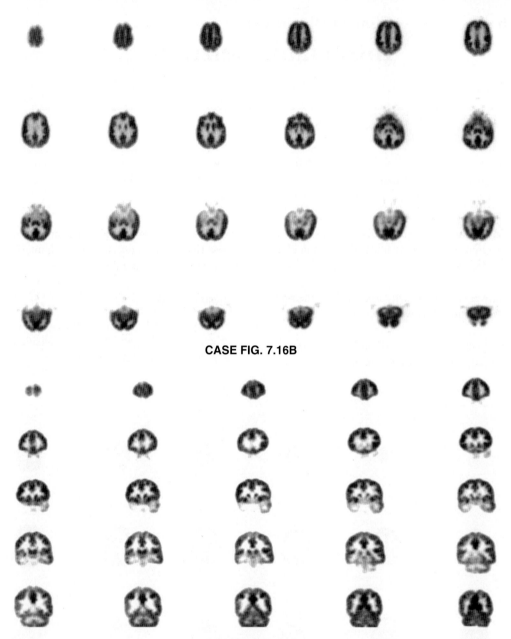

CASE FIG. 7.16B

CASE FIG. 7.16C

Clinical Diagnosis:
Seizure Disorder

CONTRIBUTORS:	IMAGING DATA:	
Ronald L. Van Heertum, M.D.,	**PET Scanner:** Siemens XACT 47	**Attenuation Correction Method:**
Betty Triantafillou, M.D.	**Tracer:** ^{18}FDG	Autoattenuation protocol
Institution: New York Presbyterian Medical Center		**Dose:** 10.33 mCi

This 35-year-old woman had a 1-year history of seizures.

Video EEG reveals interictal slowing in the right temporal region and occasional sharp waves in the right anterior temporal region. MRI reveals only mild atrophy (Case Fig. 7.17A).

Transverse- and coronal-plane ^{18}FDG PET images (Case Figs. 7.17 B,C) reveal a focal area of decreased radiotracer uptake in the right anterior temporal lobe.

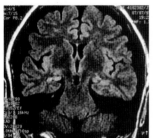
  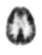
   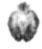

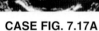
CASE FIG. 7.17A

CASE FIG. 7.17B

CASE FIG. 7.17C

CASE 7-18

Clinical Diagnosis:

Medically Refractory Seizures

<table>
<tr><td>CONTRIBUTORS:</td><td>IMAGING DATA:</td><td></td></tr>
<tr><td>Ronald L. Van Heertum, M.D.,</td><td>PET Scanner: Siemens XACT 47</td><td>Attenuation Correction Method:</td></tr>
<tr><td>Betty Triantafillou, M.D.</td><td>Tracer: [18]FDG</td><td>Autoattenuation protocol</td></tr>
<tr><td>Institution: New York Presbyterian Medical
Center</td><td></td><td>Dose: 8.58 mCi</td></tr>
</table>

This 18-year-old woman had a history of partial complex seizures since 5 years of age. Her seizures are not responding to medication.

Video EEG reveals a focal slowing over the right temporal lobe and suggests a right hemispheric focus. MRI reveals thalamic asymmetry, right smaller than left, and a subtle increase in signal intensity in the right thalamus (Case Fig. 7.18A).

Transverse- and coronal-plane [18]FDG PET images (Case Figs. 7.18 B,C) shown here reveal a decreased radiotracer uptake involving the entire right anterior and midtemporal lobe and the right thalamus. There is also mildly decreased radiotracer uptake to the entire right hemisphere.

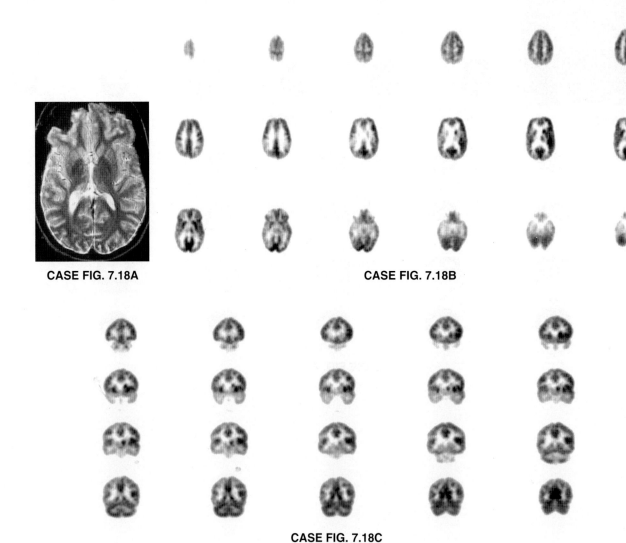

CASE FIG. 7.18A

CASE FIG. 7.18B

CASE FIG. 7.18C

Clinical Diagnosis:
Suspected Temporal Lobe Epilepsy

CONTRIBUTORS:

James M. Mountz, M.D., Ph.D.,
Elmer C. San Pedro, M.D.
Institution: The University of Alabama at
   Birmingham Medical Center

IMAGING DATA:

Camera: Picker PRISM 3000 XP ADAC
   MCD Vertex Plus operating in
   coincidence made with no
   collimator
Tracer: ^{99m}Tc HMPAO, ^{18}FDG

Collimator: low-energy, high-resolution,
   parallel-hole
Dose: 24 mCi
Dose: 4.8 mCi

This 30-year-old man had suspected temporal lobe epilepsy.

^{99m}Tc HMPAO SPECT interictal scans (Case Fig. 7.19) in the transverse and coronal plane shows only a slight asymmetry; there is slightly decreased radiotracer uptake on the left as compared to the right (*top row*). An interictal ^{18}FDG coincidence image scan (*bottom row*) shows significant tracer decrease in the left medial and lateral aspects of the temporal lobe (*arrows*).

^{18}FDG coincidence image scans can show the hypometabolism associated with temporal lobe epilepsy when compared to scans obtained with ^{99m}Tc HMPAO.

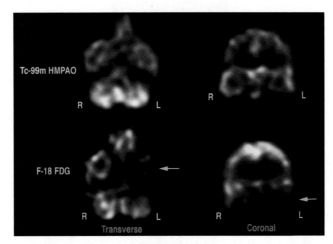

CASE FIG. 7.19

Clinical Diagnosis:
Refractory Seizures

CONTRIBUTOR:	IMAGING DATA:	
Ronald L. Van Heertum, M.D.	**PET Scanner:** Siemens XACT 47	**Attenuation Correction Method:**
Institution: New York Presbyterian Medical Center	**Tracer:** [18]FDG	Autoattenuation protocol
		Dose: 9.7 mCi

This 19-year-old man had refractory seizures.

The MRI reveals encepholomalacia involving the left mesial inferofrontal cortex (Case Fig. 7.20A).

Transverse, coronal, and sagittal-plane PET images (Case Fig. 7.20 B–D) reveal absent radiotracer uptake in the left mesial inferofrontal region, corresponding to the MRI findings.

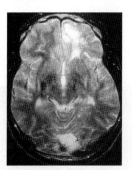

CASE FIG. 7.20A

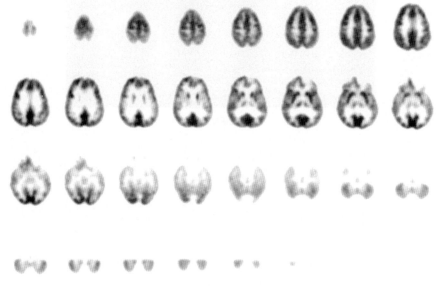

CASE FIG. 7.20B

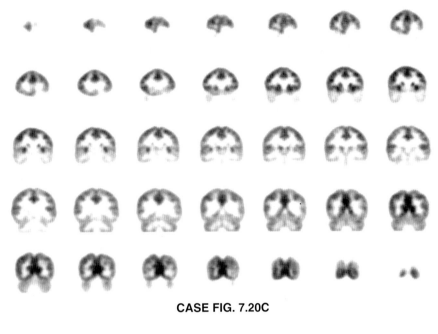

CASE FIG. 7.20C

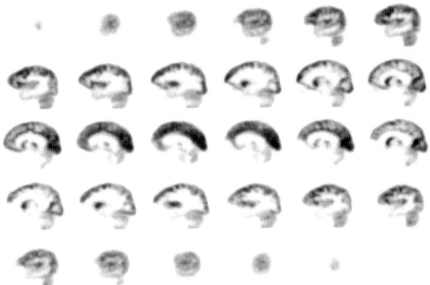

CASE FIG. 7.20D

Clinical Diagnosis:
Postsurgical Epilepsy

CONTRIBUTORS:

Ronald S. Tikofsky, Ph.D.,
Chaitali Bagchi, M.D.
Institution: Columbia University/Harlem
Hospital Center

IMAGING DATA:

Camera: Picker PRISM 3000
Tracer: ^{99m}Tc ECD

Collimator: Ultra-high-resolution fan-beam
Dose: 25 mCi

This 46-year-old woman developed seizures, empyema, and menigitis following evacuation of a subdural hematoma.

The MRI shows encephalomalacic changes in the left frontal lobe without mass effect (Case Fig. 7.21A).

SPECT ECD images were obtained in the transverse, coronal, and sagittal planes (Case Figs. 7.21 B–D). There is near absent perfusion in the region of the left superior frontal cortex near the midline. These findings correspond to the region of encephalomacia seen on CT, which probably represents the region of seizure focus.

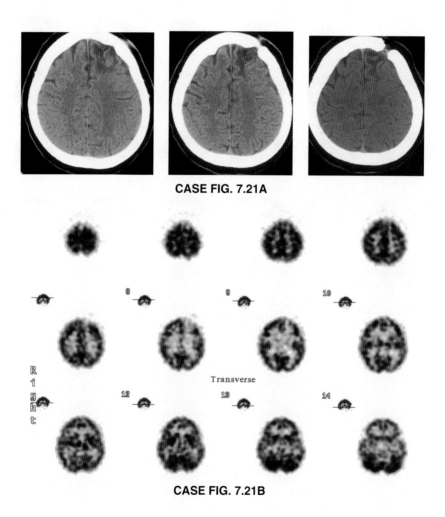

CASE FIG. 7.21A

CASE FIG. 7.21B

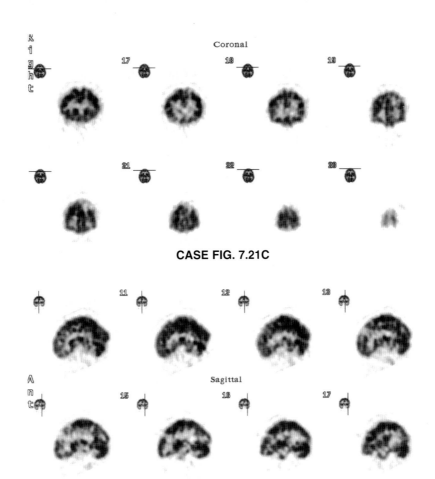

CASE FIG. 7.21C

CASE FIG. 7.21D

Clinical Diagnosis:
Complex Partial Seizure Disorder

CONTRIBUTOR:	IMAGING DATA:	
Kastytis Karvelis, M.D.	**Camera:** ADAC Genesys	**Collimator:** High-resolution
Institution: Henry Ford Hospital	**Tracer:** ^{99m}Tc HMPAO	**Dose:** 20 mCi

This 35-year-old man with known complex partial seizures of uncertain etiology was referred for further evaluation. Specifically, the patient was referred to determine if the seizures originated in the temporal lobe.

An MRI scan (Fig. 7.22A) demonstrated a subarachnoid cyst in the superior aspect of the right parietal occipital lobe.

An HMPAO SPECT study (Fig. 7.22B) in the transaxial plane revealed a focus of absent radiotracer activity corresponding to the subarachnoid cyst seen on MRI.

Teaching Point:

In this case, without an accompanying MRI study, the region of absent tracer activity could easily have been interpreted as evidence of an area of infarction. When there is no history of cerebrovascular disease or hemorrhage, anatomic imaging such as CT or MRI is essential in order to establish a correct diagnosis. This case demonstrates a good correlation between SPECT and MRI with respect to lesion locus.

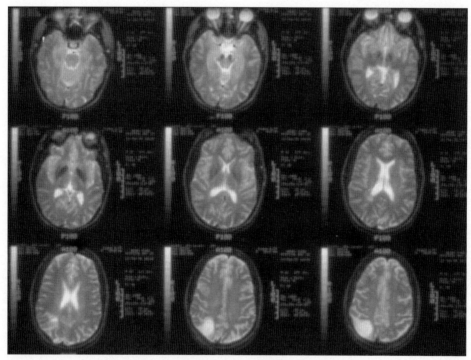

CASE FIG. 7.22A

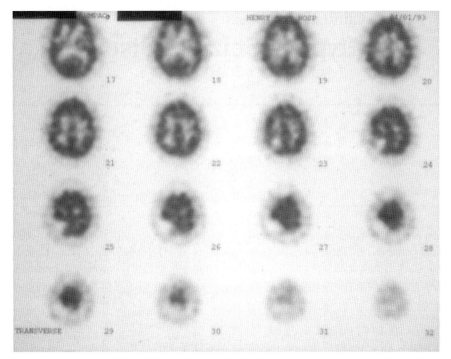

CASE FIG. 7.22B

Clinical Diagnosis:
Atypical Seizure Disorder

CONTRIBUTORS:

S. Askienazy, M.D.,
M.O. Habert, M.D.
Institution: C.H. Sainte-Anne/Service
   Medicine Nucleaire (Paris)

IMAGING DATA:

Camera: SOPHY
Tracer: 99mTc HMPAO

Collimator: Ultra-high-resolution
Dose: 25 mCi

This 56-year-old woman presented with a history of recurrent episodes of left-hand hemiparesis. Three years prior to her current presentation, she had sustained a traumatic contusion of the right temporal lobe. At present, neurologic examination revealed a left lateral homonymous hemianopsia. Scalp EEG demonstrated the presence of permanent lateralized epileptiform discharges (PLEDs). After 1 week of antiepileptic therapy, a follow-up scalp EEG demonstrated the disappearance of PLEDs.

The CT scan (Case Fig. 7.23A) revealed a hypodensity in the right temporal lobe consistent with prior trauma to the temporal lobe.

The initial HMPAO SPECT study (Case Fig. 7.23B), in the transaxial (1) and coronal (2) planes revealed increased radiotracer activity in the right posterior temporal lobe. A follow-up HMPAO SPECT scan (Case Fig. 7.23C), in the transaxial (1) and coronal (2) planes, showed a decrease in radiotracer activity in the right temporal lobe following treatment with anticonvulsants.

> **Teaching Point:**
>
> Cerebral SPECT imaging can be a useful tool in the assessment of epilepsy patients not only for the localization of the seizure focus, but also for establishing the diagnosis of epilepsy, when the patient's clinical presentation is atypical.

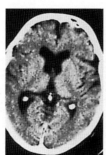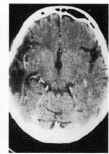

CASE FIG. 7.23A

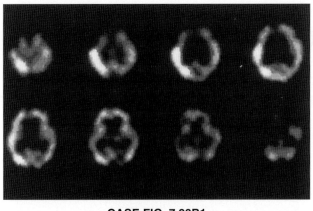

CASE FIG. 7.23B1

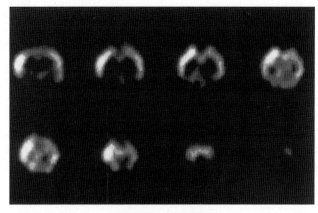

CASE FIG. 7.23B2

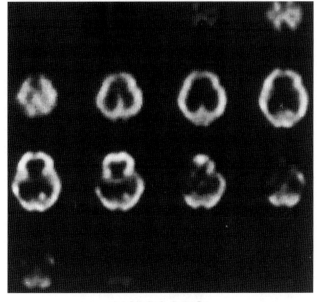

CASE FIG. 7.23C1

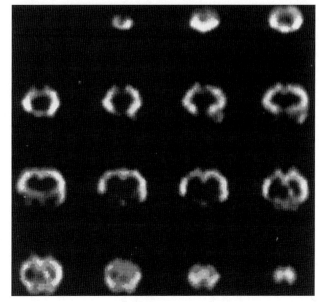

CASE FIG. 7.23C2

Clinical Diagnosis:
Intractable Complex Partial Seizures

CONTRIBUTORS:	IMAGING DATA:	
Ronald L. Van Heertum, M.D.,	**PET Scanner:** Siemens XACT 47	**Attenuation Correction Method:**
Angela Lignelli, M.D.	**Tracer:** [18]FDG	Autoattenuation protocol
Institution: New York Presbyterian Medical		**Dose:** 10.47 mCi
Center		

This 30-year-old woman had been suffering from intractable complex partial seizures for approximately 2 1/2 years. The seizures are described by the patient as simple and also grand mal seizures. The "simple seizures" are associated with auditory symptoms.

Video EEG study demonstrated a single left temporal seizure focus; an MRI study was interpreted as negative.

No region of increased or decreased focal tracer was observed (Case Fig. 7.24A,B). The PET scan was interpreted as negative.

Teaching Point:

Interictal PET and MRI are often diagnostic but may be non-contributory in select cases, as in this patient.

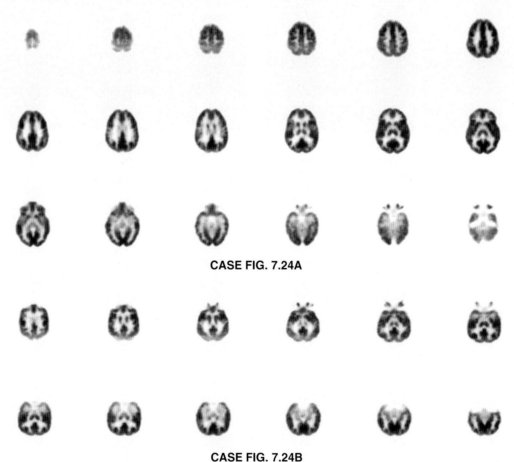

CASE FIG. 7.24A

CASE FIG. 7.24B

Clinical Diagnosis:
Complex Partial Seizures

CONTRIBUTOR:

William H. Theodore, M.D.

Institution: National Institute of
Neurological Disorders and
Stroke, National Institutes of
Health

IMAGING DATA:

PET Scanner: Scanditronix 1024-7B
Tracer: ^{15}O-H$_2$O (bolus)

Attenuation Correction Method:

GA 68 transmission

Dose: 50 mCi for each study (ictal/
interictal)

This patient had a history of complex partial seizures and was a candidate for temporal lobe resection.

An EEG revealed a left temporal focus; mesial temporal sclerosis was found at surgery.

Transverse ^{15}O-H$_2$O PET studies revealed decreased radiotracer activity in the left temporal region (Case Fig. 7.25, *arrow*) on the interictal study. The ictal study revealed increased cerebral blood flow bilaterally and involved the thalamus.

Reproduced by permission from Theodore WH, Balish MB, Leiderman DB, et al. The effect of seizures on cerebral blood flow measured with ^{15}O-H$_2$O and positron emission tomography. *Epilepsia* 1996;37:796–802.

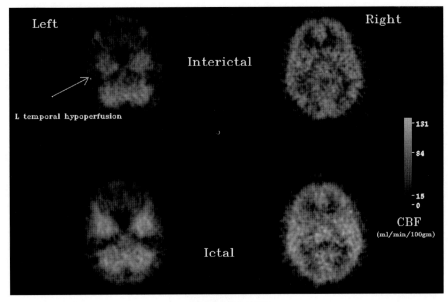

CASE FIG. 7.25

Functional Cerebral SPECT and PET Imaging, Third Edition,
edited by R.L.Van Heertum and R.S. Tikofsky,
Lippincott Williams & Wilkins, New York © 2000.

CHAPTER 8

Trauma

Ronald S. Tikofsky and Ronald L. Van Heertum

There has not been a significant drop in the number of persons who have experienced traumatic brain injury (TBI) since the last edition of this book. Head injury remains a major medical management problem in the United States. According to Julien Dilks, president of the JMA Foundation, Inc./National Brain Injury Research Group, Inc. (personal communication), there is one head injury per minute per day. According to the National Head Injury Foundation, over 1,190,000 of the 2 million yearly head injuries survive. There are approximately 300,000 hospitalizations per year for minor head injury, and 34% of this group are unable to return to work after 3 months. These epidemiologic data confirm that head trauma is a major cause of disability in the United States. Structural brain imaging, particularly computed tomography (CT) and magnetic resonance imaging (MRI), is extremely useful in the evaluation of acute and chronic head trauma. Unfortunately, structural imaging techniques, particularly in minor head trauma, do not always correlate with the clinical deficits that these patients manifest. However, a 1996 report by the Therapeutics and Technology Assessment Subcommittee of the Academy of Neurology (1) still considered brain single-photon-emission computed tomography (SPECT) in head trauma to be investigational.

There continues to be a stream of research testing hypotheses regarding the relationship of functional brain imaging findings to neurobehavioral "abnormalities" as a consequence of TBI. These studies incorporate single-photon-emission computed tomography (SPECT) imaging and, more recently positron-emission tomography (PET), as part of their research protocols (2–7).

Regional cerebral blood flow (rCBF/SPECT) imaging in

patients with closed cranial trauma is becoming recognized as a clinically useful evaluation procedure (8–12). There is a growing body of literature describing SPECT findings associated with various types of clinical sequelae resulting from closed cranial and other trauma to the brain (13–18).

SPECT/PET imaging does not replace CT or MRI for the identification of major structural lesions or the presence of intracerebral hemorrhages, subdural hematoma, or edema. However, functional imaging can contribute to evaluating alterations in perfusion and/or metabolism in the cerebral cortex, basal ganglia, and thalamus that may result from TBI (19–23).

Although most of the attention in the functional brain imaging community has been on closed cranial trauma and its sequelae, SPECT/PET may also have a role in evaluating other types of brain injury. Penetrating wounds to the head and brain typically produce focal lesions, often due to missiles that penetrate the skull and enter the brain. CT and MRI can often track the path of the missile through the brain. However, SPECT/PET may be useful in detecting perfusion deficits secondary to the primary lesion. Neuropsychological changes resulting from, for example, gunshot wounds to the head may be related to both the structural damage detected by CT/MRI and the surrounding perfusion defects seen with functional brain imaging. Penetrating lesions of the brain tend to be focal in nature. On the other hand, closed head injuries resulting from vehicular accidents, falls, or other blows to the head are frequently more diffuse. In many cases of closed head injury (CHI), the resulting brain damage is a combination of focal and diffuse brain damage. Even when there is diffuse injury, the frontal, temporal, and basomesial areas appear to be the most vulnerable to damage (24). Some recent reports (9,25,26) suggest that basal ganglia and thalamus may also show altered perfusion, with secondary changes in the cortex suggesting a "disconnection" process. Thus, SPECT studies on this patient population can be expected to reveal regions of absent tracer uptake that will cor-

R. S. Tikofsky: Department of Radiology, Columbia University College of Physicians and Surgeons, Harlem Hospital Center, New York, New York 10032.

R. L. Van Heertum: Department of Radiology, Columbia University College of Physicians and Surgeons, New York, New York 10032.

relate with sites of structural damage seen on anatomic imaging.

Wilson (26) notes that abnormalities seen by the use of neuroimaging techniques may be classified by type, locus, extent, and persistence after injury. Hematomas—which may be extradural, subdural, or intracerebral—may produce secondary changes in the brain, including contusion, compression, necrosis, and edema. In some cases, evacuation of the hematoma will be followed by cortical atrophy. CT is an excellent tool for the detection of hematomas. Functional brain imaging, on the other hand, may be more useful in identifying perfusion/metabolic deficits following evacuation of the hematoma. Data from Oder et al. (27) and Cusumano et al. (28) suggest that SPECT brain imaging may be useful in predicting outcome in severely injured and comatose patients.

Because SPECT scans can detect alterations in perfusion, the technique is particularly useful in identifying regions of contrecoup injury. These alterations in perfusion, suggesting impaired neural function, can often account for a patient's clinical presentation when no structural lesions are found with CT or MRI. This is of particular importance in evaluating patients with "minor" head trauma who may experience only brief periods of unconsciousness and leave the emergency room with no overt neurologic impairment but who later return with complaints of visual, cognitive, or behavioral changes. Recent reports in the SPECT and PET literature (12,16) suggest that these techniques may be useful in establishing the presence of brain injury in minor head trauma. However, it is important to note that current research does not show a direct or strong correlation between diffuse perfusion deficits and specific neurobehavioral impairments.

With the availability of stable radiopharmaceuticals, it is possible to inject patients in the ER. Comatose patients can then be imaged after they have been stabilized or, in the case of minor trauma, after all the other examinations including CT or MRI have been completed. Based on the currently available data, SPECT/PET studies should not be performed on every patient with minor head trauma. Alexander (29) argues that functional imaging should not be performed in the immediate postacute state and that it should be used for patients with persistent behavioral, cognitive, psychiatric symptoms after a reasonable recovery period (approximately 6 months) with or without treatment.

Children are particularly susceptible to head injury. There are now a few studies using PET and SPECT to evaluate children and adolescents (10,25,30). Results are still sketchy, but it appears that SPECT showed altered perfusion, thus suggesting brain impairment in symptomatic children when CT showed no impairment. Worley et al. (30) report that routine PET in children and adolescents with severe TBI is not any more predictive of recovery than CT or MRI. Early PET scans did correlate significantly with outcome. More research with this population is needed before the role of functional brain imaging in children with TBI can be adequately assessed.

Wilson's (26) 1990 comment that, the "new functional tomographic" methods (PET, SPECT) "present exciting, as yet largely untapped, opportunities for the future" requires only slight modification. Research studies on functional imaging in TBI are increasingly demonstrating the value of these procedures in this patient population. When used appropriately and with conservative interpretation, SPECT and PET can play an important part in the clinical evaluation of patients with traumatic brain injury.

The cases presented in this section represent the range of images associated with various types of head trauma.

REFERENCES

1. Report of the Therapeutics and Technology Assessment Subcommittee of the American Academy of Neurology. *Neurology* 1996;46:278–285.
2. Abu-Judeh HH, Singh M, Maseu JC, Abdel-Dayem HM. Discordance between FDG uptake and technetium-99m-HMPAO brain perfusion in acute traumatic brain injury. *J Nucl Med* 1998;39:1357–1359.
3. Umile EM, Plotikin RC, Sandel ME. Functional assessment of mild traumatic brain injury using SPECT and neuropsychological testing. *Brain Inj* 1998;12:577–594.
4. Ruff R, Crouch J, Troster A, et al. Selected cases of poor outcome following minor brain trauma: comparing neuropsychological and positron emission tomography assessment. *Brain Inj* 1994;8:297–308.
5. Bicik I, Radanov BP, Schafer N, et al. PET with 18 fluorodeoxyglucose and hexamethylpropylene amine oxime SPECT in late whiplash syndrome. *Neurology* 1998;59:345–350.
6. Laatsch L, Jobe T, Sychra J, et al. Impact of cognitive rehabilitation therapy on neuropsychological impairments as measured by brain perfusion SPECT: a longitudinal study. *Brain Inj* 1997;11:851–853.
7. Ruff RM, Crouch JA, Troster AI, et al. Selected cases of poor outcome following a minor brain trauma: comparing neuropsychological and positron emission tomography assessment. *Brain Inj* 1994;8:297–308.
8. Reid RH, Gulenchyn KY, Ballinger JR, Ventureyra ECG. Cerebral perfusion imaging with technetium-99m-HMPAO following cerebral trauma: initial experience. *Clin Nucl Med* 1990;15:383–388.
9. Goldenberg G, Oder W, Spatt J, Podreka I. Cerebral correlates of disturbed executive function and memory in survivors of severe closed head injury: a SPECT study. *J Neurol Neurosurg Psychiatry* 1992;55:362–368.
10. Emanuelson IM, von Wendt L, Bjure J, et al. Computed tomography and single-photon emission computed tomography as diagnostic tools in acquired brain injury among children and adolescents. *Dev Med Child Neurol* 1997;39:502–507.
11. Nedd K, Sfakianakis G, Ganz W, et al. ^{99m}Tc-HMPAO SPECT of the brain in mild to moderate traumatic brain injury patients: compared with CT—a prospective study. *Brain Inj* 1993;4:469–479.
12. Masdeu JC, Van Heertum RL, Kleiman A, et al. Early single-photon emission computed tomography in mild head trauma: a controlled study. *J Neuroimag* 1994;4:177–181.
13. Oder W, Goldenberg G, Podreka I, Deecke L. HM-PAO SPECT studies in persistent vegetative state after head injury: prognostic indicator of the likelihood of recovery? *Intens Care Med* 1991;17:149–153.
14. Gray BG, Ichise M, Chung D-G, et al. Technetium-99m-HMPAO SPECT in the evaluation of patients with a remote history of traumatic brain injury: a comparison with x-ray computed tomography. *J Nucl Med* 1992;33:52–58.
15. Ichise M, Chung D-G, Wang P, et al. Technetium-99m-HMPAO SPECT, CT, and MRI in the evaluation of patients with chronic traumatic brain injury: a correlation with neuropsychological performance. *J Nucl Med* 1994;35:217–226.
16. Varney NR, Bushnell MD, Kahn D, et al. NeuroSPECT correlates of disabling mild head injury: preliminary findings. *J Head Trauma Rehabil* 1995;10:18–28.
17. Jacobs A, Put E, Ingels M, et al. One year follow-up of technetium-99m-HMPAO SPECT in mild head injury. *J Nucl Med* 1996;37:1605–1609.
18. Kant R, Smith-Seemiller L, Isaac G, Duffy J. Tc-HMPAO SPECT in persistent post-concussion syndrome after mild head injury: comparison with MRI/CT. *Brain Inj* 1997;11:115–124.

19. Roper SN, Mena I, King WA, et al. An analysis of cerebral blood flow in acute closed-head injury using technetium-99m-HMPAO SPECT and computed tomography. *J Nucl Med* 1991;34:1684–1687.
20. Varney NR, Bushnell D. NeuroSPECT findings in patients with post-traumatic anosmia: a quantitative analysis. *J Head Trauma Rehabil* 1998;13:63–72.
21. Choksey MS, Costa DC, Iannoti F, et al. 99TCm-HMPAO SPECT studies in traumatic intracerebral haematoma. *J Neurol Neurosurg Psychiatry* 1991;54:6–11.
22. Prayer L, Wimberger D, Oder W. Crainal MR imaging and cerebral 99mTc-HM-PAO-SPECT in patients with subacute or chronic severe closed head injury and normal CT examinations. *Acta Radiol* 1993;34:593–599.
23. Ito H, Ishii K, Onum, et al. Cerebral perfusion changes in traumatic diffuse brain injury; IMP SPECT studies. *Ann Nucl Med* 1997;11: 167–172.
24. Adams JH. Head injury. In: Adams JH, Corsellis JAN, Duchen LW, eds. *Greenfield's neuropathology, 4th ed.* London: Edward Arnold, 1984:85–124.
25. Goshen E, Zwast ST, Shahar E, Tadmor R. The role of 99Tcm-HM-PAO brain SPET in paediatric traumatic brain injury. *Nucl Med Commun* 1996;17:418–422.
26. Wilson, JTL. Review: the relationship between neuropsychological function and brain damage detected by neuroimaging after closed head injury. *Brain Inj* 1990;4:349–363.
27. Oder W, Goldenberg G, Podreka I, Deecke L. HM-PAOSPECT studies in persistent vegetative state after head injury: prognostic indicator of the likelihood of recovery. *Intens Care Med* 1991;17:149–153.
28. Cusumano S, Paolin A, Di Paola F, et al. Assessing brain in post-traumatic coma by means of bit-mapped SEPs, BAEPs, SPET and clinical scores: prognostic implications. *Electroencephalogr Clin Neurophysiol* 1992;84:499–514.
29. Alexander MP. In the pursuit of proof of brain damage after whiplash injury. (editorial). *Neurology* 1998;51:336–340.
30. Worley G, Hoffman JM, Paine SS, et al. 18-Fluorodeoxyglucose positron emission tomography in children and adolescents with traumatic brain injury. *Dev Med Child Neurol* 1995;37:213–220.

SUGGESTED READINGS

Abdel-Dayem HM, Ab-Judeh H, Kumar M, et al. SPECT brain perfusion abnormalities in mild or moderate traumatic brain injury. *Clin Nucl Med* 1998;23:309–317.
Lewis DH. Functional brain imaging with cerebral perfusion SPECT in cerebrovascular disease, epilepsy, and trauma. *Neurosurg Clin North Am* 1997;8:337–344.
Mitchner A, Wyper DJ, Patterson J, et al. SPECT, CT, and MRI in head injury: acute abnormalities followed up at six months. *J Neurol Neurosurg Psychiatry* 1997;62:633–636.
Tikofsky RS, Ichise M, Seibyl JP, Verhoeff NPLG. Functional brain SPECT imaging: 1999 and beyond. In: LM Freeman ed. *Nuclear Medicine Annual.* New York: Lippincott Williams & Wilkins. 1999;193–264.

Clinical Diagnosis:
Intracranial Gunshot Injury

CONTRIBUTORS:

Robert S. Hellman, M.D.,
Ronald S. Tikofsky, M.D.
Institution: Medical College of Wisconsin

IMAGING DATA:

Camera: GE 400 AC/T;STAR
Tracer: [123]I IMP

Collimator: High-resolution
Dose: 5.0 mCi

This 23-year-old man was referred for evaluation of a left hemiparesis and loss of cognitive function after sustaining a gunshot wound to the head.

An initial CT scan showed hyperdense hematomas in the right frontal and deep right parietal lobes, which appeared hyperdense on a follow-up CT scan.

A cerebral SPECT study (Case Fig. 8.1) in the transaxial **(A)**, coronal **(B)**, and sagittal **(C)** planes revealed a marked decrease in tracer deposition throughout the right cerebral hemisphere plus an absence of tracer activity in the right basal ganglia and the frontal lobes; tracer activity was less reduced in the right parietal lobe. The defect shown by SPECT study was of a larger area than that noted on the CT scan. The pattern of abnormal tracer deposition appreciated by the SPECT study clearly delineated the trajectory of the bullet.

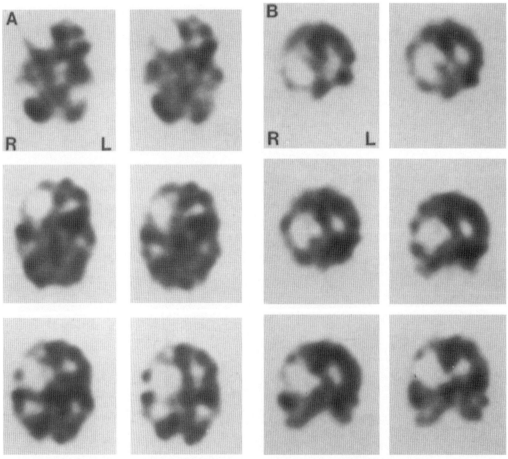

CASE FIG. 8.1A   CASE FIG. 8.1B

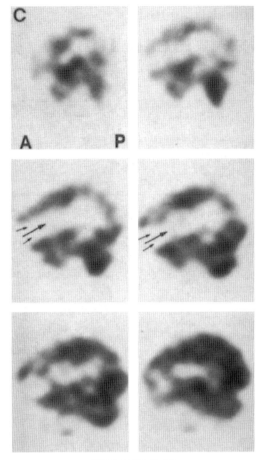

CASE FIG. 8.1C

Clinical Diagnosis:

Open Head Injury (Gunshot Wound)

CONTRIBUTORS:

S. Tzila Zwas, M.D.,
Elinor Goshen, M.D.
Institution: Chaim Sheba Medical Center
(Ramat-Gan, Israel)

IMAGING DATA:

Camera: Elscint Dual-Head Helix
Tracer: ^{99m}Tc-ECD

Collimator: Fan-beam
Dose: 30 mCi

Two months before imaging, this 43-year-old man sustained a severe open head injury due to a gunshot wound (Glasgow Coma Scale score = 3). He presented with a right hemiparesis and hemianopsia, status post left craniotomy for evacuation of a parietooccipital hematoma.

After hematoma drainage and debridement, a CT scan (Case Fig. 8.2A) revealed brain herniation and edema.

The Technetium 99m-hexamethylpropyleneamine-oxime (^{99m}Tc-HMPAO) SPECT study (Case Fig. 8.2B) in the

transaxial plane reveals an extensive left parietal perfusion defect with herniation, corresponding to the CT findings. In addition, decreased perfusion was observed in the left temporal and occipital cortex and the contralateral right cerebellum.

Teaching Point:

Brain SPECT may be helpful in demonstrating the perfusion pattern in herniated brain and after severe open head injury.

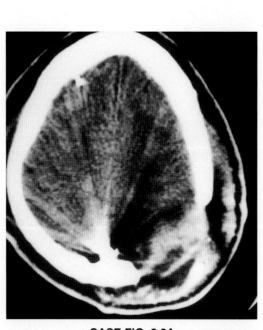

CASE FIG. 8.2A

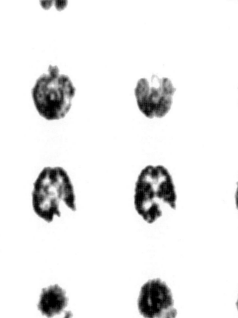

CASE FIG. 8.2B

CASE 8-3

Clinical Diagnosis:

Large Right Subdural Hematoma

CONTRIBUTOR:	IMAGING DATA:	
Joji Nagawara, M.D.	**Camera:** Shimadzu Headtome Set-031	**Collimator:** High-resolution
Institution: Nakamura Memorial Hospital	**Tracer:** ^{123}I IMP	

This 65-year-old man was referred for evaluation of right-sided headaches and a left hemiparesis. Two months previously, he had sustained head trauma.

On a CT scan, a subdural hematoma was noted on the right side.

An initial cerebral SPECT study (Case Fig. 8.3A) in the transaxial plane revealed decreased peripheral tracer depo-sition in the right cerebral hemisphere *(arrows)*. In addition, crossed cerebellar diaschisis was observed *(arrowhead)*.

A week after the subdural hematoma was drained, a follow-up cerebral SPECT study (Case Fig. 8.3B) showed significantly improved tracer deposition in the periphery of the right cerebral hemisphere.

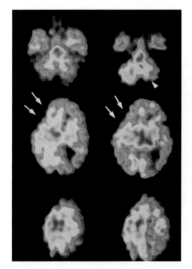

CASE FIG. 8.3A

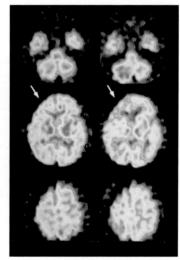

CASE FIG. 8.3B

Clinical Diagnosis:
Chronic Subdural Hematoma

CONTRIBUTOR:	IMAGING DATA:	
Ronald L. Van Heertum, M.D.	**Camera:** Picker PRISM 3000	**Collimator:** Ultra-high-resolution fan-beam
Institution: Columbia-Presbyterian Medical Center	**Tracer:** ^{99m}Tc HMPAO	**Dose:** 20.4 mCi

This 74-year-old man was referred for evaluation of progressive confusion. The patient stated that he had in the past sustained head trauma without loss of consciousness, which he said was minor and without obvious sequelae.

A CT scan (Case Fig. 8.4A) revealed diffuse cerebral atrophy and bilateral subdural hematomas that were predominantly frontal in location.

An HMPAO SPECT study (Case Fig. 8.4B) in the transaxial plane revealed an extrinsic conical deformity in the contour of the cerebral cortex (predominantly frontal) secondary to the bilateral subdural hematomas seen on the CT scan. In addition, bilateral focal areas of absent tracer were seen in the occipital lobes. This latter finding was felt to be due to an associated contrecoup intraparenchymal brain injury.

Published with permission from Van Heertum RL, Miller SH, Mosesson R. Brain SPECT imaging in neurologic disease. *Radiol Clin North Am* 1993;31:881–907.

Teaching Point:

Cerebral SPECT imaging, as shown in this case, may be complementary to CT and MRI in the evaluation of acute and remote head trauma.

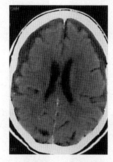

CASE FIG. 8.4A

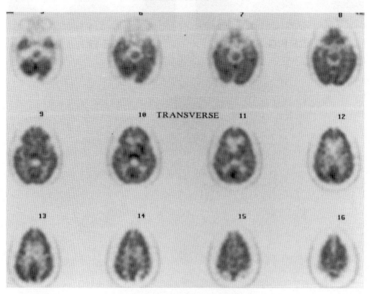

CASE FIG. 8.4B

CASE 8-5

Clinical Diagnosis:
Traumatic Brain Injury

CONTRIBUTORS:

Ronald L. Van Heertum, M.D.,

Angela Lignelli, M.D.

Institution: The Kreitchman PET Center,
New York Presbyterian Hospital

IMAGING DATA:

PET Scanner: Seimens XACT 47

Tracer: [18]FDG

Attenuation Correction Method:
Autoattenuation

Dose: 9.37 mCi

This 28-year-old man had been involved in a motor vehicle accident approximately 1 1/2 years prior to presentation. At the time, he sustained a left orbital fracture and bilateral subdural hematomas. Since the accident, the patient has been suffering from headaches, dizziness, short-term memory loss, and word-finding difficulty.

A follow-up CT scan of the brain was reported to be without evidence of abnormality.

Transverse, and oblique-angle [18]fluprodeoxyglucose ([18]FDG) PET images (Case Figs. 8.5A,B) reveal a focal area of decreased radiotracer uptake in the left orbitofrontal region. In addition, a focal area of decreased radiotracer uptake is observed in the left temporal lobe. This pattern, although not specific, may be seen with postraumatic brain injury.

Teaching Point:

PET imaging may be of some value in the evaluation of patients after trauma, particularly if characteristic regional metabolic abnormalities are visualized.

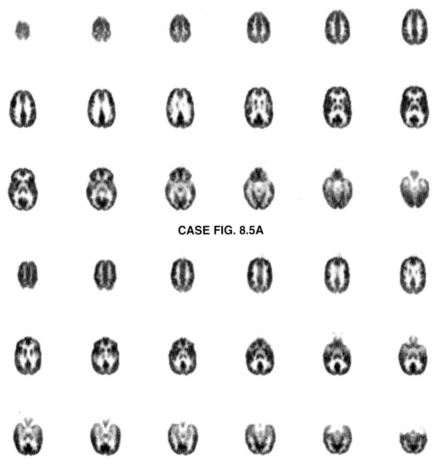

CASE FIG. 8.5A

CASE FIG. 8.5B

Clinical Diagnosis:
Closed Cranial Trauma

CONTRIBUTORS:

Ronald L. Van Heertum, M.D.,
Angela Lignelli, M.D.
Institution: The Kreitchman PET Center,
New York Presbyterian Hospital

IMAGING DATA:

PET Scanner: Seimens XACT 47
Tracer: [18]FDG labeled

Attenuation Correction Method:
Autoattenuation
Dose: 9.13 mCi

This 48-year-old man sustained a subdural hematoma due to a fall from a roof. He developed generalized and petit mal seizures; later the same year, he sustained significant head trauma following a motor vehicle accident.

Video-electroencephalography (EEG) revealed a probable left frontotemporal focus. MRI showed extensive posttraumatic encephalomalacia involving the the inferior frontal and temporal lobes and the medial right occipital lobe.

FDG PET images in the transverse, coronal, and sagittal planes (Case Figs. 8-6A–C) show decreased radiotracer uptake in the right and left orbitofrontal lobes, more pronounced on the left. Decreased radiotracer uptake is also observed in the right temporal lobe laterally, extending to the right occipital lobe.

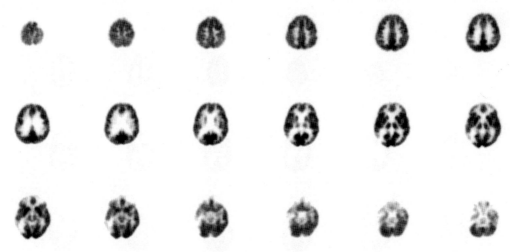

CASE FIG. 8.6A

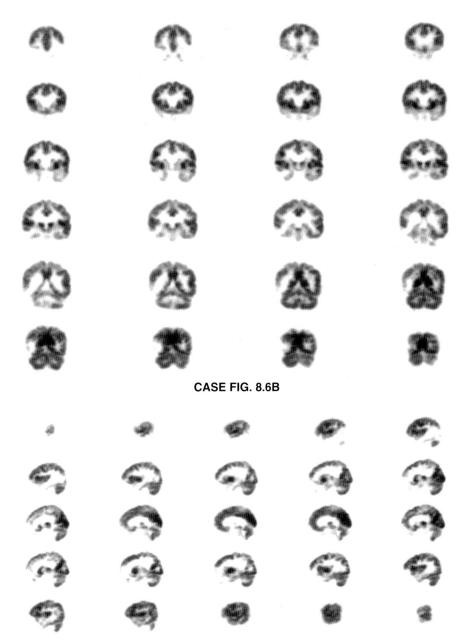

CASE FIG. 8.6B

CASE FIG. 8.6C

Clinical Diagnosis:
Traumatic Subarachnoid Hemorrhage

CONTRIBUTOR:	IMAGING DATA:	
Stefanie Jacobs, M.D.	**Camera:** GE Neurocam	**Collimator:** Ultra-high-resolution
Institution: Columbia-Presbyterian Medical Center	**Tracer:** ^{99m}Tc HMPAO	**Dose:** 21.3 mCi

This 64-year-old woman with a known history of hypertension was admitted for further assessment and treatment of a depressed level of consciousness and aphasia following a generalized seizure. At the time of the seizures, the patient sustained an injury to the left side of her head. An EEG revealed a diffuse slowing of brain activity with a focus in the left temporal lobe.

An initial CT scan (Fig. 8.7A,B) revealed a localized subarachnoid hemorrhage primarily confined to the left posterior parietotemporal lobe.

HMPAO SPECT (Fig. 8.7 C,D) in the transaxial (C), and coronal (D), planes revealed decreased radiotracer uptake throughout the left temporal lobe, which was felt to be most consistent with an area of contusion.

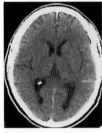 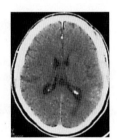

CASE FIG. 8.7A   **CASE FIG. 8.7B**

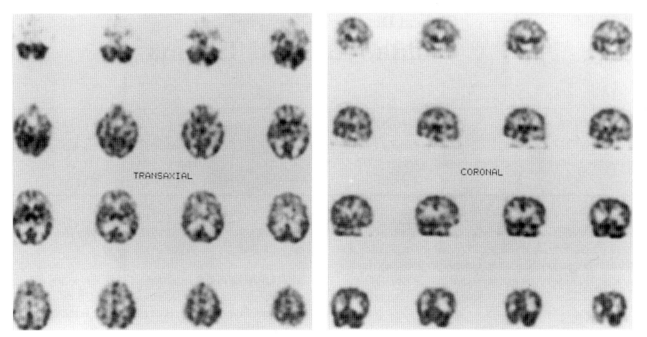

CASE FIG. 8.7C

CASE FIG. 8.7D

Clinical Diagnosis:
Childhood Head Trauma

CONTRIBUTOR:	IMAGING DATA:	
Ronald L. Van Heertum, M.D.	**Camera:** GE-3000 XCT	**Collimator:** Ultra-high-resolution
Institution: Columbia-Presbyterian Medical Center	**Tracer:** ^{99m}Tc HMPAO	**Dose:** 20.5 mCi

This 35-year-old woman (a transsexual), with a long history of polysubstance abuse was referred for evaluation and treatment of pseudoseizures, paranoid ideations, and auditory hallucinations. The patient stated that she thought she had sustained head trauma (left frontoparietal) in early childhood.

A CT scan (Case Fig. 8.8A) revealed an area of localized atrophy and hypodensity in the left frontal and anterior temporal lobes that was felt to be secondary to head trauma in childhood.

An HMPAO SPECT scan (Case Fig. 8.8B) in the transaxial plane revealed relative decreased tracer deposition in the left frontotemporal lobes, corresponding to the area of abnormality on CT.

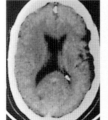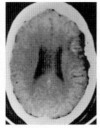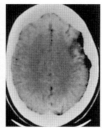

CASE FIG. 8.8A

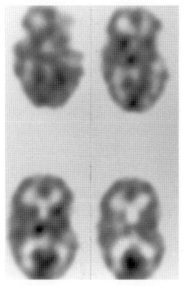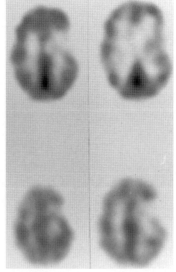

CASE FIG. 8.8B

Clinical Diagnosis:
Mild Head Trauma

CONTRIBUTOR:	IMAGING DATA:	
Ronald L. Van Heertum, M.D.	**PET Scanner:** Siemens XACT 47	**Attenuation Correction**
Institution: The Kreitchman PET Center,	**Tracer:** [18]FDG	**Method:** Autocorrection
New York Presbyterian Hospital		**Dose:** 8.43 mCi
Center		

This 34-year-old woman sustained head trauma due to an auto accident a year before she was seen for imaging. Since her injury, she has had persistent headaches and dizziness.

A CT scan of the brain from an outside hospital was negative.

[18]FDG PET images in the transverse and coronal planes (Case Figs. 8.9A,B) reveal decreased radiotracer uptake in the left anteroinferior frontal lobe. In addition, there is slightly decreased [18]FDG uptake in the left anterior temporal lobe (*see arrows*).

Teaching Point:

FDG-PET imaging may be a useful diagnostic adjunct in select patients after mild head trauma.

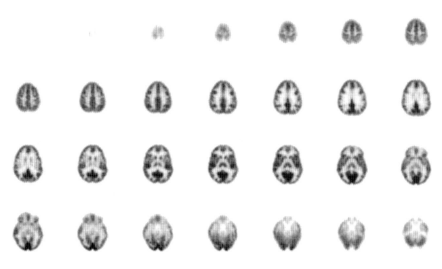

CASE FIG. 8.9A

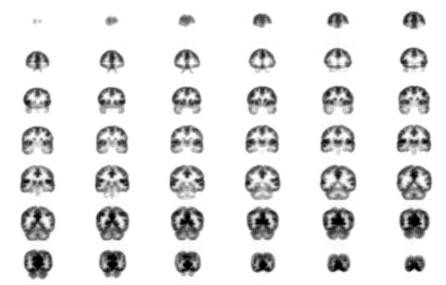

CASE FIG. 8.9B

Clinical Diagnosis:
Traumatic Brain Injury

CONTRIBUTOR:	IMAGING DATA:	
Hussein M. Abdel-Dayem, M.D.	**Camera:** Trionix	**Collimator:** High-resolution
Institution: Nuclear Medicine Service, St. Vincent's Hospital and Medical Center	**Tracer:** ^{99m}Tc HMPAO	**Dose:** 20.5 mCi

This 28-year-old left-handed woman sustained head trauma 6 days earlier with a few seconds' loss of consciousness. She now complains of persistent headaches.

A CT scan of the head was normal (Case Fig. 8.10A).

Tranverse-plane HMPAO images (Case Fig. 8.10B) reveal decreased uptake in the left posterior frontal and parietal cortex and the temporal lobes bilaterally.

Teaching Point:

After head trauma, a SPECT scan of the brain may be helpful in explaining the patient's symptoms.

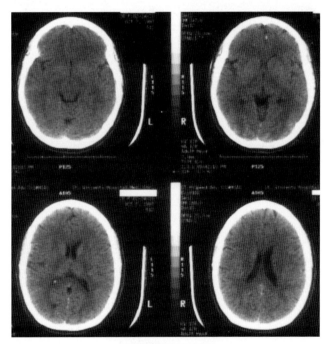

CASE FIG. 8.10A

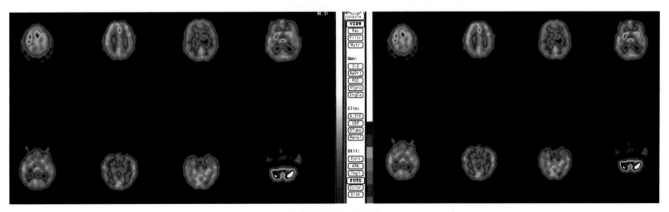

CASE FIG. 8.10B

CASE 8-11

Clinical Diagnosis:
Mild Head Trauma

CONTRIBUTOR:	**IMAGING DATA:**

Hussein M. Abdel-Dayem, M.D.
Institution: Nuclear Medicine Service, St.
Vincent's Hospital and Medical
Center

Camera: Trionix
Tracer: ^{99m}Tc ECD

Collimator: High-resolution
Dose: 25 mCi

This 23-year-old woman was seen shortly after experiencing head trauma with a transient (1 sec) loss of consciousness.

A CT scan of the head was normal.

^{99m}Tc-ECD SPECT images in the transverse plane (Case Fig. 8.11) reveal a focal perfusion defect involving the left inferior frontal lobe.

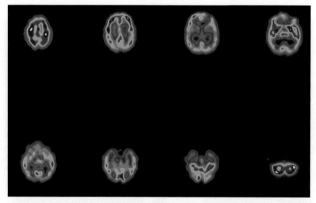

CASE FIG. 8.11

Clinical Diagnosis:
Trauma; Motor Vehicle Accident

CONTRIBUTORS:	IMAGING DATA:	
Robert S. Hellman, M.D.,	**Camera:** Neurocam	**Collimator:** High-resolution
Ronald S. Tikofsky, M.D.	**Tracer:** ^{99m}Tc HMPAO	**Dose:** 30.7 mCi
Institution: Medical College of Wisconsin		

This 44-year-old man, who was involved in a motor vehicle accident 3 weeks prior to admission, presented with the chief complaints of recurrent headaches and lethargy. His past history was significant for substance abuse.

An admission CT showed a large space-occupying lesion in the left frontal lobe with a hyperdense rim, which was thought to be due to a large subacute hematoma with surrounding edema or a cerebral abscess (Case Fig. 8.12A). There was also a moderate midline shift from left to right with asymmetric compression of the left lateral ventricles and impending transtentorial herniation on the left as well as subarachnoid hemorrhage.

An MRI study (Case Fig. 8.12B) revealed a large left frontal intracerebral abscess secondary to acute frontal sinusitis. In addition, an apparent defect in the posterior wall of the left frontal sinus was evident.

An HMPAO SPECT study (Case Fig. 8.12C) in the transaxial plane showed a large zone of absent perfusion in the left frontal region, extending across the midline, that correlated with the MRI and CT findings. A smaller zone of decreased perfusion in the right posterior parietal region was felt to be due to contrecoupe injury.

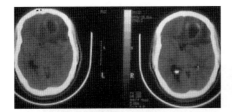

CASE FIG. 8.12A

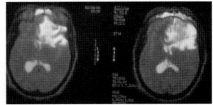

CASE FIG. 8.12B

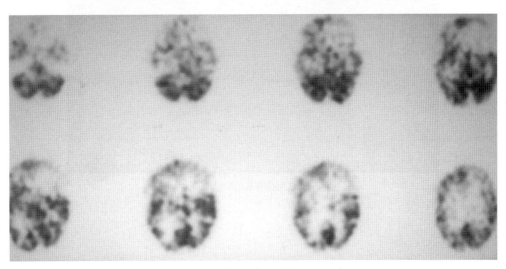

CASE FIG. 8.12C

Clinical Diagnosis:
Traumatic Brain Injury

CONTRIBUTORS:

James M. Mountz, M.D., Ph.D.,
Elmer C. San Perdo, M.D.
Institution: The University of Alabama at
        Birmingham Medical Center

IMAGING DATA:

Camera: ADAC MCD Vertex Plus
Tracer: ^{99m}Tc HMPAO (SPECT);
        ^{18}FDG-labeled (SPECT)

Collimator: High-resolution
Dose: ^{18}FDG 10 mCi; HMPAO 20 mCi

This 33-year-old man sustained head trauma during a motor vehicle accident. He presented with frontal lobe psychiatric symptoms but was not compensated for his claim because the anatomic imaging studies were interpreted as normal.

CT and MRI scans were reported as negative.

Both the ^{99m}Tc HMPAO and ^{18}FDG-labeled FDG SPECT scans (Case Fig. 8.13) show blood flow and metabolic defects in the left frontal cortex (*arrows*).

Teaching Points:

1. Cortical neuronal damage and diffuse axonal shearing (DAS) can produce significant neurological and/or functional and psychiatric abnormalities in posttraumatic brain injury.

2. Routine anatomic imaging, CT or MRI, does not reveal these injuries.

3. Because of the functional nature of the abnormality, often a physiologic scan using perfusion tracers such as ^{99m}Tc HMPAO, ^{99m}Tc ECD, or metabolic tracers such as ^{18}F-labeled ^{18}FDG can identify the focal cerebral abnormality.

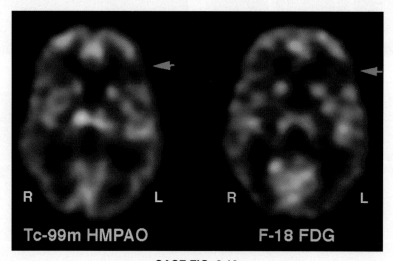

CASE FIG. 8.13

Clinical Diagnosis:
Traumatic Brain Injury

CONTRIBUTOR:

Masanori Ichise, M.D.
Institution: Mt. Sinai Hospital (Toronto)

IMAGING DATA:

Camera: Picker PRISM 3000
Tracer: ^{99m}Tc-ECD

Collimator: Ultra-high resolution fan-beam
Dose: 20 mCi

This 39-year-old man presented with a 20-h history of right facial weakness and an expressive aphasia after a motor vehicle accident.

A digital subtraction angiogram (DSA) revealed complete occlusion of the left internal carotid artery secondary to a traumatic dissection (Case Fig. 8.14A).

^{99m}Tc-ECD SPECT images in the transverse plane (Case Fig. 8.14B) reveal decreased radiotracer activity in the left frontotemporal cortex, including Broca's speech area.

Teaching Point:

Traumatic injury to the neck may cause brain perfusion abnormalities as seen in this case. Despite the occlusion of left internal carotid artery, partial perfusion to the left hemisphere is maintained secondary to collateral circulation from the contralateral hemisphere.

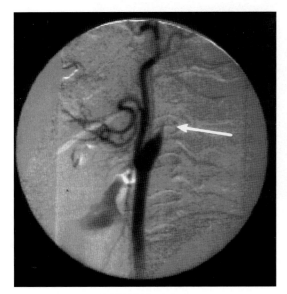

CASE FIG. 8.14A

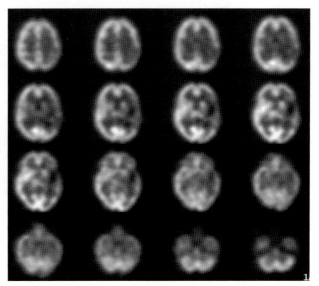

CASE FIG. 8.14B

Clinical Diagnosis:
Traumatic Brain Injury

CONTRIBUTOR:

Masanori Ichise, M.D.
Institution: Mt. Sinai Hospital, Toronto,
        Canada

IMAGING DATA:

Camera: Picker PRISM 3000
Tracer: ^{99m}Tc-ECD

Collimator: Ultra-high resolution fan-beam
Dose: 20 mCi

This 52-year-old man was hit by a truck while walking on the street. He lost consciousness for 30 min. After this trauma, he developed severe depression. ECD SPECT was done 6 months after injury.

A CT scan of the brain showed a questionable contusion in the inferior orbital region of the left frontal lobe.

Transverse ^{99m}Tc-ECD SPECT images (Case Fig. 8.15) performed 6 months posttrauma showed a well-defined cor-

tical perfusion defect in the inferior orbital region (*arrow*) of the left frontal lobe.

Teaching Point:

Traumatic brain injury in which sudden acceleration-deceleration forces are involved may result in brain contusion of the base of the brain anteriorly.

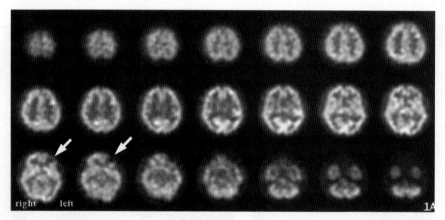

CASE FIG. 8.15

CASE 8-16

Clinical Diagnosis:
Trauma

CONTRIBUTORS:	IMAGING DATA:	
Robert S. Hellman, M.D.,	**Camera:** GE Neurocam	**Collimator:** High-resolution
Ronald S. Tikofsky, M.D.	**Tracer:** ^{99m}Tc HMPAO	**Dose:** 33 mCi
Institution: Medical College of Wisconsin		

This 57-year-old left-handed woman presented to the emergency room after having sustained severe head trauma at the time of a motor vehicle accident. Upon presentation to the emergency room, the patient was observed to be unresponsive. The initial workup revealed that she had sustained a right temporal skull fracture with an associated pneumocephalus.

An admission CT showed a large subarachnoid hemorrhage and a right intracerebral frontal-temporal-parietal hematoma with marked midline (right to left) shift. In addition, intraventricular hemorrhage was evident.

An emergency craniotomy was performed to evacuate the intracerebral hematomas. Following surgery, the patient remained comatose for 16 days. In the postcoma period, the patient was found to be severely aphasic. In addition, the patient manifested multiple episodes of inappropriate behavior.

A follow-up CT scan (Case Fig. 8.16A,B) after surgery showed a decrease in the size of the hematomas, an evolving cerebral contusion of the right temporal lobe, persistent mass effect, and a decrease in the subarachnoid hemorrhage.

An HMPAO SPECT study (Case Fig. 8.16C) in the transaxial plane, performed following evacuation of the subdural hematoma, revealed a large area of absent tracer activity in the posterior and mid-right frontal lobe extending deep into the right basal ganglia. In addition, decreased tracer uptake in the right temporal lobe, corresponding to the area of contusion seen on CT, was observed.

Teaching Point:

This patient illustrates the importance of ascertaining handedness. In this case of a left-handed patient with right hemispheric dominance, a right-sided lesion was associated with significant aphasia.

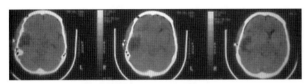

CASE FIG. 8.16A

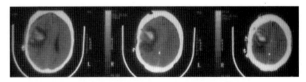

CASE FIG. 8.16B

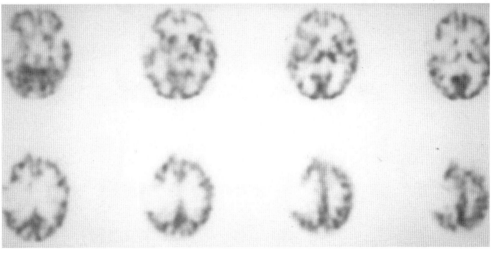

CASE FIG. 8.16C

251

Clinical Diagnosis:

Head Trauma Secondary to Sky Diving

CONTRIBUTOR:

Ronald L. Van Heertum, MD
Institution: The Kreitchman PET Center,
New York Presbyterian Hospital

IMAGING DATA:

PET Scanner: Siemens XACT 47
Tracer: ^{18}FDG

Attenuation Correction Method:
Autoattenuation
Dose: 7.73 mCi

This 21-year-old man sustained a severe closed head injury while sky diving when his parachute failed to open properly.

CT scan of the brain revealed frontal and temporal contusions (Case Figs. 8.17A,B).

An ^{18}FDG PET scan in the transverse plane (Case Fig. 8.17C) reveals a large focal area of decreased tracer activity involving the right temporal lobe and the mesial right frontal lobe (Case Fig. 8.17C).

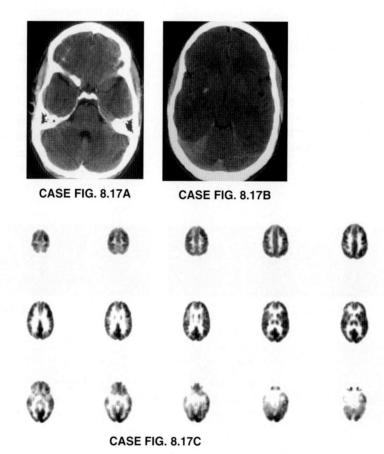

CASE FIG. 8.17A   CASE FIG. 8.17B

CASE FIG. 8.17C

Clinical Diagnosis:
Closed Cranial Trauma

CONTRIBUTORS:

S. Tzila Zwas, M.D.,
Elinor Goshen, M.D.

Institution: Chaim Sheba Medical Center

IMAGING DATA:

Camera: Elscint Dual-Head Helix
Tracer: ^{99m}Tc-ECD

Collimator: Fan-beam
Dose: 30 mCi

This 51-year-old man sustained a severe left frontal head injury following a motor vehicle accident 30 years earlier. He did not suffer any significant functional impairment and was gainfully employed. Immediately prior to the SPECT scan, he developed an obsessive-compulsive disorder (OCD), which at the time of the scan was not being treated.

A CT scan of the brain revealed chronic changes corresponding to known left frontal trauma.

The ^{99m}Tc-ECD SPECT study (Case Figs. 8.18A,B) in the transverse and coronal planes reveals a significant perfusion defect in the left frontal and temporal regions consistent with the CT findings.

CASE FIG. 8.18A   CASE FIG. 8.18B

Functional Cerebral SPECT and PET Imaging, Third Edition,
edited by R.L.Van Heertum and R.S. Tikofsky,
Lippincott Williams & Wilkins, New York © 2000.

CHAPTER 9

Psychiatric Disorders

Dolores Malaspina and Ariela Berman

It has long be accepted that schizophrenia, mood disorders, and other psychiatric diseases are biological disorders, but it is only recently that imaging technology has permitted the *in vivo* study of the brain. Although the pathophysiology of most medical conditions is well described, the inaccessibility of the skull-encased brain had precluded such research in mental illnesses. Now, the rapidly evolving technologies of radiologic science offer promising opportunities to explore the nature of brain-behavior relationships. Advances in structural brain imaging permit the resolution of smaller and smaller brain regions, and we may soon be able to explore neuroanatomy at the cellular level. Functional imaging techniques, such as positron-emission tomography (PET), single-photon-emission computed tomography (SPECT), and functional magnetic resonance imaging (fMRI) reveal neurophysiologic activity during specified behavioral conditions, showing networks of coordinated brain activity that underlie different mental operations. Other imaging research paradigms used in psychiatry include neuroreceptor and neurochemical characterization studies as well as cognitive, emotional, and pharmacologic challenge studies.

Although the use of neuroimaging to make psychiatric diagnoses is premature, imaging research has begun to suggest the neural underpinnings of several mental disorders, such as schizophrenia, affective disorders, anxiety, developmental disorders, and substance abuse. Associations among neural substrates and disease correlates, such as symptoms, illness onset, cognitive impairment, severity, and responsiveness to treatment are presently being examined. Nonetheless, variable and even contradictory results hinder the interpretation

of imaging data for many psychiatric disorders. This variability may be in part due to technologic limitations as well as clinical variables, including patient variability, illness state, neuroactivation differences, medication effects, and choice of comparison groups. Furthermore, sample sizes are often small, given the presumed heterogeneity of most psychiatric disorders. With improving technologies, variable findings may converge. As an example, 80% of studies using high-resolution MRI of slices of 1.5 mm or less have been able to identify hippocampal abnormalities in patients with schizophrenia, whereas only about 50% of studies using MRI slices greater than 1.5 mm have been able to identify these abnormalities.

This chapter highlights some of the imaging findings for several psychiatric illnesses to date. The sections are divided by specific disorder and organized by type of imaging technology. Pertinent experimental findings from a number of paradigms are reviewed and clinical applications for the radiologist are discussed.

SCHIZOPHRENIA

Structural Imaging

The largest amount of psychiatric imaging research has been directed at elucidating the illness of schizophrenia. Although it was recognized as a distinct disease a century ago, it is still the most enigmatic mental illness. The initial speculation by Kraepelin in 1919 (1) that the "frontal areas of the brain, the central convolutions, and the temporal lobes" were damaged in schizophrenia is being borne out in modern imaging studies.

The first computed tomography (CT) study in schizophrenia (2) demonstrated enlarged ventricular brain ratios (VBR), a finding now confirmed in over 50 studies, and present in up to three-fourths of patients in variable severity (3–5). The third ventricle—which surrounds the thalamus, hypothalamus, and fornix—may also be enlarged (6), as are

D. Malaspina: Columbia University College of Physicians and Surgeons and New York State Psychiatric Institute, New York, New York 10032.

A. Berman: Psychiatry Department, Columbia University College of Physicians and Surgeons and New York State Psychiatric Institute, New York, New York 10032.

the cortical sulci, the latter possibly being more specific to schizophrenia versus bipolar disorder with psychotic features (7,8). Reduced gray-matter volumes are likely to account for the diminished cortical volumes (9). Despite the nonspecificity of VBR widening, it provided the first clear evidence of neuropathology in schizophrenia. This ventriculomegaly exists without gliosis, which first suggested a neurodevelopmental etiology for schizophrenia, since later brain damage would be associated with scarring.

Despite these documented abnormalities, most structural images of schizophrenia patients are clinically read as "within normal limits," a consequence of the variability in neuroanatomy among normal subjects and the subtlety of the findings in schizophrenia. When groups of schizophrenia patients and controls are contrasted, differences between the schizophrenic and normal subject groups are revealed. With the ideal matched control for genetic background variability (monozygotic twins discordant for schizophrenia), increased ventricular size and diminished volume of medial temporal lobe structures are almost always more prominent in the affected as compared to the unaffected cotwin (10). Since these twins share all of their genes, the neuroanatomic differences between affected and unaffected cotwins are presumed to reflect the neuropathology of schizophrenia. Many MRI studies have focused specifically on the temporal lobes because of the abnormalities in language that accompany the disorder. Temporal lobe volume reductions, particularly of medial temporal lobe structures (hippocampus and amygdala), are common (10,11), even in patients with first-episode psychosis (12).

Volume reductions are also variably reported for total brain, cerebellum, thalamus, and corpus callosum (13–15). Findings of enlarged basal ganglia volumes in schizophrenia are now attributed to medication treatment effects (16,17). There is no consensus that structural findings are related to specific symptoms, treatment response, or illness features, although such data are expected with advancements in imaging and refinements in diagnosis.

Functional Imaging

Decreased frontal brain blood flow (hypofrontality) was the first reported metabolic abnormality in schizophrenia (18). Although it was replicated in some studies (19,20), others have found no differences from control subjects (21–23) or even increased frontal flow (24,25). These inconsistent results have been attributed to the use of "resting" baseline conditions that do not control cognitive activity. Using specified cognitive tasks has reduced the variability among imaging results and has led to more consistent reports of decreased regional cerebral blood flow (rCBF) in the prefrontal cortex in patients with schizophrenia (26,27). Functional MRI has likewise demonstrated decreased frontal cortical activation for schizophrenia patients' performance on tasks such as word production (28). Finally, task-related hy-

pofrontality is present at illness onset, even in neuroleptic-naive patients (29).

Besides the frontal cortex, abnormal functional activity in the temporal lobes, thalamus, and medial temporal lobe has also been identified. Despite the abnormal function in several sites, no primary site of pathologic function has been designated. It is becoming evident that the brain dysfunction in schizophrenia involves multiple neural dimensions. Defects in neurotransmitter modulation of networks, abnormal structure or function in specific network nodes, and dysfunctional connectivity could all account for the observed abnormalities. One theory of schizophrenia concerns a disruption of the normal connectivity of the frontal cortex and the medial temporal lobe (30). The integration of results from multiple studies suggests that dysfunction in the frontostriatal-thalamic circuit might underlie schizophrenia (31). This disturbed circuitry could account for the sensory overload, disturbed thinking, and psychosis of schizophrenia.

Attempts to relate specific symptoms to cerebral blood flow have most consistently associated low frontal flow with deficit and negative symptoms (27,32). Liddle et al. (33) found pre-frontal loci of altered perfusion associated with both psychomotor poverty and disorganization syndromes. In contrast, positive symptoms, such as hallucinations, seem related to increased cerebral blood flow (13). In particular, positive symptoms are reported to accompany hypermetabolism in medial temporal lobe (33,34), left temporal lobe, and Broca's area (35).

Neuroreceptors

The postulated hyperactivity of the neurotransmitter dopamine in schizophrenia has made it a focus of many studies. Although the data are still contradictory, they seem increasingly consistent with both pre- and postsynaptic alterations of dopamine transmission. Meanwhile, other neuroreceptor research in schizophrenia focuses on glutamate. The effects of neuroleptics on glucose metabolism in the brain has been explored using PET and an association between neuroleptic treatment and an increase in basal ganglia glucose metabolism has been demonstrated. In addition, using PET to explore relationships between neuroreceptor occupancy (D2 and 5-HT$_{2A}$) and neuroleptic blood levels has provided promising evidence for the mechanisms of neuroleptic action (36,37). In the future, it is anticipated that brain imaging will be used as an objective measure to determine rational pharmacotherapy for individuals with schizophrenia.

AFFECTIVE DISORDERS

Structural Imaging

Major depression is a heterogenous disorder, and its study has proven to be a challenge for investigators. Despite this limitation, specific structural abnormalities are consistently described in certain subsets of patients, particularly those who have a late-age onset, psychosis, or bipolar illness. Some variance in imaging results is attributed to clinical factors, with permanent anatomic changes associated with chronic illness, such as reduced gray-matter density in the left temporal cortex, including the hippocampus.

Reduced frontal cortical volumes are reported for some unipolar depressed patients (38,39), but not in bipolar patients (40). Other studies have shown that some patients with depression have significantly smaller caudate and putamen basal ganglia volumes (38,41). Inconsistent results examining amygdala volumes have also been reported. Finally, evidence has been found that both unipolar and bipolar patients have significantly smaller cerebellar volumes. Unlike studies of schizophrenia, most studies of patients with depression have not found global atrophy, larger cortical sulci, or increased VBRs.

Depression can arise secondarily due to damage to the neocortex and basal ganglia as a result of injury or stroke. In particular, late-life onset of depression may be caused by comorbid vascular disorders. These patients often show focal abnormalities and increased small, deep, white-matter lesions called periventricular hyperintensities, consistent with arteriosclerosis and silent cerebral infarction, providing further support for the concept of vascular depression.

For bipolar depression, as in elderly unipolar depressives, there are increased rates of subcortical white matter and periventricular hyperintensities (42,43). Enlarged third ventricles, along with decreased ventricular size, is reported for bipolar patients (44–48). The temporal lobe of patients with bipolar disorder has also received significant attention from investigators. One study found smaller temporal lobe volumes bilaterally (49), another found increased left temporal lobe volume (50), and yet another found no difference in temporal lobe volumes (51).

Strakowski et al. (52) found that patients with bipolar disorder had enlarged amygdalas (as well as other structures) compared to matched controls. In line with imaging findings, two brain circuits of mood regulation have been proposed: amygdala-thalamus-prefrontal cortex and limbic system-striatum-pallidum-thalamus. Despite the limitations to structural imaging data, such as small sample size and methodologic variances, it is a tenable hypothesis that pathology in localized regions may disrupt the neural systems that underlie mood regulation.

Functional Imaging

While brain function is not globally disturbed in affective illness, there appears to be disturbed activity in specific circuits; in some cases these are reversible state dependent changes and in other cases the dysfunction is presumably related to underlying structural abnormalities. The most consistent findings in resting state studies using both PET and SPECT are hypometabolism in the caudate (53), cingulate (54), and frontotemporal regions (55,56). Activation studies have demonstrated abnormalities in the prefrontal cortex as well as the cingulate cortices and amygdala. PET and SPECT studies have also found increased blood flow or glucose metabolism in the ventral prefrontal cortex and decreased blood flow/glucose metabolism in the dorsal prefrontal cortex in depressed patients versus controls.

Reversible, clinical state–dependent functional abnormalities are described in networks that subserve emotional processing in major depression. Abnormal metabolism in the left prefrontal cortex is related to severity of depression as gauged by the Hamilton Depression Scale. Depression accompanied by cognitive impairment has been related to decreased rCBF in the left medial frontal gyrus and an increased blood flow in the cerebellar vermis (57,58). Multiple studies have shown that blood flow normalizes in the prefrontal cortex, amygdala, ventral prefrontal cortex, and medial thalamus following treatment and paralleling improvement in depressive symptoms (59,60). The amygdala, the prefrontal cortex, and hippocampus appear to be involved in a key neural circuit that is implicated in depression. The normalization of glucose metabolism accompanying symptom improvement is related to both pharmacologic as well as nonpharmacologic treatments, including electroshock therapy (ECT), sleep deprivation, and cognitive behavioral therapy (61,62).

In bipolar depression, a PET study comparing manic to depressed states showed that global glucose metabolism was significantly increased in the manic state (53). Another study also comparing manic versus depressed states found increased rCBF, particularly in the left inferior frontal region, in manic patients and controls compared to depressed patients (63).

Neuroreceptors

A wave of receptor studies in patients with depression has begun. Serotonin is the most promising candidate based on the biology and pharmacology of depression (64). Many ligands are being synthesized and tested for their specific serotonin receptor subtype.

PANIC DISORDER

No gross neuroanatomic abnormalities have been identified in the structures implicated in panic disorder. However, PET and SPECT studies have demonstrated dysfunction in the temporal cortex, orbitofrontal cortex, thalamus, and amygdala. The amygdala plays a significant role in mediating fear and anxiety behaviors. A neuronal network between the hippocampus, cortical structures, and amygdala is theorized to be involved in developing cognitive attributions about fearful stimuli to enhance memory function and facilitate adaptive responses (65).

Panic attacks during imaging induced with yohimbine were associated with decreased rCBF in the frontal cortex in patients but not in healthy controls (66). Panic attacks induced with lactate caused decreased bilateral hippocampal and increased inferior frontal cortex in a right-left asymmetry (67). In a ^{18}FDG-PET study using an auditory continuous performance (discrimination) task, patients with panic disorder showed lower left-right hippocampal ratios and lower metabolic rates in the left inferior parietal lobule compared to controls (68). Another ^{18}fluorodeoxyglucose (^{18}FDG)-PET study of panic patients at rest showed increased left hippocampal and parahippocampal metabolism and decreased metabolism in the right inferior parietal and right superior temporal regions compared to controls (69).

Neuroreceptors

Benzodiazepine receptor imaging has also been used to explore the neurobiology of panic disorder. In a PET study using the benzodiazepine antagonist 1231-RO16-0154 (iomazenil), Schlegel and colleagues (70) showed a global reduction in the benzodiazepine binding in occipital, frontal, and temporal cortices compared to control subjects. Malizia et al. (71) also showed a global reduction in the benzodiazepine site using flumazenil radiolabeled with carbon 11.

SUBSTANCE ABUSE

Brain imaging has also been used to study the neuroanatomic and neurochemical nature of substance abuse. Substance abuse is a broad and heterogenous category of disorders. Given the direct and indirect neurotoxicity of many drugs of abuse, it is difficult to interpret whether neuroabnormalities are predisposing factors or consequences of abuse. The necessary longitudinal and high-risk studies have yet to be conducted. Abnormalities in the prefrontal cortex of substance abusers are a common finding. Higher glucose metabolism in the orbitofrontal cortex has been reported in polysubstance abusers (72) as well as in cocaine abusers (73). Alcoholic subjects show volume reductions in the frontal lobe (74) and polysubstance abusers who had been drug-free for 15 days had significantly smaller frontal lobe volumes (left and right hemispheres) compared to controls (75).

Glucose metabolism was reduced when cocaine was administered to subjects with histories of intravenous cocaine abuse (76). Pearlson and Marsh (77) found significant decreases in rCBF in frontal and basal ganglia regions when cocaine was administered to abstinent cocaine users. This decrease in rCBF was negatively correlated with subjective feelings of "high" and "rush." Likewise, abstinent cocaine abusers have been demonstrated to have decreased glucose metabolism in several frontal regions, particularly the orbitofrontal cortex and cingulate gyrus (78). These changes were related to decreased D2 receptor availability, which also correlated with years of cocaine abuse.

AUTISM ABNORMALITIES

A number of brain MRI studies have been conducted in subjects with autism compared to normal controls. The specific area of the posterior cerebellum has been studied extensively but has yielded inconsistent findings (79–81). A number of MRI studies have found significantly smaller volumes of the corpus callosum in patients versus controls (82,83), and increased brain volume is also reported (84). Other data are consistent with frontal lobe abnormalities, which correlates with the known frontal lobe deficits as measured by neuropsychological tests in patients with autism. Area 24 of the anterior cingulate may also be smaller and metabolically less active in autistic patients relative to normal controls (85).

Most or all of these studies are limited by small and heterogenous sample sizes. Furthermore, many of these studies examined high-functioning autistic subjects as opposed to more impaired or low-functioning subjects.

These advances in imaging technology may directly reveal the aberrant neurobiology that underlies the major mental disorders, allowing rapid diagnosis and guiding effective treatment for these patients. Currently, psychiatric diagnoses are based solely on the presence and longitudinal course of observable symptoms and behaviors, which are examined in diagnostic algorithms, such as those of the *Diagnostic and Statistical Manual of Mental Disorders,* 4th ed. (DSM-IV). Although reference to brain biology (lesions, other abnormalities, etc.) is not incorporated into this modern classification system, it seems feasible that future psychiatric diagnostic criteria may include neuroimaging data.

ACKNOWLEDGMENT

This work was supported by the G. Harold and Leila Mathers Foundation.

REFERENCES

1. Kraepelin E. Dementia praecox and paraphrenia. In: *Morbid anatomy.* Reprinted facsimile. New York: Robert E. Krieger Publishing, 1971:213–223.
2. Johnston EC, Crow TJ, Frith CD, et al. Cerebral ventricle size and cognitive impairment in chronic schizophrenics. *Lancet* 1976;2:924–926.
3. Raz N, Raz S, Bigler ED. Ventriculomegaly in schizophrenia: the role of control groups and the perils of dichotomous thinking. *Psychiatr Res* 1988;26:245–248.
4. Lewis SW. Computerized tomography in schizophrenia 15 years on. *Br J Psychiat* 1990;157:16–24.
5. Pfefferbaum A, Lim KO, Rosenbloom M, et al. Brain magnetic resonance imaging: approaches for investigating schizophrenia. *Schizophr Bull* 1990;16:453–476.
6. Boronow J, Pickar D, Ninan RP, et al. Atrophy limited to the third ventricle only in chronic schizophrenic patients: reports of a controlled series. *Arch Gen Psychiatry* 1985;42:266–271.
7. Pfefferbaum A, Zipursky RB, Lim KO, et al. Computed tomographic evidence for generalized sulcal and ventricular enlargement in schizophrenia. *Arch Gen Psychiatry* 1988;45:633–640.
8. Harvey I, Ron MA, DuBoulay G, et al. Reduction in cortical volume in schizophrenia on magnetic resonance imaging. *Psychol Med* 1993;23:591–604.
9. Zipursky RB, Lim KO, Sullivan EV, et al. Widespread grey matter volume deficits in schizophrenia. *Arch Gen Psychiatry* 1992;49:195–205.

10. Suddath RL, Chrisitson GW, Torrey EF, et al. Anatomical abnormalities in the brains of monozygotic twins discordant for schizophrenia. *N Engl J Med* 1990;322:789–794.

11. Barta PE, Pearlson GD, Powers RE, et al. Auditory hallucinations and smaller superior temporal lobe gyrus volume in schizophrenia. *Am J Psychiatry* 1990;147:1457–1482.

12. Velakoulis D, Pantelis C, McGorry PD, et al. Hippocampal volume in first-episode psychoses and chronic schizophrenia a high-resolution magnetic imaging study. *Arch Gen Psychiatry* 1999;56:133–141.

13. Gunther W, Petsch R, Steinberg R, et al. Brain dysfunction during motor activation and corpus callosum alterations in schizophrenia measured by cerebral blood flow and magnetic resonance imaging. *Biol Psychiatry* 1991;29:535–555.

14. Woodruff PW, Pearlson GD, Geer MJ, et al. A computerized magnetic resonance imaging study of corpus callosum morphology in schizophrenia. *Psychol Med* 1993;23:45–56.

15. Gur RE, Mozley PD, Shtasel DL, et al. Clinical subtypes of schizophrenia: differences in brain and CSF volume. *Am J Psychiatry* 1994;151:3.

16. Chakos MH, Mayerhoff DI, Loebel AD, et al. Incidence and correlates of acute extrapyramidal symptoms in first episode of schizophrenia. *Psychopharmol Bull* 1992;28:81–86.

17. Bilder RM, Wu H, Chakos MH, et al. Cerebral morphometry and clozapine treatment in schizophrenia. *J Clin Psychiatry* 1994;55(suppl B):53–56.

18. Ingvar DH, Franzen G. Abnormalities of cerebral blood flow distribution in patients with chronic schizophrenia. *Acta Psychiatr Scand* 1974;50:452–462.

19. Buchsbaum MS. The frontal lobes, basal ganglia, and temporal lobes as sites for schizophrenia. *Schizophr Bull* 1990;16:379–389.

20. Rubin E, Sackeim HA, Nobler MS, Moelle JR. Brain imaging studies of antidepressant treatment. *Psychiatr Ann* 1994;24:653–658.

21. Early TS, Reiman EM, Raichle ME, et al. Left globus pallidus abnormality in never-medicated patients with schizophrenia. *Proc Natl Acad Sci USA* 1987;84:561–563.

22. Jernigan TL, Sargent T, Pfefferbaum A, et al. 18-Fluorodeoxyglucose PET in schizophrenia. *Psychiatry Res* 1985;16:317–329.

23. Gur RE, Resnick SM, Alavi A, et al. Regional brain function in schizophrenia: I. A positron emission tomography study. *Arch Gen Psychiatry* 1987;44:119–125.

24. Szechtman H, Nahmias C, Garnett S, et al. Effect of neuroleptics on altered cerebral glucose metabolism in schizophrenia. *Arch Gen Psychiatry* 1988;45:523–532.

25. Cleghorn JM, Garnett ES, Nahmias C, et al. Regional brain metabolism during auditory hallucinations in chronic schizophrenia. *Brit J Psychiatry* 1990;157:562–570.

26. Weinberger DR, Berman KF, Zec RF. Physiologic dysfunction of dorsolateral prefrontal cortex in schizophrenia: I. Regional cerebral blood flow evidence. *Arch Gen Psychiatry* 1986;43:114–124.

27. Andreason NC, Rezai K, Alliger R, et al. Hypofrontality in neuroleptic-naive patients and in patients with chronic schizophrenia. *Arch Gen Psychiatry* 1992;49:943–958.

28. Yurgelun-Todd DA, Renshaw PF, Waternaux CM, et al. H-MRS of n-acetyl aspartate (NAA) in the temporal lobes in schizophrenia. *Biol Psychiatry* 1993;33:45A.

29. Catafau AM, Parellada E, Lomena FJ, et al. Prefrontal and temporal blood flow in schizophrenia: resting and activation technetium-99m-HMPAO SPECT patterns in young neuroleptic-naive patients with acute disease. *J Nucl Med* 1994;35:935–941.

30. Friston KJ, Firth CD. Schizophrenia: a disconnection syndrome? *Clin Neurosci* 1995;3:89–97.

31. Buchsbaum MS, Hazlett EA. Positron emission tomography studies of abnormal glucose metabolism in schizophrenia. *Schizophr Bull* 1998;24:343–364.

32. Weinberger DR, Gibson R, Coppola R, et al. The distribution of cerebral muscarinic acetylcholine receptors in vivo in patients with dementia. *Arch Neurol* 1991;48:169–175.

33. Liddle PF, Friston KJ, Frith CD, et al. Patterns of cerebral blood flow in schizophrenia. *Brit J Psychiatry* 1992;160:179–186.

34. Musalek M, Poderka I, Walter H, et al. Regional brain function in hallucinations: a study of regional cerebral blood flow with 99m-Tc-HM-PAO-SPECT in patients with auditory hallucinations, tactile hallucinations, and normal controls. *Comp Psychiatry* 1989;30:99–108.

35. McGuire PK, Shah GM, Murray RM. Increased blood flow in Broca's area during auditory hallucinations in schizophrenia. *Lancet* 1993;342:703–706.

36. Nyberg S, Nilsson U, Okubo Y, et al. Implications of brain imaging for the management of schizophrenia. *Int Clin Psychopharmacol* 1998;13(suppl 3):S15–S20.

37. Kapur S, Zipursky RB, Remington G, et al. 5-HT2 and D2 receptor occupancy of olanzapine in schizophrenia: a PET investigation. *Am J Psychiatry* 1998;155:921–928.

38. Krishnan KR, McDonald WM, Escalona PR, et al. Magnetic resonance imaging of the caudate nuclei in depression: preliminary observations. *Arch Gen Psychiatry* 1992;49:553–557.

39. Coffey CE, Wilkinson WE, Weiner RD, et al. Quantitative cerebral anatomy in depression: a controlled magnetic resonance imaging study. *Arch Gen Psychiatry* 1993;50:7–16.

40. Schlaepfer TE, Harris GJ, Tien AY, et al. Decreased regional cortical grey matter volume in schizophrenia. *Am J Psychiatry* 1994;151:842–848.

41. Husain MM, McDonald WM, Doraiswamy PM, et al. A magnetic resonance imaging study of putamen nuclei in major depression. *Psychiatry Res* 1991;40:95–99.

42. Swayze VW, Andreasen NC, Alliger RJ, et al. Subcortical and temporal structures in affective disorder and schizophrenia: a magnetic resonance imaging study. *Biol Psychiatry* 1992;31:221–240.

43. Figiel GS, Krishnan KRR, Rao VP, et al. Subcortical hyperintensities on brain magnetic resonance imaging: a comparison of normal and bipolar subjects. *J Neuropsychiatr Clin Neurosci* 1991;3:18–22.

44. Jacoby RJ, Levy R. Computed tomography in the elderly: Part 3. Affective disorder. *Br J Psychiatry* 1980;136:270–275.

45. Rieder RO, Mann LS, Weinberger DR, et al. Computed tomographic scans in patients with schizophrenia, schizoaffective, and bipolar affective disorder. *Arch Gen Psychiatry* 1983;40:735–739.

46. Targum SD, Rosen LN, DeLisi LE, et al. Cerebral ventricular size in major depressive disorder: association with delusional symptoms. *Biol Psychiatry* 1983;18:329–336.

47. Schlegel S, Kretzschmar K. Computed tomography in affective disorders: Part 1. Ventricular and sulcal measurements. *Biol Psychiatry* 1987;22:4–14.

48. Dewan MJ, Haldipur CV, Lane EE, et al. Biopolar affective disorder: I. Comprehensive quantitative computed tomography. *Acta Psychiatr Scand* 1988;77:670–676.

49. Altshuler LL, Conrad A, Hauser P, et al. Reduction of temporal lobe volume in bipolar disorder: a preliminary report of magnetic resonance imaging. *Arch Gen Psychiatry* 1991;48:482–483.

50. Harvey I, Persaud R, Ron MA, et al. Volumetric MRI measurements in bipolars compared with schizophrenics and healthy controls. *Psychol Med* 1994;24:689–699.

51. Johnstone EC, Owens DGC, Crow TJ, et al. Temporal lobe structure as determined by nuclear magnetic resonance in schizophrenia and bipolar affective disorder. *J Neurol Neurosurg Psychiatry* 1989;52:736–741.

52. Strakowski SM, DelBello MP, Sax KW, et al. Brain magnetic resonance imaging of structural abnormalities in bipolar disorder. *Arch Gen Psychiatry* 1999;56:254–260.

53. Baxter LR Jr., Phelps ME, Mazziotta JC, et al. Cerebral metabolic rates for glucose in mood disorders. *Arch Gen Psychiatry* 1985;42:441–447.

54. Dolan RJ, Grasby PM, Bench C, et al. Pharmacological challenge and PET imaging of serotonin-2 receptors in depression (abstr). *Psychiatry Res* 1992;15:216.

55. Post RM, DeLisi LE, Holcomb HH, et al. Glucose utilization in the temporal cortex of affectively ill patients: positron emission tomography. *Biol Psychiatry* 1987;22:545–553.

56. Dolan RJ, Grasby PM, Bench C, et al. Pharmacological challenge and PET imaging. *Clin Neuropharmacol* 1992;15(suppl 1, pt A):216A–217A.

57. Bench RM, Fristson KJ, Brown RG, et al. Regional cerebral blood flow in depression measured by positron emission tomography: the relationship with clinical dimensions. *Psychol Med* 1993;23:579–590.

58. Bench RM, Frackowiak RSJ, Dolan RJ. Changes in regional cerebral blood flow on recovery from depression. *Psychol Med* 1995;25:247–251.

59. Drevets WC, Raichle ME. Neuroanatomical circuits in depression: implications for treatment mechanisms. *Psychopharmacol Bull* 1992;26:261–274.

60. Drevets WC, Price JL, Simpson JS, et al. State-and trait-like neuroimaging abnormalities in depression: effects of antidepressant treatment (abstr). *Soc Neurosci* 1996;22:266.

61. Sackheim HA, Prohovnik I, Moeller JR, et al. Regional cerebral blood flow in mood disorders. *Arch Gen Psychiatry* 1990;40:60–70.

62. Rubin E, Sackheim HA, Nobler MS, Moeller JR. Brain imaging studies of antidepressant treatment. *Psychiatr Ann* 1994;24:653–658.

63. Rubin RT, Phillips JJ, Sadow TF, McCracken JT. Adrenal gland volume in major depression: increase during the depressive episode and decrease with successful treatment. *Arch Gen Psychiatry* 1995;52:213–218.

64. D'haenen H, Bossuyt A, Mertens J, et al. SPECT imaging of serotonin-2 receptors in depression. *Psychiatry Res* 1992;45:227–237.

65. Goddard AW, Charney DS. Toward an integrated neurobiology of panic disorder. *J Clin Psychiatry* 1997;58(suppl 2):4–11.

66. Woods SW, Koster K, Krystal JK, et al. Yohimbine alters regional cerebral blood flow in panic disorder (letter). *Lancet* 1988;2:678.

67. DeCristofaro MT, Sessarego A, Pupi A, et al. Brain perfusion abnormalities in drug-naive, lactate-sensitive panic patients. *Biol Psychiatry* 1993;33:505–512.

68. Nordahl TE, Semple WE, Gross M, et al. Cerebral glucose metabolic differences in patients with panic disorder. *Neuropsychopharmacol* 1998;46:243–250.

69. Bisaga A, Katz JL, Antonini A, et al. Cerebral glucose metabolism in women with panic disorder. *Am J Psychiatry* 1998;155:1178–1183.

70. Schlegel S, Steinert H, Bockisch A, et al. Decreased benzodiazepine receptor binding in panic disorder measured by iomazenil-SPECT. *Eur Arch Psychiatry Clin Neurosci* 1994;244:49–51.

71. Malizia AL, Cunningham VJ, Bell CJ, et al. Decreased brain GABA(A)-benzodiazepine receptor binding in panic disorder: preliminary results from a quantitative PET study. *Arch Gen Psychiatry* 1998;55:715–720.

72. Stapelton JM, Morgan MJ, Phillips RL, et al. Cerebral glucose utilization in polysubstance abuse. *Neuropsychopharmacol* 1995;13:21–31.

73. Volkow ND, Fowler JS, Wolf AP, et al. Changes in brain glucose metabolism in cocaine dependence and withdrawal. *Amer J Psychiatry* 1991;148:621–626.

74. Pfefferbaum A, Sullivan EV, Mathalon DH, et al. Frontal lobe volume loss observed with magnetic resonance imaging in older chronic alcoholics. *Alcohol Clin Exp Res* 1997;21:521–529.

75. Liu X, Matochik JA, Cadet J, London ED. Smaller volume of prefrontal lobe in polysubstance abusers: a magnetic resonance imaging study. *Neuropsychopharmacology* 1998;18:243–252.

76. London ED, Cascella NG, Wong DF, et al. Cocaine induced reduction of glucose utilization in human brain. *Arch Gen Psychiatry* 1990;47:567–574.

77. Pearlson GD, Marsh L. Magnetic resonance imaging in psychiatry. *Rev Psychiat* 1993;12:347.

78. Volkow ND, Fowler JS, Wang GL, et al. Decreased dopamine D2 receptor availability is associated with reduced frontal metabolism in cocaine abusers. *Synapse* 1993;14:169–177.

79. Courchesne E, Townsend J, Saitoh O. The brain in infantile autism: posterior fossa structures are abnormal. *Neurology* 1994;44:215–222.

80. Priven J, Nehme E, Simon J, et al. Magnetic resonance imaging in autism: measurement of the cerebellum, pons, and fourth ventricle. *Biol Psychiatry* 1992;31:491–504.

81. Kleiman MD, Neff S, Rosman NP. The brain in infantile autism: is the cerebellum really abnormal (abstr). *Ann Neurol* 1992;26:442.

82. Priven J, Bailey J, Ransom BJ, et al. An MRI study of the corpus callosum in autism. *Am J Psychiatry* 1997;154:1051–1056.

83. Egaas B, Courchesne E, Saitoh O. Reduced size of the corpus callosum in autism. *Arch Neurol* 1995;52:794–801.

84. Priven J, Arndt S, Bailey BS, et al. An MRI study of brain size in autism. *Am J Psychiatry* 1995;152:1145–1149.

85. Haznedar MM, Buchsbaum MS, Metzger M. Anterior cingulate gyrus volume and glucose metabolism in autistic disorder. *Am J Psychiatry* 1997;154:1047–1050.

Clinical Diagnosis:

Schizoaffective Disorder

CONTRIBUTORS:	IMAGING DATA:	
Prof. Hans Biersack, E. Klemm, M.D.	**Camera:** ADAC-Genesys	**Collimator:** Ultra-high-resolution
Institution: University of Bonn	**Tracer:** 99mTC	**Dose:** 20 mCi

This 49-year-old patient with a known schizoaffective disorder was referred for further evaluation. At the time of the SPECT study, he was on an antidepressant and a benzodiazepine.

An hexamamethypropyleneamine-oxime (HMPAO)-SPECT study (Case Fig. 9.1) in the transaxial (*upper row*), coronal (*middle row*), and sagittal (*lower row*) planes revealed decreased radiotracer in the left temporal region.

Teaching Point:

This is another example of the types of temporal lobe asymmetries that may be seen in psychosis.

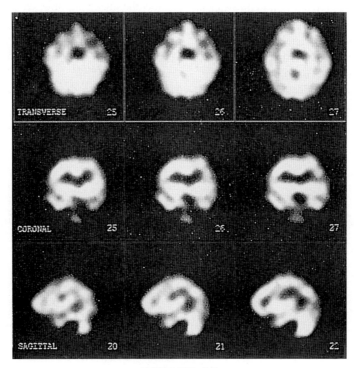

CASE FIG. 9.1

Clinical Diagnosis:

Acute Paranoid Schizophrenia: Follow-up During Treatment

CONTRIBUTOR:	IMAGING DATA:	
Ronald L. Van Heertum, M.D.	**Camera:** GE 400AC/T;STAR II	**Collimator:** High-resolution
Institution: St. Vincent's Hospital and Medical Center	**Tracer:** [123]I IMP	**Dose:** 3.0 mCi

This 30-year-old man was referred for evaluation of an acute psychosis characterized by paranoid delusions, auditory hallucinations, and destructive behavior that had become progressively worse over the preceding 2 years. An electroencephalography (EEG) and a CT scan were normal. The clinical diagnosis was acute paranoid schizophrenia.

At the time of the initial SPECT study, the patient was receiving a total daily dose of 100 mg of loxapine (an antipsychotic medication). The initial cerebral SPECT study (Case Fig. 9.2A) in the transaxial (**A**), coronal (**B**), and sagittal (**C**) planes revealed an increased tracer deposition in the caudate nuclei, along with a mild decrease of tracer activity in the cortex of the frontal lobes. Two weeks later, a follow-up cerebral SPECT study was performed. At that time, the patient was much improved clinically. The follow-up study (Case Fig. 9.2B) demonstrated a significant but partial decrease of tracer activity in the caudate nuclei. A slight focal increase in tracer deposition was noted in the right temporal lobe. This later finding may have been related to the patient's medication lowering the seizure threshold.

Published with permission from Van Heertum RL, O'Connell RA. The evaluation of psychiatric disease with IMP cerebral SPECT Imaging. *Adv Functional Neuroimaging* 1988;1:4–11.

> *Teaching Point:*
>
> As the preceding three cases illustrate, the pattern of increased tracer activity in the caudate nuclei (with or without decreased tracer uptake in the frontal lobe) may be seen in patients with acute psychoses.

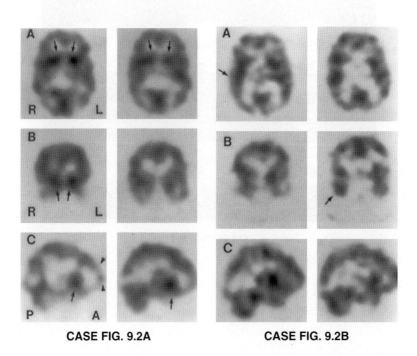

CASE FIG. 9.2A   CASE FIG. 9.2B

Clinical Diagnosis:
Acute Paranoid Schizophrenia: Change in Treatment

CONTRIBUTOR:	IMAGING DATA:	
Ronald L. Van Heertum, M.D.	**Camera:** GE 400AC/T;STAR II	**Collimator:** High resolution
Institution: St. Vincent's Hospital and Medical Center	**Tracer:** ^{123}I IMP	**Dose:** 3.0 mCi

This 41-year-old woman, known to have paranoid schizophrenia, was referred for evaluation of threatening auditory hallucinations. An EEG and a CT scan (Case Fig. 9.3A) were normal. At the time of the cerebral SPECT examination, she had been receiving trifluoperazine, 50 mg daily, and benztropine, 1 mg daily.

The cerebral SPECT study (Case Fig. 9.3B) in the transaxial (**A**) and sagittal (**B**) planes revealed increased tracer activity in the caudate nuclei, with focal increased uptake of tracer in the right temporal lobe. As a result of her continuing hallucinations and the cerebral SPECT finding of increased temporal lobe activity, the patient's medication was modified to include an anticonvulsant (carbamazepine).

Following modification of her medication, the patient showed a dramatic improvement, with a marked decrease in the frequency of auditory hallucinations.

Published with permission from Notardonato H, Gonzalez-Avila A, Von Heertum RL, O'Connell RA, Yudd AP. The pudential valve of serial cerebral SPECT Scanning in the evaluation of psychiatric illness *Clin Nucl Med* 1989;14:319–322.

Teaching Point:

As this case demonstrates, the cerebral SPECT study may reveal useful information that is not demonstrable on other studies such as the EEG or CT scan.

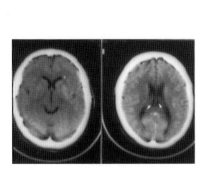

CASE FIG. 9.3A

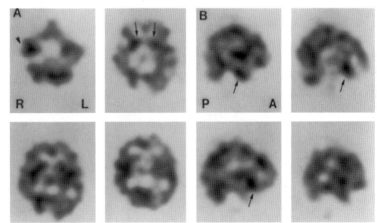

CASE FIG. 9.3B

CASE 9-4

Clinical Diagnosis:
Bipolar Disorder—Depressed

CONTRIBUTOR:

Ronald L. Van Heertum, M.D.
Institution: Columbia-Presbyterian Medical
Center

IMAGING DATA:

Camera: Picker PRISM 3000
Tracer: ^{99m}TC HMPAO

Collimator: Ultra-high-resolution fan-beam
Dose: 21.3 mCi

This 30-year-old man was referred for evaluation of severe depression.

CT scan was reported to be within normal limits.

HMPAO SPECT (Case Fig. 9.4) in the transverse **(A),** coronal **(B)** and sagittal **(C)** planes revealed a global decrease in radiotracer uptake that was most marked in the frontal lobes.

Teaching Point:

Cerebral SPECT may be helpful in the evaluation of patients with mood disorders, in particular depression.

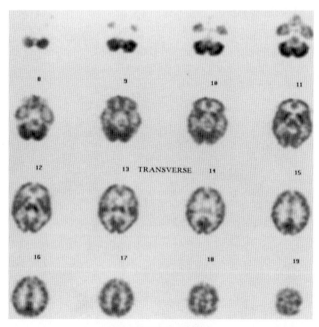

CASE FIG. 9.4A

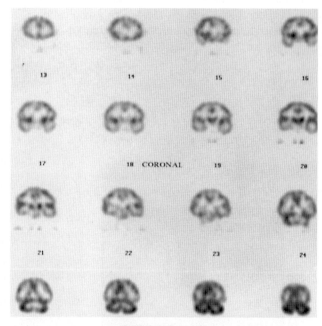

CASE FIG. 9.4B

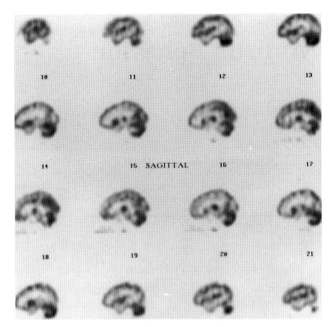

CASE FIG. 9.4C

CASE 9-5

Clinical Diagnosis:
Autistic Behavior

CONTRIBUTOR:	IMAGING DATA:	
James Mountz, M.D., Ph.D.	**Camera:** ADAC Genesys	**Collimator:** Ultra-high-resolution
Institution: University of Alabama Hospital	**Isotope:** ^{99m}TC HMPAO	**Dose:** 13 mCi

This 10-year-old boy was referred for further evaluation of a very low IQ and a high level of autistic behavior. At the time of the SPECT study, the patient displayed unpredictable behavior and demonstrated no effectual reactions: language was limited to occasional use of gestures and signs and continuous noncommunicative vocalization.

A CT scan (Fig. 9.5A) was normal.

An HMPAO SPECT study (Fig. 9.5B), in the transaxial plane, revealed significant reduction of radiotracer uptake in the right hemisphere.

Teaching Point:

Although the patient was injected while in the fully alert autistic state, general anesthesia was administered for scanning. This demonstrates the value of using anesthesia or sedation to image severely, noncompliant patient.

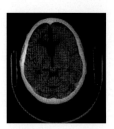

CASE FIG. 9.5A

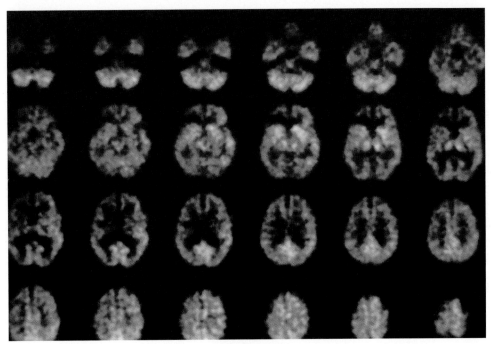

CASE FIG. 9.5B

Clinical Diagnosis:

Autism

CONTRIBUTOR:

James M. Mountz, M.D.
Institution: The University of Alabama at
Birmingham Medical Center

IMAGING DATA:

Camera: ADAC Dual Head
Tracer: ^{99m}Tc HMPAO

Collimator: High resolution
Dose: 13 mCi

This 12-year-old boy was diagnosed as having autistic disorder. He patient had social, behavioral, and language deficits, with language showing the greatest impairment.

MRI, ^{99m}Tc HMPAO SPECT, and MRI fusion images in the transverse plane are shown in Fig. 9.6. The MRI is nor-mal; however, the brain SPECT scan reveals decreased tracer activity in the left temporal lobe. These findings are in regions of the brain known to be related to language function.

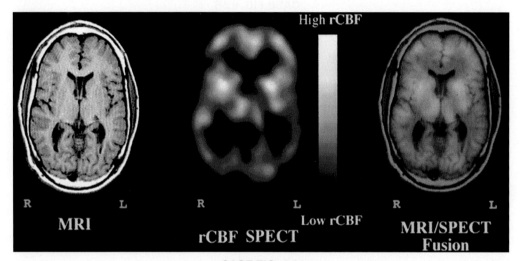

CASE FIG. 9.6

Clinical Diagnosis:

Cocaine Abuse

CONTRIBUTOR:	IMAGING DATA:	
Nora D. Volkow, M.D.	**PET Scanner:** PETT VI	**Dose:** 6–7 mCi
Institution: Brookhaven National Laboratory	**Tracer:** [^{18}F]N-methylspiroperidol	

Normal volunteer and a cocaine abuser (6-month history of use of free-base cocaine at a dose of at least 4 g/week; lack of dependence on any other drugs and lack of evidence of neurologic or psychiatric disorders other than DSM-III-R diagnostic criteria for cocaine abuse). Age range of normal volunteers: 28.1 +/− 3.0 years; cocaine abusers: 26 +/−3.5 years.

Teaching Points:

1. Dopamine is a brain neurotransmitter involved in movement, motivation, and reinforcement. It has been implicated in the reinforcing and addictive properties of cocaine.

2. PET has been used to measure dopamine receptors in the brains of cocaine abusers. PET measurement of dopamine receptor availability using the tracer [^{18}F]N-methylspiroperidol in normal human brain (Case Fig.

9.7, *top*) and in a chronic cocaine user (Fig. 9.7, *bottom*).

3. Tracer uptake occurs in the striatum, an area rich in dopamine receptors and important in the regulation of pleasure, drive, and movement.

4. This PET study shows reduced dopamine receptors in the cocaine abuser as compared to the normal subject, possibly due to down-regulation of receptors as a result of cocaine-induced increases in intrasynaptic dopamine levels.

5. This study demonstrates the ability of PET to uncover molecular mechanisms which may be deranged by the chronic abuse of cocaine.

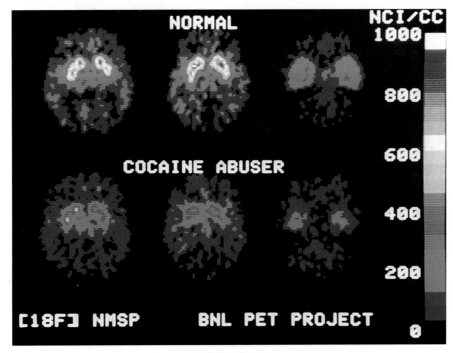

CASE FIG. 9.7

Clinical Diagnosis:
Cocaine Abuse

CONTRIBUTOR:	IMAGING DATA:	
Nora D. Volkow, M.D.	**PET Scanner:** CTI 931	**Dose:** 6-8 mCi
Institution: Brookhaven National Laboratory	**Tracer:** [18]FDG	

Normal volunteers and a cocaine abuser (6-month history of use of free-base cocaine at a dose of at least 4 g/week; lack of dependence on any other drugs, and lack of evidence of neurologic or psychiatric disorders other than DSM-III-R diagnostic criteria for cocaine abuse). Age range of normal volunteers: 28.1 +/− 3.0 years; cocaine abusers: 26 +/−3.5 years.

Teaching Points:

1. Glucose is the main source of energy for the human brain; thus, the measurement of glucose utilization provides a map of functional activity in the human brain.

2. PET was used to measure regional brain glucose metabolism using [18]FDG in a normal subject (Case Fig. 9.8, *top row*) and a chronic cocaine user studied at 10 days (Fig. 9.8, *middle row*) and at 100 days (Fig. 9.8, *bottom row*) 10 days and 100 days after the last cocaine dose. These decreases are most prominent in the frontal areas of the brain, which are important in planning and organizing activities, abstract thinking, and regulating impulsive and repetitive behavior.

3. The fact that these changes persist after 100 days of cocaine detoxification provide evidence of the long-lasting effects of chronic cocaine use on the living human brain.

4. The reduced metabolism is correlated with the amount of cocaine used.

5. These decreases in metabolism are seen in subjects who have no evidence of neurologic or neuropsychological symptoms.

6. This study demonstrates the sensitivity of the PET technique in revealing abnormalities in brain metabolism that cannot be uncovered with other currently available techniques.

Image reproduced with permission from Voliow, et al. Long term frontal brain metabolic changes in cocaine a busers. *Synapse* 1992;11:184–190.

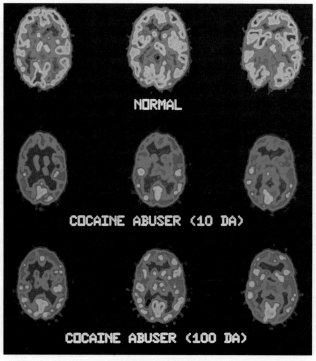

CASE FIG. 9.8

Clinical Diagnosis:
AIDS Encephalopathy/Dementia

CONTRIBUTOR:	IMAGING DATA:	
Feza Tunc, M.D.	**PET Scanner:** PRISM 3000	**Collimator:** LEUHR fan-beam
Institution: New York Presbyterian Medical Center	**Tracer:** ^{99m}Tc HMPAO	**Dose:** 13 mCi

This 14-year-old girl was known to be HIV-seropositive. Her progressive encephalopathy was felt to be secondary HIV disease.

An MRI (Case Fig. 9.9A) shows moderate diffuse atrophy with increased signal in the perviventricular white matter.

Transverse-plane HMPAO brain SPECT images (Case Fig. 9.9B) reveal marked global hypoperfusion and diffuse cortical heterogeneous perfusion. There is also markedly decreased radiotracer activity in the periventricular white matter, disproportionate to the ventricular size noted on MRI. These latter findings are felt to be secondary to diffuse white-matter disease.

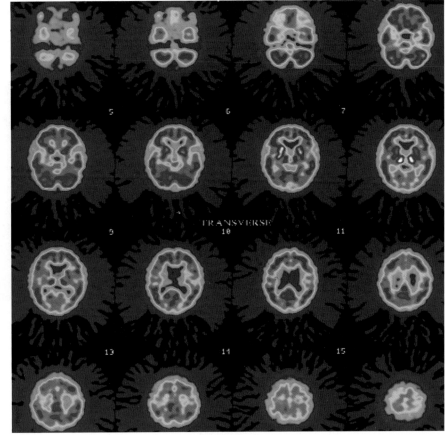

CASE FIG. 9.9A

CASE FIG. 9.9B

CASE 9-10   **Clinical Diagnosis:**
Lesch-Nyhan Disease

CONTRIBUTOR:

Monique Ernst, M.D., Ph.D.
Institution: National Institutes of Health,
National Institute on Drug
Abuse

IMAGING DATA:

PET Scanner: Scanditronix   **Dose:** 5 mCi
Tracer: [18]FDG

This 20-year-old man has Lesch-Nyhan disease (a rare X-linked recessive disorder of purine synthesis, whose clinical presentation includes hyperuricemia and neuropsychiatric findings of choreoathetosis, dystonia, aggression, and self-injurious behavior). For comparison, an image of a 20-year-old healthy man who served as volunteer control is also shown.

Transverse plane [18]FDG PET images (Case Fig. 9.10) at the level of the basal ganglia reveal marked loss of radiotracer activity bilaterally in the basal ganglia of the patient

with Lesch-Nyhan disease, with only a remnant of activity in the caudate nuclei compared to the normal volunteer.

Teaching Points:

The findings shown here, of significant reductions of tracer activity in the basal ganglia, are typical of those for all subjects with Lesch-Nyhan disease.

Image reproduced with permission from Ernst, Zametkin AJ, Matochik JA et al. Presynaptic dopaminergic deficits in Lesch-Nyhan disease. *N Engl J Med* 1996;334:1568–1572.

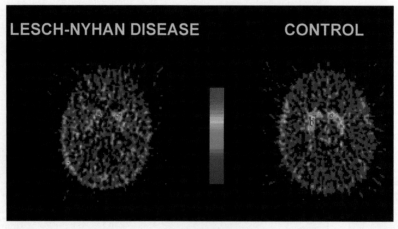

CASE FIG. 9.10

Healthy volunteers age 24–86 years. Subjects had a PET scan with [¹¹F]Raclopride to assess dopamine D2 receptor availability and they also had tests of motor performance and cognitive performance.

CONTRIBUTOR:

Nora D. Volkow, MD

Institution: Brookhaven National
                Laboratory

IMAGING DATA:

PET Scanner: CTI 931   **Dose:** 4-10 mCi
Tracer: [¹¹F] Raclopride

Teaching Points:

1. The brain dopamine system is one of the most vulnerable neurotransmitter systems in the brain.

2. The PET images (Case Fig. 9.11) show that dopamine receptors decline with age. These scans were taken from a study with 30 normal volunteers who also were assessed for cognitive and motor performance. The resulting PET scans showed that declines in dopamine receptors were significantly associated with declines in motor performance (finger tapping test) and declines in performance of tasks involving frontal brain regions including measures of abstraction and mental flexibility (Wisconsin Card Sort Test) and attention and response inhibition (Stroop Color-Word Test, interference score). This study suggests that interventions that enhance dopamine activity may improve performance and quality of life for the elderly.

Image reproduced with permission from: Volkow ND, Wang GJ, et al. Association between decline in brain dopamine activity with age and cognitive and motor impairment in healthy individuals. *Am J Psychiatry* 1998;155:344–349. Reprinted by permission from the American Psychiatric Association.

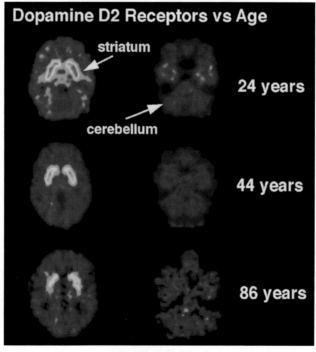

CASE FIG. 9.11

CASE 9-12

Clinical Diagnosis:
Acute Psychosis After Acute Head Trauma

CONTRIBUTOR:

Ronald L. Van Heertum, M.D.

Institution: St. Vincent's Hospital and Medical Center

IMAGING DATA:

Camera: GE 3000 XCT

Tracer: ^{99m}TC HMPAO

Collimator: Ultra-high resolution

Dose: 19.5 mCi

This 25-year-old man was referred for evaluation and treatment following two suicide attempts. Six months prior to admission, he had sustained a severe traumatic brain injury at the time of a fall from a three-story building. At that time, the patient was found to have a left frontal lobe hematoma, which was evacuated during emergency craniotomy. Over the previous several months, the patient had been noted to be increasingly delusional, suffering from insomnia, and experiencing auditory hallucinations.

A follow-up CT scan (Case Fig. 9.12A) revealed a craniotomy defect in the left frontal region with an underlying area of focal hypodensity corresponding to the site where the left frontal intracerebral hematoma had been evacuated.

An HMPAO SPECT study (Case Fig. 9.12B) in the transaxial (1), coronal (2), and sagittal (3) planes revealed absent radiotracer activity in the left posterior frontal lobe. The area of absent tracer activity, which extended deep into the adjacent white matter, was significantly larger than the site of the evacuated hematoma noted on CT scan.

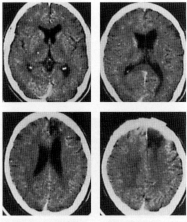

CASE FIG. 9.12A

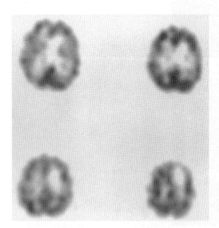

CASE FIG. 9.12B1

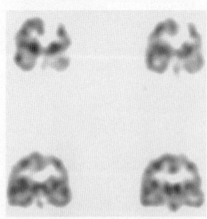

CASE FIG. 9.12B2

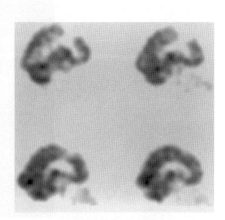

CASE FIG. 9.12B3

274

Functional Cerebral SPECT and PET Imaging, Third Edition,
edited by R.L.Van Heertum and R.S. Tikofsky,
Lippincott Williams & Wilkins, New York © 2000.

CHAPTER 10

Brain Tumors, Other Diseases, and Activation

Ronald L. Van Heertum and Ronald S. Tikofsky

Cerebral single-photon-emission computed tomography (SPECT) position emission tomography (PET) imaging may prove to be useful in a wide variety of other disease states in addition to cerebrovascular disease, dementia, epilepsy, head trauma, and psychiatric disorders. These disorders include brain tumors, anoxic states, toxic encephalopathy, substance abuse, tinnitus, and Lyme disease. Moreover, both PET and SPECT have been used in activation studies. This chapter presents a series of SPECT and PET images that reflect these developments in functional brain imaging. The first section is devoted to brain tumors, followed by a variety of images reflecting disease states less commonly seen in clinical practice. The last section provides some examples of activation studies.

BRAIN TUMORS

Imaging with SPECT/PET is gaining increasing currency as a viable technique in the evaluation of patients suspected of having brain tumors. These imaging procedures are also proving useful for determining tumor viability following radiation or chemotherapy. Brain scintigraphy using ^{99m}Tc pertechnetate was, until the mid-1970s, the only imaging technique for studying brain tumors (1). These procedures were eclipsed by the introduction of computed tomography (CT) and magnetic resonance imaging (MRI). However, SPECT and PET continue to play an important role in the clinical evaluation of brain tumors. The use of SPECT imaging with ^{99m}Tc sestamibi and ^{201}Tl chloride has been show to be of value in resolving questions of tumor recurrence, viability, and the effects of radiation therapy is now well docu-

mented (2–4). Mountz et al. (5) provide an excellent review of this subject. Taken together, the results of these studies show that ^{201}Tl SPECT brain imaging of tumors can aid in differentiating high- from low-grade gliomas; evaluating for recurrent tumor vs. postsurgical or radiation changes (sequential follow-up scans can be used to assess efficacy of therapy), and determining the presence of residual tumor following therapy.

Schwartz et al. (6) report that their dual-isotope technique correlates with the pathologic findings in 14 of 15 cases studied. These findings for ^{201}Tl are similar to those reported by others. Patients with high ^{201}Tl uptake in treated tumor beds had local tumor recurrence, and those with low uptake showed only radiation changes and no evidence of solid tumor. However, in those patients with an intermediate level of ^{201}Tl uptake in the tumor bed, ^{99m}Tc hexamethylpropyleneamine-oxime (HMPAO) uptake permitted a differentiation of patients with active tumor from those whose tumors were not active. Schwartz et al. (6) suggest that the technique may be helpful in distinguishing sites of potential tumor growth from postradiation changes in patients being treated for malignant glioma.

It is also important to determine whether radiation or chemotherapy produces necrotic changes in cortex or if there are other cortical changes resulting from treatment. These effects, typically seen as decreased tracer activity, may indicate cortical necrosis or result from a complete or partial destruction of pathways that have been damaged by the tumor; or they may represent the effects of treatment. Thus, imaging using two agents such as HMPAO in conjunction with ^{201}Tl SPECT imaging can provide significant clinical information regarding tumor recurrence and the secondary effects of damaged pathways to cortex or treatment. ECD (^{99m}Tc-ethylcisteinate dimer) has also been used as a radiotracer for evaluating brain tumors. However, Papazyan et al. (7) demonstrated significant differences between these tracers in brain tumor imaging. They suggest that HMPAO will

R. L. Van Heertum: Department of Radiology, Columbia University College of Physicians and Surgeons, New York, New York 10032.

R. S. Tikofsky: Department of Radiology, Columbia University College of Physicians and Surgeons, Harlem Hospital Center, New York, New York 10032.

show greater radiotracer activity as compared to ECD in brain tumor imaging. Soricelli et al. (8) compared 27 brain tumor patients imaged with either ^{201}Tl or ^{99m}Tc tetrofosmin. They report that not only is ^{99m}Tc tetrofosmin a suitable agent for SPECT brain tumor imaging but that it yields a better definition of tumor margins and higher contrast between neoplastic and normal brain tissue. This agent is not in wide use at the present, and more clinical studies are needed before it will gain wide acceptance.

The interpretation of ^{201}Tl images is usually based on visual inspection. Accumulation of ^{201}Tl provides the best correlation with clinical status. The more avid the uptake of ^{201}Tl, the greater the likelihood of a high-grade tumor or tumor recurrence. However, it is possible to quantify ^{201}Tl results of tumor imaging with SPECT (3,9). The indices make it possible to use the measures described to classify brain tumors. Jinnouchi et al. (10) have developed a quantitative system using delayed uptake indices to classify meningiomas. They found that high accumulation of ^{201}Tl occurred in all types of meningiomas, but that retention rates change as a function of histologic type, with a high retention rate being indicative of the meningioma's malignant potential. A simpler method of quantification has been proposed by Schwartz et al. (6). They describe three major categories of uptake based on a ^{201}Tl lesion-to-scalp ratio: (a) high lesion-to-scalp ratio, >2; (b) moderate lesion-to-scalp ratio, $= 1$–2; and (c) low lesion-to-scalp ratio, <1. With experience, it is possible to assess visually how avidly the tracer is taken up by the tumor.

PET and coincidence imaging are also useful tools in the clinical evaluation of patients with brain tumors. Several studies (11–16) have demonstrated the viability of PET brain tumor imaging using fluorodeoxyglucose (FDG). Other tracers using PET technology have also been used to good clinical effect for brain tumor imaging. One such tracer is 11C-methionine (MET). There are now several studies comparing MET with FDG (17–20). Another promising PET tracer being evaluated for evaluating malignant brain tumors is 2-[C-11]thymidine (21). The development of coincidence imaging allows for FDG PET using modified gamma cameras. Clinical research is now under way examining the utility of this type of imaging for brain tumors (22,23). Another recent study compared 1-3-[^{123}I]iodo-alpha-methyltyrosine (IMT) SPECT and ^{18}FDG PET for detecting and grading glioma recurrence in previously treated patients (24). The findings suggest although while both procedures were comparable in most cases, IMT-SPECT and ^{18}FDG were equivalent. IMT-SPECT was did better at confirming low-grade recurrences, but ^{18}FDG was better at grading tumors than IMT-SPECT.

OTHER DISEASES

There has been increasing interest in developing new clinical applications for functional brain imaging. Several of these are described in Tikofsky et al. (25). Among the clinical areas being studied are applications in systemic lupus erythematosus (SLE) (26–28). There are also reports (29–31) demonstrating the value of functional brain imaging in patients with encephalitis. Functional brain imaging is being used with increasing frequency in the evaluation of patients with chronic Lyme encephalopathy. Several studies (32–34) have reported on the potential contribution of functional brain imaging in detecting cerebral abnormalities in this patient population. Images obtained on Lyme patients frequently have characteristics similar to those of patients whose findings are characterized by diffuse heterogenous hypoperfusion.

ACTIVATION

Functional brain imaging has played an important role in understanding the brain's response to a variety of cognitive stimuli and motor tasks. The early utilization of SPECT in this area was reviewed by Tikofsky and Hellman (35). An excellent review of the role of PET in cognitive neuroscience, focusing on learning and memory, can be found in Roland et al. (36), and there are several other sections in Gazzaniga's work on cognitive neuroscience (37) that expand on the role of functional brain imaging in studying normal cognitive function. The work in this area is continuing at a rapid pace and has attracted the attention of researchers from a wide variety of disciplines, as is evidenced in several recent studies focusing on such diverse areas as semantic and episodic memory (38), hippocampal involvement in memory (39,40), and effects of task difficulty on motor performance (41). In addition, new techniques such as statistical parametric mapping (SPM) (42) for quantifying and comparing PET/SPECT are being used with greater frequency to analyze both clinical and research data derived from studies of functional brain imaging.

REFERENCES

1. Biersack HJ, Grunwal F, Kropp J. Single photon emission computed tomography imaging of brain tumors. *Semin Nucl Med* 1991;21:2–10.
2. Mountz JM, Stafford-Schuck K, McKeever PE, et al. Thallium-201 tumor/cardiac ratio estimation of residual astrocytoma. *J Neurosurg* 1988;68:705–709.
3. Kim KT, Black KL, Marciano D, et al. Thallium-201 SPECT imaging of brain tumors: methods and results. *J Nucl Med* 1990;31:965–969.
4. Soler C, Beauchesne P, Maatougui K, et al. Technetium-99m-sestamibi brain single-photon-emission tomography for detection of recurrent gliomas after radiation therapy. *Eur J Nucl Med* 1998;25:1649–1657.
5. Mountz JM, Deutsche G, Kuzniecky R, et al. Brain SPECT: 1994 update. In: Freeman LM: *Nuclear medicine annual 1994*. New York: Raven Press 1994:1–54.
6. Schwartz RB, Carvalho PA, Alexander E III, et al. Radiation necrosis vs high-grade recurrent glioma: differentiation by using dual-isotope SPECT with 201 Tl and Tc-HMPAO. *AJNR* 1992;12:1187–1192.
7. Papazyan J-P, Delavelle J, Burkhard P, et al. Discrepancies between HMPAO and ECD SPECT imaging in brain tumors. *J Nucl Med* 1997;38:592–596.
8. Soricelli A, Cuocolo A, Varrone A, et al. Technetium-99m-tetrofosmin uptake in brain tumors by SPECT: comparison with thallium-201 imaging. *J Nucl Med* 1998;39:802–806.
9. Mountz JM, Rosenfeld SS, Li Y. Utility of 201-Tl and 99m-Tc-sestamibi SPECT for early determination of malignant brain tumor chemotherapy efficacy (abstr). *J Nucl Med* 1993;34:206P.

10. Jinnouchi S, Hosi H, Ohnishi T, et al. Thallium-201 SPECT for predicting histological types of meningiomas. *J Nucl Med* 1993;34:2091–2094.
11. Barker FG II, Chang SM, Valk PE, et al. 18-Fluorodeoxyglucose uptake and survival of patients with suspected recurrent malignant glioma. *Cancer* 1997;79:115–126.
12. Deshmukh A, Scott JA, Palmer EL, et al. Impact of fluorodeoxyglucose positron emission tomography on the clinical management of patients with glioma. *Clin Nucl Med* 1996;21:720–725.
13. Ericson K, Kihlstrom L, Mogard J, et al. Positron emission tomography using 18F-fluorodeoxyglucose in patients with stereotactically irradiated brain mestastases. *Stereotact Funct Neurosurg* 1996;66(suppl):214–224.
14. Kole AC, Nieweg OE, Pruim J, et al. Detection of unknown occult primary tumors using positron emission tomography. *Cancer* 1998;82:1160–1166.
15. Spence AM, Muszi, M, Graham MM, et al. Glucose metabolism in human malignant gliomas measured quantitatively with PET, 1-[C-11] glucose and FDG: analysis of the FDG lumped constant. *J Nucl Med* 1998;39:440–448.
16. Delbeke D. Oncological applications of FDG PET imaging: brain tumors, colorectal cancer, lymphoma and melanoma. *J Nucl Med* 1999;40:591–603.
17. Hara T, Kosaka N, Shinoura N, Kondo T. PET imaging of brain tumor with [methyl-11C]choline. *J Nucl Med* 1997;38:842–847.
18. Voges J, Herholz K, Holzer T, et al. 11C-methionine and 18F-2-fluorodeoxyglucose positron emission tomography: a tool for diagnosis of cerebral glioma and monitoring after brachytherapy with ^{125}I seeds. *Stereotact Funct Neurosurg* 1997;69:129–135.
19. Kaschten B, Stevenaert A, Sadzot B, et al. Preoperative evaluation of 54 gliomas by PET with fluorine-18-fluorodeoxyglucose and/or carbon-11-methionine. *J Nucl Med* 1998;39:778–785.
20. Sasaki M, Kuwabara Y, Yoshida T, et al. A comparative study of thallium-201 SPECT, carbon-11 methionine PET and fluorine-18-fluorodeoxyglucose PET for the differentiation of astrocytic tumors. *Eur J Nucl Med* 1998;25:1261–1269.
21. Eary JF, Mankoff DA, Spence AM, et al. 2-[C-11]thymidine imaging of malignant brain tumors. *Cancer Res* 1999;59:615–621.
22. Maria BL, Drane WE, Mastin ST, Jimenez LA. Comparative value of thallium and glucose SPECT imaging in childhood brain tumors. *Pediatr Neurol* 1998;19:351–357.
23. Delbeke D, Patton JA, Martin WH, Sandler MP. FDG PET and dual-headed gamma camera positron coincidence detection imaging of suspected malignancies and brain disorders. *J Nucl Med* 1999;40:110–117.
24. Bader JB, Samnick S, Morninglane JR, et al. Evaluation of 1-3-[123]iodo-alpha-methyltyrosine SPET and [18F]-fluorodeoxyglucose PET in the detection and grading of recurrences in patients pretreated for gliomas at follow-up: a comparative study with sterotactic biopsy. *Eur J Nucl Med* 1999;26:144–151.
25. Tikofsky RS, Ichise M, Seibyl JP, Verhoeff NPLG. Functional brain SPECT imaging: 1999 and beyond. In: Freeman LM: *Nuclear medicine annual 1999*. Philadelphia: Lippincott Williams & Wilkins, 1999:193–263.
26. Kovacs JAJ, Urowits MB, Gladman DD, Zeman R. The use of single emission computerized tomography in neuropsychiatric SLE: a pilot study. *J Rheumatol* 1995;22:218–228.
27. Lin W-Y, Wang S-J, Yen T-C, Lan J-L. Technetium-99m-HMPAO SPECT in systemic lupus erythematosus with CNS involvement. *J Nucl Med* 1997;38:1112–1115.
28. Grunwald F, Schomburg A, Badali A, et al. Eighteen FDG-PET and acetazolimide-enhanced ^{99m}Tc-HMPAO SPECT in systemic lupus erythematosus. *Eur J Nucl Med* 1995;22:1073–1077.
29. Tohyama Y, Sako K, Daita G, et al. Dissociation of ^{99m}Tc-ECD and ^{99m}Tc-HMPAO distributions in herpes simplex encephalitis. *Childs Nerv Syst* 1997;13:352–355.
30. Schmidbauer M, Podreka I, Wimberger D, et al. SPECT and MRI imaging in herpes simplex encephalitis. *J Comput Assist Tomogr* 1991;15:811–815.
31. Launes J, Siren J, Valanne MD, et al. Unilateral hyperperfusion in brain-perfusion SPECT predicts prognosis in acute encephalitis. *Neurology* 1997;48:1347–1351.
32. Bloom M, Jacobs S, Pile-Spellman J, et al. Cerebral SPECT imaging: effects on clinical management. *J Nucl Med* 1996;37:1070–1074.
33. Das S, Plutchok JJ, Liegner KB, et al. Tc-99m-HMPAO brain SPECT detection of perfusion abnormalities in Lyme disease patients with clinical encephalopathy (abstr). *J Nucl Med* 1996;37:270.
34. Logigian EL, Johnson KA, Kijewski MF, et al. Reversible cerebral hypoperfusion in Lyme encephalopathy. *Neurology* 1997;49:1661–1670.
35. Tikofsky RS, Hellman RS. Brain single photon emission computed tomography: newer activation and intervention studies. *Sem Nucl Med* 1991;21:40–57.
36. Roland PE, Kawashima R, Gulyas B, O'Sullivan B. Positron emission tomography in cognitive neuroscience: methodological constraints, strategies, and examples form learning and memory. In: Gazzaniga MS, ed. *The cognitive neurosciences*. Cambridge, MA: MIT Press, 1995:781–788.
37. Gazzaniga MS, ed. *The cognitive neurosciences*. Cambridge, MA: MIT Press, 1995.
38. Carlesimo GA, Casadio P, Sabbadini M, et al. Cortical networks implicated in semantic and episodic memory: common or unique? *Cortex* 1998;34:547–561.
39. Lepage M, Habib R, Tulving E. Hippocampal PET activations of memory encoding and retrieval: the HIPPER model. *Hippocampus* 1998;8:313–322.
40. Schacter DL, Alpert NM, Savage CR, et al. Conscious recollection and the human hippocampal formation: evidence from positron emission tomography. *Proc Natl Acad Sci USA* 1996;93:321–325.
41. Paaus T, Koski L, Stippich C, et al. Regional differences in the effects of task difficulty and motor output on blood flow response in the human anterior cingulate cortex: a review of 107 PET activation studies. *Neuroreport* 1998;9:R37–R47.
42. Friston KJ, Holmes AP, Worsley J-P, et al. Statistical parametric maps in functional imaging: a general linear approach. *Hum Brain Map* 1995;2:189–210.

CASE 10-1

Clinical Diagnosis:
Astrocytoma

CONTRIBUTORS:	IMAGING DATA:	
Robert S. Hellman, M.D.,	**Camera:** GE Neurocam	**Collimator:** High-resolution
Ronald S. Tikofsky, M.D.	**Tracer:** ^{201}Tl Chloride, ^{99m}Tc HMPAO	**Dose:** 3.0 mCi
Institution: Medical College of Wisconsin		**Dose:** 31.3 mCi

This 34-year-old woman with a known right occipital lobe astrocytoma that had been resected and treated with irradiation 6 years prior to admission was referred for evaluation of increasing drowsiness and headaches.

A CT scan showed an enhancing tumor mass at the site of the original lesion. A follow-up MRI scan (Case Fig. 10.1A) revealed a significant increase in size of the right occipital and periventricular tumor compared with the prior CT scan.

A ^{201}Tl SPECT study (Case Fig. 10.1B) in the transaxial plane revealed intense increased thallium uptake deep in the right hemisphere. This finding is consistent with viable tumor deep in the right hemisphere extending superiorly into the region of the right corpus callosum.

An HMPAO study (Fig. 10.1C) in the transaxial plane revealed extensive regions of absent activity in the right temporal, parietal, and occipital regions. In addition, absent tracer uptake was seen in the deep subcortical regions, particularly the right thalamus, corresponding to the deep right hemispheric mass identified on MRI and thallium SPECT. A mild decrease in tracer activity in the posterior right frontal lobe, possibly secondary to prior radiation therapy or diaschisis, was also noted.

Teaching Point:

Combined ^{201}Tl and ^{99m}Tc HMPAO SPECT studies are frequently more helpful than single SPECT imaging studies with either compound.

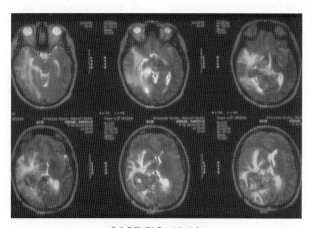

CASE FIG. 10.1A

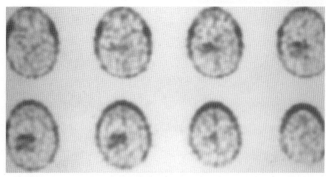

CASE FIG. 10.1B

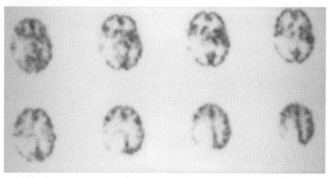

CASE FIG. 10.1C

278

Clinical Diagnosis:

Recurrent Astrocytoma: Grade III/IV

CONTRIBUTORS:	IMAGING DATA:	
Robert S. Hellman, M.D.,	**Camera:** GE Neurocam	**Collimator:** High-resolution
Ronald S. Tikofsky, M.D.	**Tracer:** ^{201}Tl chloride	**Dose:** 3.1 mCi
Institution: Medical College of Wisconsin	^{99m}Tc HMPAO	**Dose:** 32.0 mCi

This 59-year-old woman was referred for evaluation following surgical reopening of a right parietal craniotomy with microsurgical excision of a recurrent glioblastoma multiforme.

A follow-up T1- and T2-weighted MRI study (Case Fig. 10.2A,B) revealed a lesion in the right thalamus as well as a right temporal parietal mass that had increased in size when compared with prior studies. In addition, a vascular malformation was evident in the left temporoparietal lobe.

A thallium SPECT study (Case Fig. 10.2C) in the transaxial plane showed foci of increased activity in the right temporoparietal region and the right thalamus that were felt to represent recurrent tumor.

An HMPAO SPECT study (Case Fig. 10.2D) in the transaxial plane revealed a postsurgical decrease in tracer on the right side and a focus of increased activity in the right parietotemporal region, corresponding to the area of abnormality on MRI. Follow-up thallium and HMPAO SPECT studies (Case Fig. 10.12A,B) showed intense focal increased uptake of HMPAO and thallium in the right posterior temporal lobe secondary to recurrent tumor.

Teaching Point:

In this case, thallium SPECT was helpful in localizing the sites of recurrent tumor.

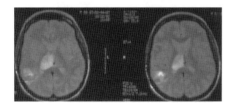

CASE FIG. 10.2A

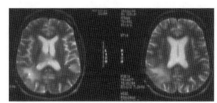

CASE FIG. 10.2B

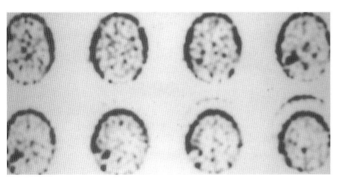

CASE FIG. 10.2C

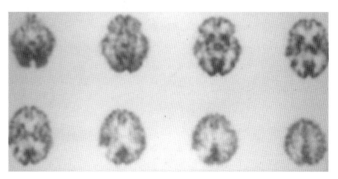

CASE FIG. 10.2D

Clinical Diagnosis:
Grade III Anaplastic Astrocytoma

CONTRIBUTORS:	IMAGING DATA:	
Ronald L. Van Heertum, M.D., Angela Lignelli, M.D. **Institution:** New York Presbyterian Medical Center	**PET Scanner:** Siemens XACT 47 **Tracer:** ¹⁸FDG	**Attenuation Correction Method:** Autoattenuation **Dose:** 9.78 mCi

This 36-year-old woman had a gross total resection of a grade III anaplastic astrocytoma followed by radiation therapy. A follow-up MRI showed contrast enhancement in the medial anterior right frontal lobe.

MRI (Case Fig. 10.3A) showed contrast enhancement in a focus within the medial anterior right frontal lobe.

PET images in the transverse, coronal, and sagittal planes (Case Fig. 10.3B–D) reveal a region absent radiotracer activity in the right anterosuperior temporal lobe. A focal area of significantly increased radiotracer activity is seen in the right inferior frontal lobe medially. This finding corresponds with the region of contrast enhancement seen on MRI and is consistent with a high-grade neoplastic process.

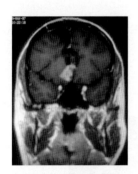

CASE FIG. 10.3A

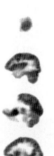 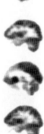 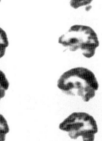 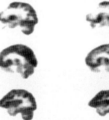 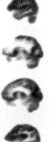 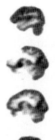

CASE FIG. 10.3B

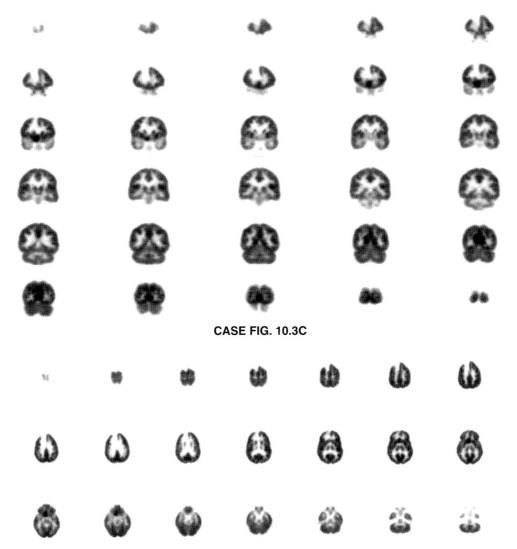

CASE FIG. 10.3C

CASE FIG. 10.3D

Clinical Diagnosis:
Low-Grade Astrocytoma

CONTRIBUTORS:	IMAGING DATA:	
Ronald L. Van Heertum, M.D.,	**PET Scanner:** Siemens XACT 47	**Attenuation Correction Method:**
Jeffrey Plutchock, M.D.	**Tracer:** [18]FDG	Autoattenuation
Institution: New York Presbyterian Medical		**Dose:** 10.08 mCi
Center		

This 42-year-old woman with a low-grade astrocytoma was treated with radiation therapy to a lesion in the left parieto-occipital region. She now presents with progressive speech difficulties on MRI.

MRI (Case Fig. 10.4A) showed an enhancing nodule within the radiation port.

PET images in the transverse, coronal, and sagittal planes (Case Fig. 10.4B–D) reveal a region of absent radiotracer activity in the region of the left parietooccipital radiation port. There is a focal area of mild hypermetabolism within the larger "cold" area corresponding to the "enhancing nodule" seen on MRI. These findings are secondary to a recurrent low-grade astrocytoma within an area of radiation necrosis.

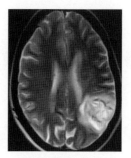

CASE FIG. 10.4A

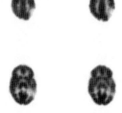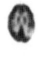
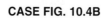

CASE FIG. 10.4B

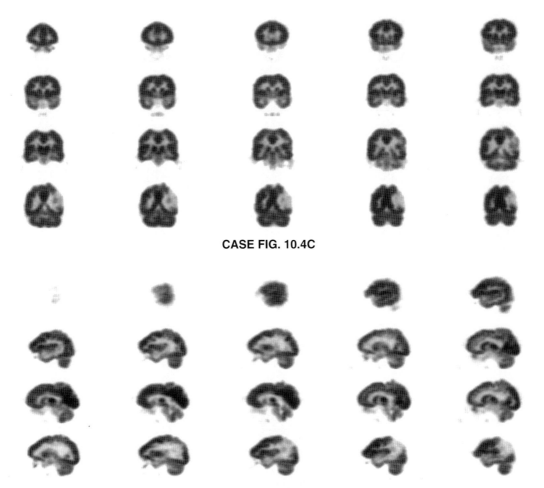

CASE FIG. 10.4C

CASE FIG. 10.4D

CASE 10-5

Clinical Diagnosis:
Grade IV Glioblastoma

CONTRIBUTORS:	IMAGING DATA:	
Ronald L. Van Heertum, M.D.,	**PET Scanner:** Siemens XACT 47	**Attenuation Correction Method:**
Jeffrey Naimen, M.D.	**Tracer:** [18]FDG	Autoattenuation
Institution: New York Presbyterian Medical		**Dose:** 10.11 mCi
Center		

This 67-year-old man had an enhancing left cerebral mass noted on MRI following a seizure.

An MRI (Case Fig. 10.5A) revealed an enhancing left cerebral mass.

FDG PET images in the transverse, coronal, and sagittal planes reveal a region of markedly increased tracer uptake in the left inferior frontotemporal region, which corresponds with the enhancing mass on MRI (Case Figs. 10.5B–D). This finding is most consistent with a malignant lesion. Decreased tracer is seen in the left cerebral cortex and in the right cerebellum. These findings are most likely due to a disconnect (diaschisis) possibly secondary to compression of the white-matter nerve tracts connecting these two areas.

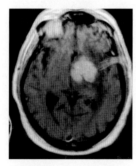

CASE FIG. 10.5A

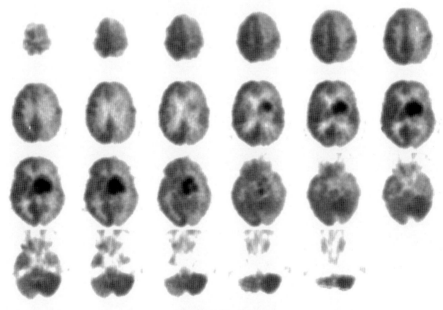

CASE FIG. 10.5B

284

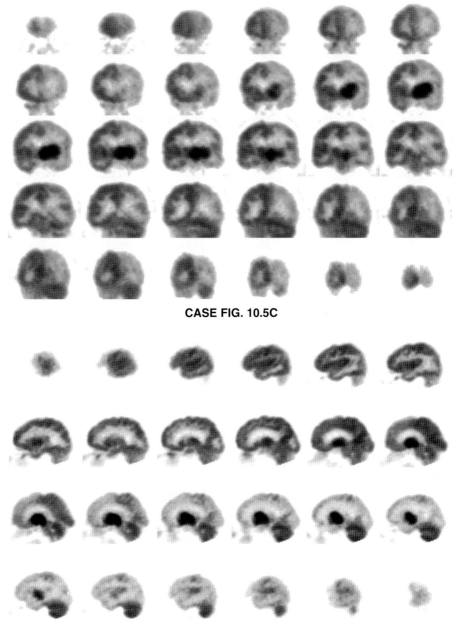

CASE FIG. 10.5C

CASE FIG. 10.5D

Clinical Diagnosis:
Glioblastoma Multiforme

CONTRIBUTORS:

Ronald L. Van Heertum, M.D.,
Jongwon Lee, M.D.
Institution: New York Presbyterian Medical
Center

IMAGING DATA:

PET Scanner: Siemens XACT 47
Tracer: [18]FDG

Attenuation Correction Method:
Autoattenuation
Dose: 9.65 mCi

This 41-year-old man had a history of glioblastoma multiforme in the right temporal lobe; he was treated surgically by resection of the tumor followed by radiation therapy.

An MRI (Case Fig. 10.6A) revealed a large mass effect due to edema in the right hemisphere with irregular enhancement in the right anterior temporal surgical bed, which appeared to be increased compared to a prior MRI.

PET images in the transverse, coronal, and sagittal planes (Case Figs. 10.6B–D) reveals a "ring-like" area of in-

creased radiotracer activity in the anterior tip of the right temporal lobe, corresponding to the ring enhancement seen in the MRI involving the meninges and anterior surgical margin. The central area of decreased radiotracer activity is due to central tumor necrosis. There is also globally decreased radiotracer activity throughout the right cerebral hemisphere, right basal ganglia, and thalamus due to prior radiation. Decreased radiotracer activity is also present in the left cerebellum, which is most compatible with crossed cerebellar diaschisis.

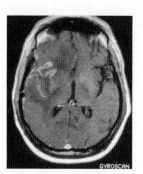

CASE FIG. 10.6A

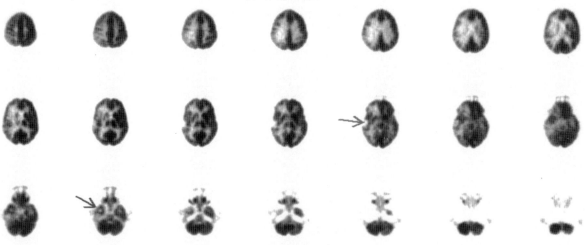

CASE FIG. 10.6B

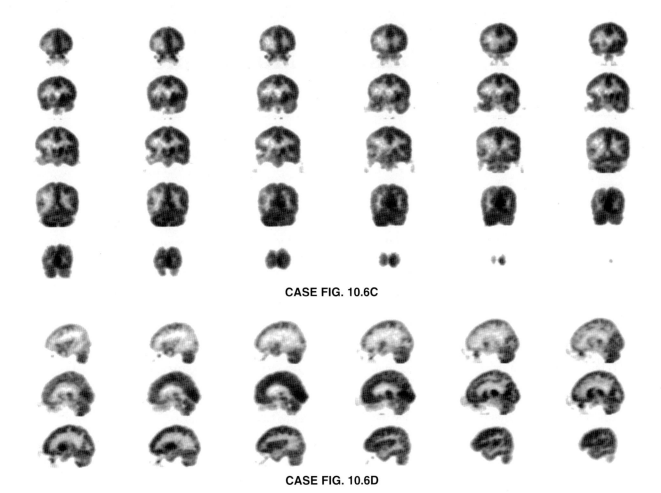

CASE FIG. 10.6C

CASE FIG. 10.6D

Clinical Diagnosis:
Glioblastoma Multiforme

CONTRIBUTORS:

James M. Mountz, M.D., Ph.D.,
Elmer C. San Pedro, M.D.
Institution: The University of Alabama at
Birmingham Medical Center

IMAGING DATA:

Camera: PRISM 3000
Tracer: ^{201}Ti, ^{99m}Tc sestamibi

Collimator: High-resolution, parallel-hole
Dose: 5 mCi, 20 mCi

This 47-year-old woman with glioblastoma multiforme previously underwent radiation therapy and chemotherapy.

MRI scan shows high signal intensity in the right cerebral hemisphere. However, the MRI image does not permit a distinction between residual viable tumor vs. radiation necrosis and edema.

The ^{201}Tl brain SPECT scan shows intense uptake indicating tumor recurrence (Case Fig. 10.7). A ^{99m}Tc sestambi (MIBI) scan also shows the intense uptake in the right hemisphere, with better anatomic delineation of the tumor boundary as noted by extension of the tumor through the anterior commissure (*green arrowhead*), whereas the thallium scan, in the same location, has less clear definition. Also note the ^{99m}Tc MIBI in the midportion of the left hemisphere, which is related to tumor uptake but due to choroid plexus secretion of the ^{99m}Tc MIBI.

Teaching Point:

Both ^{201}Tl and ^{99m}Tc MIBI are excellent for the detection of new, recurrent, or residual viable brain tumor, since both have avidity to viable tumor and both have high target-to-background uptake.

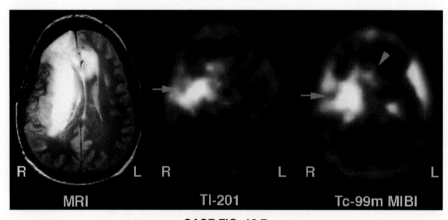

CASE FIG. 10.7

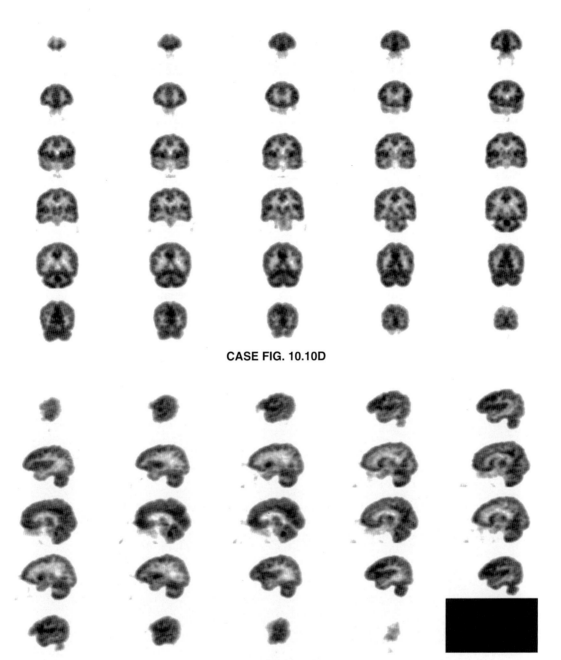

CASE FIG. 10.10D

CASE FIG. 10.10E

Clinical Diagnosis:
Recurrent Brain Tumor

CONTRIBUTORS:

James M. Mountz, M.D., Ph.D.,
Elmer C. San Pedro, M.D.
Institution: The University of Alabama at
          Birmingham Medical Center

IMAGING DATA:

Camera: ADAC MCD Vertex Plus
Tracer: [18]FDG (coincidence PET)
Dose: 5 mCi

A patient with recurrent brain tumor.

Case Fig. 10.11 shows a normal [18]FDG coincidence PET scan (*top two rows*) with normal [18]FDG distribution throughout the brain. These images are contrasted with those in the two rows below. They show recurrent brain tumor involving both the right anterior (*arrow*) and left posterior cerebral hemispheres (*arrowhead*).

Teaching Points:

[18]FDG is the standard for the detection new, recurrent, or residual viable brain tumor; in this case, it shows an example of the unambiguous high-intensity uptake due to recurrent high-grade brain tumor.

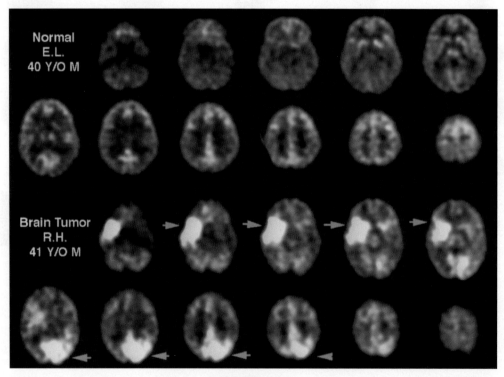

CASE FIG. 10.11

Clinical Diagnosis:
Left Frontal Meningioma

CONTRIBUTOR:	IMAGING DATA:	
Ronald L. Van Heertum, M.D.	**Camera:** GE Neurocam	**Collimator:** Ultra-high-resolution
Institution: Columbia-Presbyterian Medical Center	**Tracer:** ^{99m}Tc HMPAO	**Dose:** 21.0 mCi

This 75-year-old man with a known left frontal meningioma was referred for evaluation after several episodes of imbalance (unsteadiness).

An MRI study (Case Fig. 10.12A, B), pre- **(a)** and post- **(b)** gadolinium injection, revealed an enhancing 3-cm meningioma in the inferolateral aspect of the left frontal lobe that was connected to the meninges by a small stalk.

An HMPAO SPECT study (Case Fig. 10.12C) in the transaxial plane revealed focal increased radiotracer uptake in the left inferior frontal meningioma.

Teaching Points:

^{99m}Tc HMPAO tracer uptake in meningiomas may vary. In general, however, the tracer concentration in these lesions tends to be avid.

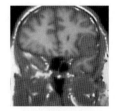

CASE FIG. 10.12A

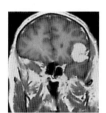

CASE FIG. 10.12B

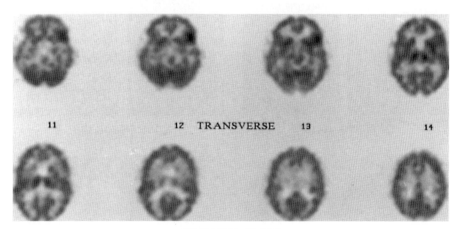

CASE FIG. 10.12C

Clinical Diagnosis:
Falx Cerebri Meningioma

CONTRIBUTOR:	IMAGING DATA:	
Ronald L. Van Heertum, M.D.	**Camera:** GE-3000 XCT	**Collimator:** Ultra-high-resolution
Institution: St. Vincent's Hospital and Medical Center	**Tracer:** 99mTc HMPAO	**Dose:** 20.0 mCi

This 66-year-old woman presented complaining of a progressively increasing "pressure sensation" involving the right side of her head.

A skull series revealed a large, predominantly lytic lesion in the right frontal bone with sclerotic margins.

A MRI examination (Case Fig. 10.13A, B) in the axial (**a**) and coronal (**b**) planes revealed a large lobular mass with intra- and extracranial components most consistent with a meningioma arising from the falx cerebri.

An HMPAO SPECT study (Case Fig. 10.13C, D) in the coronal (**c**) and sagittal (**d**) planes revealed radiotracer uptake in the mass seen on the MRI study.

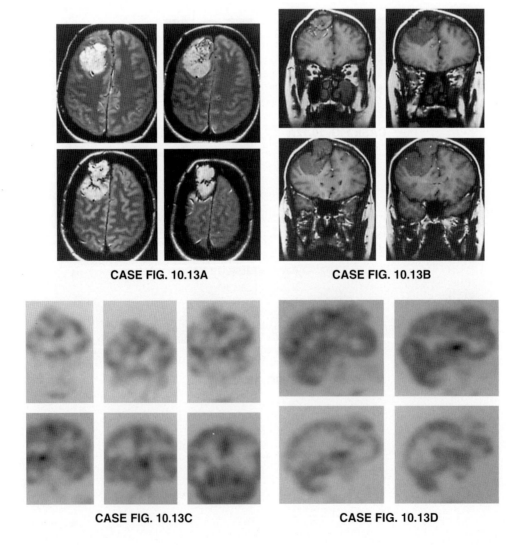

CASE FIG. 10.13A   CASE FIG. 10.13B

CASE FIG. 10.13C   CASE FIG. 10.13D

CASE 10-14

Clinical Diagnosis:
Toxic Encephalopathy

CONTRIBUTOR:

James Mountz, M.D., Ph.D.
Institution: University of Alabama Hospital

IMAGING DATA:

Camera: Adac dual-headed Genesys
Tracer: ^{99m}Tc HMPAO

Collimator: High-resolution
Dose: 25 mCi

This 52-year-old woman presented with progressive symptoms of insomnia, headaches, and dizziness of 6 years' duration. During this period, she also complained of malaise, memory loss, and weakness. The patient said that these symptoms were related to her work environment, where she was exposed to oils, coolants, solvents, fumes, and vapors. Her symptoms abated when she was not at work. Neurologic examination showed episodic numbness, dizziness, poor balance, jerky motions of the extremities, and a positive Romberg test. Her serum manganese level was very elevated, at 4.8 ng/ml.

An HMPAO SPECT study (Case Fig. 10.14) in the transaxial plane revealed reduction of tracer uptake in the basal ganglia (body of the caudate nuclei) and thalami. These findings were felt to be related to a toxic encephalopathy.

A repeat study obtained a year after the patient abstained from plant work showed significant improvement in tracer uptake to these regions. At that time, the patient's clinical status had improved significantly.

Teaching Point:

Although there appears to be a strong relation between the manganese level and reduced tracer uptake in the basal ganglia and thalamus, such findings may also be related to other environmentally toxic substances in the patient's workplace.

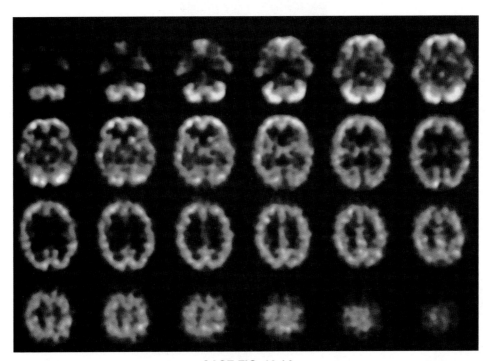

CASE FIG. 10.14

CASE 10-15

Clinical Diagnosis:
Rapidly Progressive Mental Dysfunction

CONTRIBUTORS:

Ronald L. Van Heertum, M.D.,
Jongwon Lee, M.D.
Institution: New York Presbyterian Medical
Center

IMAGING DATA:

PET Scanner: Siemens XACT 47
Tracer: [18]FDG

Attenuation Method: Autoattenuation
Dose: 9.94 mCi

This 49-year-old woman had a 5-week history of rapidly progressive mental dysfunction.

An electroencephalography (EEG) and MRI (Case Fig. 10.15A) examinations were normal.

PET images in the transverse, coronal, and sagittal planes (Case Fig. 10.15 B–D) reveal markedly decreased radio-

tracer activity in the bilateral frontal, temporal, and parietal lobes with minimal asymmetry in the region of the temporal lobes. There is also a marked decrease in radiotracer activity in the bilateral basal ganglia and thalamus with sparing of the occipital lobes. This a pattern that can be seen with diffuse encephalopathy, either drug-induced or due to inflammatory/infections.

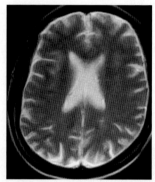

CASE FIG. 10.15A

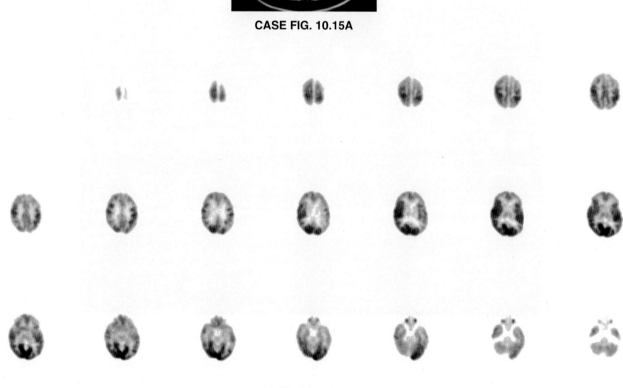

CASE FIG. 10.15B

298

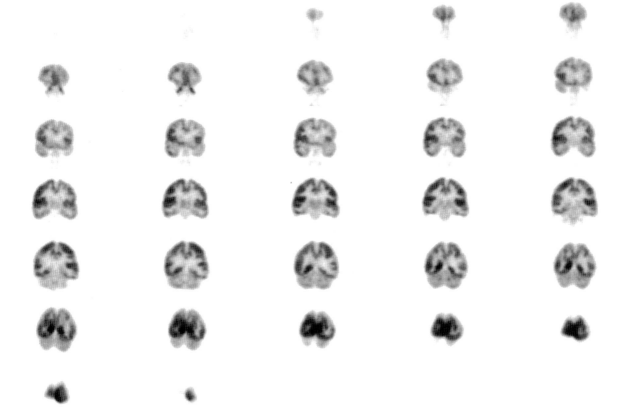

CASE FIG. 10.15C

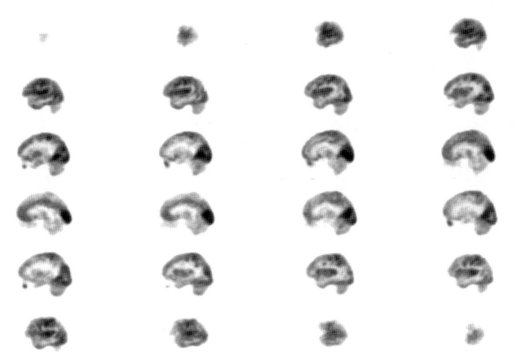

CASE FIG. 10.15D

Clinical Diagnosis:
Cerebral Microangiopathy

CONTRIBUTOR:	IMAGING DATA:	
Osama Sabri, M.D., Ph.D.	**PET/SPECT Scanner:** ECAT 953/15; dual-head ROTA gamma camera	**Collimator:** PET, none; SPECT, LEAP
Institution: Aachen University of Technology		**Tracer:** ^{18}FDG
		^{99m}Tc-HMPAO
		Dose: FDG 274 MBQ
		HMPAO 748 MBQ

This 72-year-old woman had enhanced muscle reflexes and motor paresis of the right upper extremity. Her performance on extensive neuropsychological testing was above average.

CT revealed multiple lacunar infarctions and severe leukoaraiosis without brain atrophy, suggestive of severe cerebral microangiopathy. MRI (Case Fig. 10.16) examination reveals multiple lacunar infarctions (*arrowhead*) and severe confluent deep white-matter lesions (*arrows*).

Transverse PET/SPECT images (Case Fig. 10.16) are within normal limits.

Teaching Points:

This case illustrates that neuropsychological impairment (dementia) does not correlate with the severity of white matter lesions on MRI in patients with presumed vascular dementia. These patients will often have normal findings on functional imaging studies. When there is no atrophy, but cognitive deficits are present, based on neuropsychological testing, functional imaging may show hypoperfusion and hypometabolism.

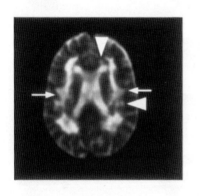
MRI

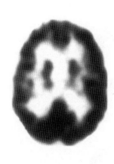
PET

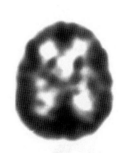
SPECT

CASE FIG. 10.16

CASE 10-17

Clinical Diagnosis:
Cerebral Microangiopathy

CONTRIBUTOR:	IMAGING DATA:	
Osama Sabri, M.D., Ph.D.	**PET/SPECT Scanner:** ECAT 953/15; dual-head ROTA gamma camera	**Collimator:** PET, none; SPECT, LEAP
Institution: Aachen University of Technology (Germany)		**Tracer:** [18]FDG
		^{99m}Tc-HMPAO
		Dose: [18]FDG 244 MBQ
		HMPAO 750 MBQ

This 73-year-old woman had left-sided hemiparesis. Neuropsychological evaluation was suggestive of dementia.

CT revealed a lacunar infarct in the right internal capsule—a morphologic sign of slight cerebral microangiopathy. MRI (Case Fig. 10.17) examination revealed broadening of the lateral sulci and interhemispheric fissure (*thin arrows*) and ventricles (*thick arrow*) as well as local atrophy in the right superior temporal region (*arrowhead*).

Transverse PET/SPECT images (Case Fig. 10.17) show reduced glucose metabolism and blood flow, matching MRI findings of atrophy.

Image reproduced with permission from Sabri O, Ringelstein EB, Helling D, et al. Neuropsychological impairment correlates with hypoperfusion and hypometabolism but not severity of white matter lesions on MRI in patients with cerebral microangiopathy. *Stroke* 1999;30:556–566.

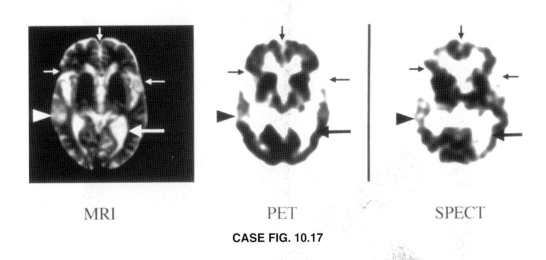

MRI   PET   SPECT

CASE FIG. 10.17

Clinical Diagnosis:
Lyme Disease

CONTRIBUTOR:	IMAGING DATA:	
David Landsnes, M.D.	**PET Scanner:** PRISM 3000	**Collimator:** LEUHR fan-beam
Institution: New York Presbyterian Medical Center	**Tracer:** ^{99m}Tc HMPAO	**Dose:** 21 mCi

This 21-year-old man with known chronic Lyme encephalopathy now presents with progressive cognitive decline.

Transverse-plane HMPAO brain SPECT images (Case Fig. 10.18) reveal moderate global hypoperfusion and cortical heterogeneity.

Teaching Points:

The brain SPECT perfusion pattern most often seen in chronic Lyme encephalopathy is not specific for Lyme disease and may be seen in a variety of other diseases, including vasculitis, encephalitis, substance abuse, and HIV encephalopathy.

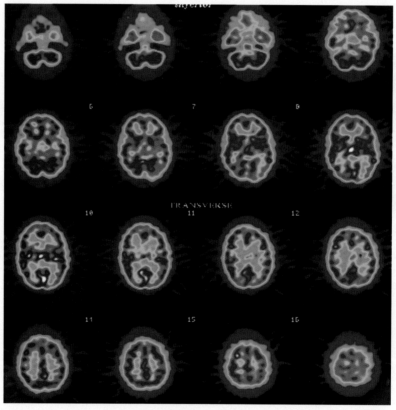

CASE FIG. 10.18

CASE 10-19

Clinical Diagnosis:
Lyme Disease

CONTRIBUTOR:	IMAGING DATA:	
David Landsnes, M.D.	**PET Scanner:** PRISM 3000	**Collimator:** LEUHR fan-beam
Institution: New York Presbyterian Medical Center	**Tracer:** 99mTc HMPAO	**Dose:** 21 mCi

This 29-year-old man had an ELISA test positive for Lyme disease and a progressive cognitive decline.

Transverse-plane HMPAO brain SPECT images (Case Fig. 10.19) reveal progression in heterogeneity and decreased perfusion.

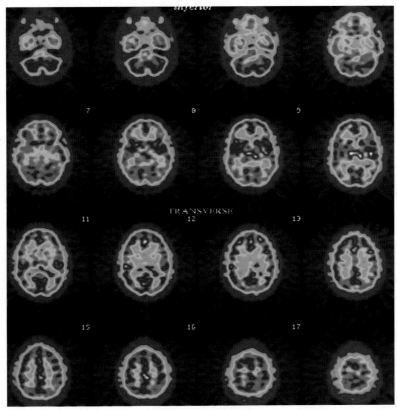

CASE FIG. 10.19

Clinical Diagnosis:
Severe Disabling Tinnitus

CONTRIBUTORS:

Abraham Schulman, M.D.,
Arnold M. Strashun, M.D.
Institution: SUNY Health Sciences Center at
Brooklyn

IMAGING DATA:

Camera: Trionix Triad
Tracer: ^{99m}Tc HMPAO

Collimator: High-resolution
Dose: 25.0 mCi

This 44-year-old man with known severe disabling tinnitus of approximately 3 years' duration was referred for further evaluation. The patient's symptoms were persistent since ear cleaning for wax removal. The tinnitus was characterized as bilateral but was greater in the left ear, with a "hiss" and "tea kettle" quality; it was constant in duration, with a tinnitus intensity index of 7 on a scale of 0–7 (7 maximum). The patient additionally noted intermittent ear blockages (left greater than right) and episodes of dysequilibrium. He also noted a past history of major depression with hospitalization on two occasions and a sleep disorder. The patient's tinnitus gradually increased in severity with associated loss of hearing but no additional signs of neurologic disease.

Neuropsychological testing revealed a question of cognitive impairment and borderline visual spatial dysfunction.

A CT scan revealed mild diffuse cortical atrophy.

An HMPAO SPECT study (Case Fig. 10.20) in the transaxial **(A)**, coronal **(B)**, and sagittal **(C)** planes revealed reduced radiotracer activity in the bilateral inferior frontal as well as the mesial and midposterior temporal (left greater than right) regions. Overall, the subcortical regions were relatively spared.

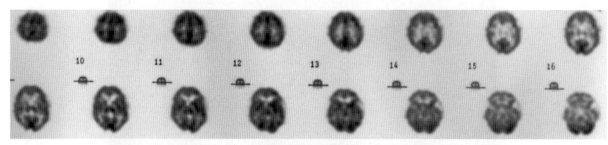

CASE FIG. 10.20A

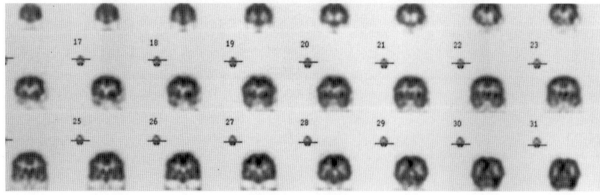

CASE FIG. 10.20B

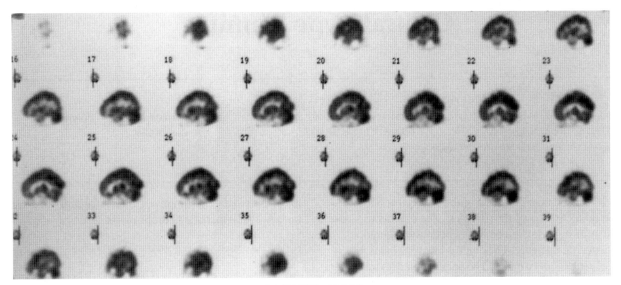

CASE FIG. 10.20C

Central-Type Tinnitus

CONTRIBUTORS:	IMAGING DATA:	
Abraham Schulman, M.D.,	**Camera:** Trionix Triad	**Collimator:** High resolution
Arnold M. Strashun, M.D.	**Tracer:** ^{99m}Tc HMPAO	**Dose:** 25.0 mCi
Institution: SUNY Health Sciences Center at Brooklyn		

This 72-year-old man presented with tinnitus that had increased in intensity over the past year. The tinnitus was described as a "high ring" in both ears of constant duration and fluctuating intensity. The tinnitus intensity index was 6 on a 0–7 scale (7 maximum). The patient noted an associated bilateral hearing loss (left greater than right), early memory dysfunction, and positional dysequilibrium. Subsequent workup identified the tinnitus to be predomitral in type with a bilateral cochlear component (left greater than right) and a presumptive clinical diagnosis of a secondary endolymphatic hydrops on the left.

A head CT scan was reported to be negative.

An HMPAO SPECT study (Case Fig. 10-21) in the transaxial plane revealed an overall decrease in cortical tracer activity than was most marked in the bilateral frontal, temporal, and right parietal lobes and to a lesser degree subcortically.

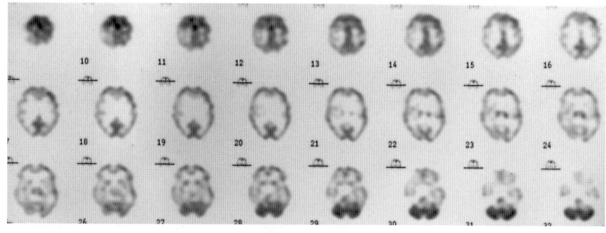

CASE FIG. 10-21

Normal Visual Activation Paradigm

CONTRIBUTOR:	IMAGING DATA:	
Thomas C. Hill, M.D.	**Camera:** Strichman SME 810	**Collimator:** High-resolution
Institution: Deaconess Hospital	**Tracer:** ^{99m}Tc ECD	**Dose:** 20 mCi

This 43-year-old right-handed normal male volunteer was studied at baseline with eyes open, ears unplugged, in a dark room, sitting at a computer console during a visual activation with full-field visual stimulation (flashing checkerboard).

Baseline ethylcysteinate dimer (ECD) SPECT study (Case Fig. 10.22A) in the transaxial plane (*top*) reveals a normal tracer distribution. Activation ECD SPECT (Case Fig. 10.22B), in the transaxial plane (*bottom*), injected at the time of visual stimulation revealed enhanced radiotracer uptake primarily in the region of the visual cortex.

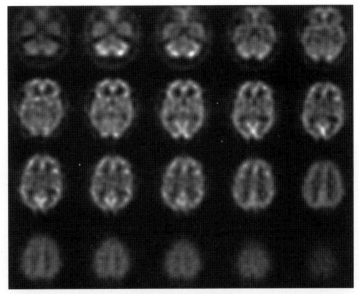

CASE FIG. 10.22A

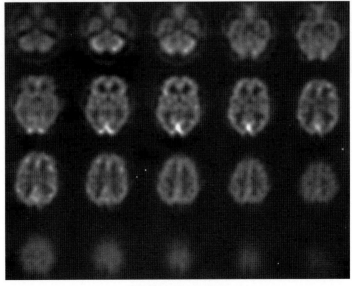

CASE FIG. 10.22B

Studies of right- and left-handed normal volunteer subjects superimposed on an averaged MRI brain atlas

CONTRIBUTOR:	IMAGING DATA:
Ferruccio Fazio, M.D.	**PET Scanner:**
Institution: Universita'Di Milano—Polo H.S. Raffaele, Instituto D Scienze Radiologiche, Cattedra Di Medicina Nucleare	**Tracer:**
	Other (activation, pharmacologic challenge, etc.): Subjects watched a video during the first 80 min of tracer uptake.

These PET studies demonstrate a functional hemispheric asymmetry in bimanual coordination. In right-handers, portions of the motor and premotor areas are more active in the left as opposed to the right hemisphere. The converse pattern is evident in left-handers. These results suggest that some components of the neural processing involved in bimanual coordination may be carried out only in the dominant hemisphere. Between-hands asynchrony may then reflect the time for dispatching the result of processing to the contralateral hemisphere (Case Fig. 10.23).

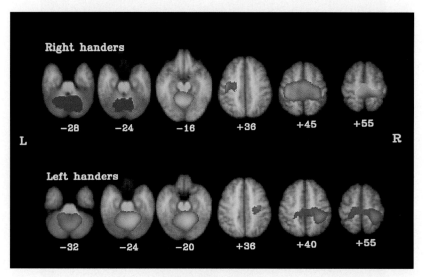

CASE FIG. 10.23

Clinical Diagnosis:
Right-Handed Normal Subject During Movement Activation

CONTRIBUTOR:	IMAGING DATA:
Ferruccio Fazio, M.D.	PET Scanner:
Institution: Universita'Di Milano- Polo H.S.	**Tracer:** $^{15}O\ H_2O$
Raffaele, Instituto D Scienze	**Other (activation, pharmacologic challenge,**
Radiologiche, Cattedra Di	**etc.):**
Medicina Nucleare	

A normal right-handed volunteer was studied during movement activation.

In vivo PET study of regional cerebral blood flow using $^{15}O\ H_2O$ during the execution of opening-closing of the right hand. Activated areas overlapped to a 3D MRI (EMPI RAGE) of the same subject. Case Figure 10.24 shows several activated areas, including not only the right-hand primary motor area in the left precentral gyrus but also other regions of the left frontal cortex related to movement preparation and planning, which form a specific functional circuit.

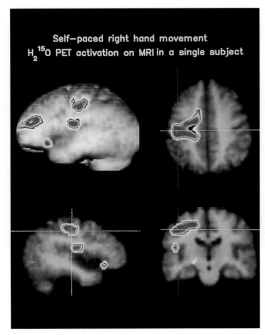

CASE FIG. 10.24

Clinical Diagnosis:
Rest–Activation

CONTRIBUTORS:

Gerg Deutsch, Ph.D.,

James M. Mountz, M.D.

Institution: The University of Alabama at

      Birmingham Medical Center

IMAGING DATA:

Camera: PRISM 3000

Tracer: ^{133} Xe

Other (Diamox, pharmacologic challenge, etc.):

Collimator: Custom ^{133}xe LE parallel hole

Dose: 22 mCi, 60 sec

This is a normal volunteer.

Coronal-plane ^{133}Xe brain SPECT images were obtained using the ^{133}Xe inhalation method. These images compare resting state (Case Fig. 10.25, *top row*) with a left-hand-finger oppositional task (Case Fig. 10.25, *bottom row*) The figure reveals increased radiotracer activity in the right cerebral somatomotor region during the task.

Teaching Points:

^{133}Xe is a useful tracer for studying functional activation. Differences between resting and activation states can also be quantified using this tracer.

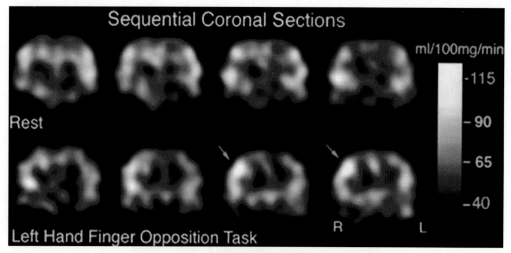

CASE FIG. 10.25

Clinical Diagnosis:
Activation Mental Rotation Task

CONTRIBUTORS:

Gerg Deutsch, Ph.D.,

James M. Mountz, M.D.

Institution: The University of Alabama at
　　　　　　　Birmingham Medical Center

IMAGING DATA:

Camera: PRISM 3000

Tracer: ^{133}Xe

This is a normal volunteer.

Transverse fMRI image obtained using the BOLD technique (measuring the difference between oxyhemoglobin and deoxyhemoglobin content) demonstrates an activation response primarily in the right hemisphere (Case Fig. 10.26, *right image, primarily posterior regions*).

Transverse-plane ^{133}Xe brain SPECT images were obtained using the ^{133}Xe inhalation method (Case Fig. 10.26, *left image, arrows*) reveals a similar pattern of activation.

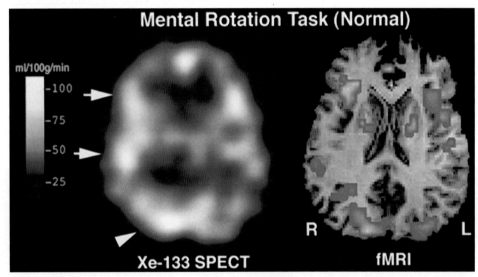

CASE FIG. 10.26

Subjects were normal women volunteers: a 48-year-old nonsmoker and a 51-year-old smoker

CONTRIBUTOR:

Joanna S. Fowler, Ph.D.
Institution: Brookhaven National
Laboratory

IMAGING DATA:

PET Scanner: CTI 931
Tracer: [^{11}C]L-deprenyl-D2

Dose: 6–8 mCi

Teaching Points:

1. These transverse brain PET images (Case Fig. 10.27) and those of other volunteers showed that smokers had an average 40% lower brain monoamine oxidase B (MAO B) than nonsmokers.

2. Though smoking is a major public health problem, little is known about the pharmacologic effects of smoke on the human brain.

3. MAO B is an enzyme that breaks down neurotransmitters like dopamine. Reduced MAO B could imply elevated brain dopamine and reduced amounts of hydro-gen peroxide, a potential source of free radicals and oxidative stress.

4. Inhibition of brain MAO B by tobacco smoke may account for the reduced risk of Parkinson's disease in smokers and the high rate of smoking in individuals with depression and individuals who are addicted to other substances.

Reproduced with permission from: Fowler JS, Volkow ND, Wang GJ, et al. Inhibition of monamine oxidase B in the brains of smokers. *Nature* 1996;379:733–736.

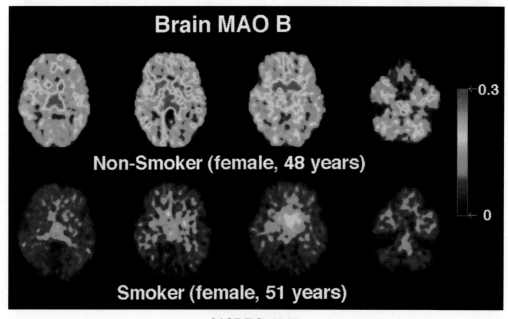

CASE FIG. 10.27

Subject Index

Page numbers followed by "t" represent information found in tables.